Constructive Conversations About Health

Poli... and values

Learning Centre

Edited by

Marsh...

Radcliffe Publishing
Oxford • Seattle

Radcliffe Publishing Ltd
18 Marcham Road
Abingdon
Oxon OX14 1AA
United Kingdom

www.radcliffe-oxford.com
Electronic catalogue and worldwide online ordering facility.

British Library Cataloguing in Publication Data

A catalogue record for this book is available from the British Library.

ISBN-10 1 84619 033 9
ISBN-13 978 1 84619 033 9

Typeset by Anne Joshua & Associates, Oxford
Printed and bound by TJI Digital, Padstow, Cornwall

Contents

About the editor

Marshall Marinker began his career in the 1960s as a general practitioner; subsequently he was Foundation Professor of Community Health, University of Leicester School of Medicine, and Director, the MSD Foundation UK, concerned with the post-graduate development of doctors in general practice. In recent years he has been visiting Professor at GKT, King's College London; Chair, the National Advisory Group on Forensic Mental Health R&D; and co-Chair, the Department of Health's Medicines Partnership Task Force. He has published widely on the theory of medical generalism, the relationship of the arts to medical science and practice, medical education, health policy, and medical ethics.

About the contributors

Per Carlsson is Professor of Health Technology Assessment, Centre for Medical Technology Assessment, Linköping University, and Director of the National Centre for Priority Setting in Health Care. He is a member of the National Pharmaceutical Benefits Board, the SBU Alert Advisory Board, and the Swedish Council on Technology Assessment in Health Care. His research interests include health technology assessment, policy implications of the diffusion of health innovations, and priority setting in healthcare.

Marc Danzon was first elected as WHO Regional Director for Europe in 1999, and was re-elected to a second term in 2004. In 1974, following his medical training, he joined the French Committee for Health Education and served as Director from 1989–1992. At the Regional Office for Europe of WHO (1985–1989) Dr Danzon organised the first European Conference on Tobacco Policies. He returned as Director of the new Department for Country Health Development in 1992, and implemented the EUROHEALTH programme for Central and Eastern Europe. Prior to his appointment as WHO Regional Director, he served as Director for Public Health in France's National Federation of Mutual Insurance Societies.

Isabelle Durand-Zaleski is Professor of Public Health, Henri Mondor Hospital and University Paris XII. She obtained her medical degree from Paris University School of Medicine in 1985, and had additional training in economics and political science at the Institut d'Etudes Politiques de Paris, from which she graduated in 1985. She moved to Boston, USA, obtained a Masters degree in public health at Harvard University, and subsequently worked in the Division of Clinical Decision Making at the New England Medical Center. She returned to France and worked as a resident in Paris hospitals, obtaining a PhD in economics from Paris University in 1991. Her work focuses on health economics and the evaluation of professional practice.

Josep Figueras is Head of Secretariat and Research Director of the European Observatory on Health Care Systems and Head of the WHO European Centre On Health Policy. A medical doctor by training, he has a PhD in health planning and financing, and is Honorary Fellow of the UK Faculty Of Public Health Medicine, and former Lecturer in health services management at the London School of Hygiene and Tropical Medicine. He is co-editor of the European Observatory series published by Open University Press and has published several volumes on health systems and health policy in European countries.

Julio Frenk has been Minister of Health, Mexico, since 2000. Previously he served as Executive Director, Evidence and Information for Policy, at the World Health Organization, where he contributed to the design and application of a comprehensive framework for the assessment of health system performance. He was Founding Director General of the National Institute of Public Health of Mexico; Founding Director of the Centre for Public Health Research; Executive

Vice President, the Mexican Health Foundation, and Director of its Centre for Health and the Economy; and Adjunct Professor at the Faculty of Medicine of the National University of Mexico. He has been awarded the position of National Researcher in Mexico. He has published widely on health matters, and is a member of numerous editorial boards and international health-related committees.

Peter Garpenby is Associate Professor in Health Policy Analysis, Centre for Medical Technology Assessment, Linköping University, and Project Manager at the National Centre for Priority Setting in Health Care in Linköping. His research interests include health policy, international comparisons in the field of health, and procedural justice in priority setting in healthcare.

David J Hunter is Professor of Health Policy and Management at Durham University. Prior to taking up this post in 1999 he was Director of the Nuffield Institute for Health at the University of Leeds. He has also held posts at the University of Aberdeen and the King's Fund, London. He is currently Chair of the UK Public Health Association. His current research interests lie in public health implementation. He has published widely on health policy and management.

Ilona Kickbusch is a political scientist with a PhD from the University of Konstanz, Germany. She works as an independent global health consultant and serves as senior health policy adviser to the Swiss Federal Office for Public Health. She became Head of the Division of Global Health at Yale University School of Medicine, following a distinguished career with the World Health Organization where she initiated the OTTAWA Charter for Health Promotion and headed a range of innovative programmes such as Healthy Cities and Health Promoting Schools. She is a sought-after speaker and adviser on policies and strategies to promote health at the national and international level, with a focus on new challenges to health governance. She has published widely and has received many prizes and honours.

Mihály Kökény is Government Commissioner for Public Health Coordination, Hungary. He was formerly a practising physician at the National Institute of Cardiology, later joining the Ministry of Health, where his responsibilities included organising health programmes. As Department Head at the Office of the Council of Ministers, he was in charge of elaborating the first ever Hungarian health promotion strategy. In 1994 he was elected Member of Parliament. He served as Parliamentary Secretary of State at the Ministry of Welfare from 1994; Minister of Welfare, 1996–1998; and Chairman of Parliament's Health and Social Affairs Committee, 1998–2002. He served as State Secretary, and again as Health Minister, 2002–2004.

Suszy Lessof is the Project Manager of the European Observatory on Health Systems and Policies and is involved in supporting policy makers to bring evidence to bear on decision making in practice. Prior to joining the Observatory Suszy worked on national standards in public health for the NHS Executive of England and Wales, for the EUPHA/ASPHER consortia evaluating the European Commission's Europe Against Cancer programme, and at the London School of Hygiene & Tropical Medicine where she was the project manager of capacity-building initiatives in Romania, taught organisational management, and was the

Course Organiser for the Health Services Management MSc. She also contributed to the work of WHO's Health Systems Analysis Unit in the run up to the Ljubljana conference on healthcare sector reform. Suszy's background is in community economic development and urban regeneration. She has an MBA from City University, London.

Graham Lister is senior associate, the Judge Business School, Cambridge, and was previously senior associate, the Nuffield Trust. He has served as Chair of the College of Health and on several national and regional health policy committees. He led the Coopers and Lybrand health consulting team, and has advised on health futures, health policy and management for the WHO and in the UK, Australia, Cambodia, China, Denmark, Hungary, Italy, Kenya, Lithuania, Spain, Sweden, Tanzania and the Czech Republic. He coordinated the Nuffield Trust Programme 'Global Health: A Local Issue', and edits the website at www. ukglobalhealth.org.

Martin McKee is Professor of European Public Health, London School of Hygiene and Tropical Medicine. He directs the European Centre on Health of Societies in Transition, a WHO Collaborating Centre at the London School of Hygiene and Tropical Medicine. He is also a research director at the European Observatory on Health Systems and Policies. A medical doctor by training, he has published over 350 papers in scientific journals, as well as over 20 books, many on health and health policy in Central and Eastern Europe.

Giovanni Moro is Director of Active Citizenship Network (www.activecitizen ship.net), a programme aimed at involving citizens' organisations from European Union member states, and candidate countries, in European policy making. A political sociologist by training, he was, from 1989 to 2002, General Secretary of the Italian citizens' movement 'Cittadinanzattiva'.

Miquel Porta is Head of the Clinical & Molecular Epidemiology of Cancer Unit, IMIM, Barcelona, Professor of Preventive Medicine & Public Health, Universitat Autònoma de Barcelona; Adjunct Professor, School of Public Health, University of North Carolina. His research interests include clinical and molecular epidemiology; diagnostic delay in cancer; and the social impact of persistent organic pollutants. In addition to his research papers he has published on music and genome metaphors, the bibliographic impact factor and scientific journals, and the roles of scientific associations.

Suzanne Rameix, an alumna of the Ecole Normale Supérieure, is Associate Professor at the University of Paris XII, and Head of the Department of Medical Ethics. Her research focuses on moral and political philosophy applied to the field of the patient–doctor relationship. She has published on autonomy, decision making, genetic information, quality of life, statute of body parts, and the theory of justice in healthcare systems. She is a member of the Ethics Commission of the French Society of Intensive Care Medicine. In 1996 she won the Maurice Rapin Ethics Prize for her book *The Philosophical Foundations of Medical Ethics*.

Jennifer Prah Ruger is Assistant Professor, Division of Global Health, Yale School of Public Health. Her research interests focus on the political economy of health and include economic evaluation of addiction programmes and emergency and humanitarian services; health, health finance and development; and health and social justice. Professor Ruger received a Masters degree from Oxford University, and a doctoral degree from Harvard University. Following a post-doctoral fellowship at Harvard's Center for Population and Development Studies, she served on the health and development satellite secretariat of World Health Organization Director-General's Transition Team and co-authored a report examining the economic linkages between health and development.

Constantino T Sakellarides is Professor of Health Policy and Management at the National School of Public Health, New University of Lisbon; President, the Scientific Council of the National School of Public Health; founding member of the Portuguese Health Systems Observatory; President of the Portuguese Public Health Association. He was the first Academic Director of the Escuela Andaluza de Salud Pública in Granada, Spain, 1985–87, Director for Health Policy and Services of WHO/Europe in Copenhagen, 1990–1995, Chairman of the Management Board of Lisbon Health Region, 1996, and Director General of Health of Portugal, 1997–99. In the early stages of his career he practised as a rural doctor in Mozambique, and later contributed to the launch of general medical practice in Portugal.

Divya Srivastava is Research Officer at the European Observatory on Health Systems and Policies. An economist by training, Divya's current research focuses on public health policies in Europe and their implications for policy development, implementation and good governance. Her other research interests include the effect of pharmaceutical policy on market competition. Divya obtained her MSc in International Health Policy from the London School of Economics and Political Science and was the recipient of the Brian Abel-Smith Award for best dissertation. Before joining the Observatory, she worked for the Canadian government in the Ministry of Finance and the Ministry of Health.

Hans Stein is a lawyer by training. He is German Section Head at the European Public Health Centre, consultant on European Union health policy to various national and international institutions, and has acted as Head of the 'General Health Policy and Public Health Research', and 'European Health Policy' Divisions at the German Ministry of Health. He has represented his country on many European Union Council and Commission committees, and has published on EU health policy, health targets, monitoring of policy, public health research and international cooperation.

Morton Warner is Professor of Health Strategy and Policy, and Founding Director, Welsh Institute for Health and Social Care, University of Glamorgan. Since 1992 he has led a WHO Collaborating Centre for Regional Health Strategy and Management Development in Europe. He holds a PhD in Medical Sociology (University of Wales) and is Fellow of the Institute of Healthcare Management, and Fellow of the Faculty of Public Health Medicine, The Royal College of Physicians, London. In recent years he has had wide experience as Visiting Professor in a number of European universities, and as health policy adviser to various health institutions in Lithuania, Hungary, Bulgaria, Russia and Sweden.

Derek Yach was Professor of Public Health, Head of the Division of Global Health, Yale School of Public Health, and became Head of Global Health at the Rockefeller Foundation in 2006. Between 1995 and 2004 he worked at the World Health

Organization where he had responsibility for developing a new global 'Health For All' policy. His current research interests include studying the impacts of globalisation on health and chronic disease prevention and control. He serves on several international health advisory committees.

Acknowledgements

I have many people to thank. In 1997 an Academic Advisory Board was brought together by Merck & Co., Inc., Whitehouse Station, New Jersey, USA,* to give independent advice to, and oversee, its European Health Targets Research Grant Programme. I was invited to chair the Board, the current members of which are: Professor Arpo Aromaa (Finland); Professor Isabelle Durand-Zaleski (France); Dr George France (Italy); Professor Dr Klaus-Dirk Henke (Germany); Professor Ilona Kickbusch (Switzerland); Professor Morton Warner (UK); Professor Stipe Ores-kovic (Croatia); Professor Miquel Porta (Spain); and Professor Andrzej Rys (Poland). It was from discussions at the meetings of this Board, and many associated international workshops and conferences, that the ideas that inspired the production of this book originated. Its publication coincides with my retirement – from the Board and all other professional activities. It is therefore a particular pleasure to thank these good friends for their fellowship, and for the tolerant way in which, over the past nine years, they have undertaken the often daunting task of trying to educate their chairman.

I thank all the authors – for their generous responses to my invitation to write, for meeting the deadlines, for their tolerance of my editorial pernicketiness, for the quality of their contributions, and for the sheer pleasure of our exchanges in the course of meetings and editing.

The book has been generously supported by an unrestricted educational grant from Merck & Co., Inc. I want to thank Dr Jeffrey L Sturchio (Vice President, External Affairs, Human Health Intercontinental) for his stimulating insights on health policy, and his unfailing encouragement and enthusiasm. Melinda Hanisch (Manager, External Affairs, Europe, Middle East & Africa) has been unfailingly supportive of the work of the Board and the production of this book; her compendious knowledge of the European health field, and her shrewd judgement, have been invaluable to me.

Finally, I should like to thank Gillian Nineham, Editorial Director, Radcliffe Publishing Ltd., for her enthusiastic support from the earliest days of the book, and her ever-helpful colleagues, Lisa Abbott, Paula Moran, Gregory Moxon and Susan Rabson.

Marshall Marinker
January 2006

* Merck & Co., Inc., Whitehouse Station, New Jersey, USA, operates in most countries outside North America as Merck, Sharp & Dohme, or MSD.

Chapter 1

Health policy and the constructive conversationalist

Marshall Marinker

In Lewis Carroll's classic children's story *Through the Looking Glass*, Alice encounters Humpty Dumpty.[1]

> 'When *I* use a word,' Humpty Dumpty said in rather a scornful tone, 'it means just what I choose it to mean – neither more nor less.'
>
> 'The question is,' said Alice, 'whether you *can* make words mean so many different things.'
>
> 'The question is,' said Humpty Dumpty, 'which is to be master – that's all.'

Humpty Dumpty issues a sharp challenge to those who advocate constructive conversation about health, with which this book is concerned. The literature on health policy is vast. On offer are models of health services, economic theory, management theory, disquisitions on ethical principles, social analyses, literally thousands of publications. In a globalised and electronically networked world, this literature has already generated its own particular language, a policy jargon replete with terms that look deceptively familiar, terms which will be much in evidence in what now follows, terms whose meanings require our closest attention.

Although I acknowledge the force of Humpty Dumpty's relativism, my aim will be to limit some of the damage caused by a systemic ambiguity in the way we talk about health. When we choose a word it cannot mean just what we choose it to mean, although it will almost always mean both more and less. Humpty Dumpty's assertion is the dilemma that lies at the heart of constructive conversation about health.[2]

In 1847 Rudolph Virchow, who famously averred that medicine was a social science, was asked to investigate the causes and containment of a typhus epidemic among immigrant Polish workers in Silesia. He recommended ameliorating the hardships and injustices experienced by the workers, improving their education, increasing their income, involving them in local politics, and permitting them to use Polish for official purposes.[3]

Some 40 years later Robert Koch was to demonstrate the bacterial causes of the infectious diseases. Yet more than a century after Koch, and a century and a half after Virchow, Victor Rodwin[4] describes the cities of the West, citing New York, London, Paris and Tokyo, as socially infected breeding grounds for both disease and urban terrorism, and implies an overlapping of causes. He links a failure to deal adequately with fresh epidemics of infectious diseases, including AIDS and

TB, with problems of water and air pollution, homelessness, poverty, the exclusion of ethnic minority groups, and terrorism.

What is the link, in Rodwin's analysis, between TB and AIDS, which can be described in terms of a biological model, and urban terrorism which cannot? What model of disease could possibly have connected the severity of the typhus outbreak to the denial of use of a mother tongue? How are we to understand the full meaning of the public health?

Marc Danzon (Chapter 2) observes that 'health seems to be universally recognised as the hard currency of modern times'. The word has been so often defined, by philosophers, politicians, poets. What does health mean to the individual, to the citizens in whose name all health policy is made?

The following quotation is ascribed to the novelist Katherine Mansfield, written in a letter when, as a young woman, she was already dying of tuberculosis. The words, or some version of them, appear in a number of contexts, such that perhaps the feelings expressed were thematic throughout her writing and life. 'By health I mean the power to live a full, adult, living, breathing life in close contact with what I love . . . the earth and the wonders thereof – the sea – the sun . . . I want to be *all that I am capable of becoming.*' I italicise those seven words because they resonate with the capabilities approach of Amartya Sen and others.[5] In Bismarck's terms, health was a means to a public end – the productive capacity of Prussia's workforce and the fighting capacity of its soldiery. Referring to Sen and others, Jennifer Prah Ruger (Chapter 4) observes that '. . . the degree to which individuals have the capability actively to participate in their work, social and political life, to be well-educated . . . are ends in themselves'.

In the early 1960s I was a general practitioner. One of my patients was a child (I will call her Helena) born with multiple congenital abnormalities – microcephaly (small head size with incomplete development of the cerebral hemispheres), a deeply cleft soft palate with micrognathia (failure of the lower jaw to develop), transverse limb deficiencies (the arms and legs were stumps with vestigial hand- and foot-like structures). She was doubly incontinent, communicated by piercing screams, moved by scuttling along the floor, and suffered occasional epileptic seizures. This was the most extreme example of congenital damage in a surviving child that I had ever seen. With no hesitation, the young parents, supported by their own parents and neighbouring siblings, declared that they would look after the child at home.

One morning, when Helena was five years old, I was called to see her. This in itself was unusual; the parents rarely asked for a home visit and were stoically self-reliant. A brief examination revealed some small spots, like grains of salt, on the palate: she was developing measles and I explained that the rash would appear the following day. As I left the house her mother turned to me and said, 'I hesitated to bother you, but yesterday I just knew she was not well.'

Down the years those words have continued to disturb and shock. Helena 'was not well' that day. What do we mean by 'well'? What do we mean by 'health'? How are we to communicate across the yawning gap of words? In this opening chapter I will present the Madrid Framework, an array of the issues in health policy and governance – their scope, processes, aims, principles and the values that underpin them. I will be concerned both with the elements of health policy, and since all policy begins in discourse, I shall say something about words and how we use them.

The Madrid Framework

The language of health targeting was given international currency by the World Health Organization,[6] and has since dominated the literature and practice of health policy. Targets, in the new lexicon, were to be specific, quantifiable and measurable objectives designed to improve the health of individuals and families, communities, and regional and national populations.

Thenceforward 'targeting' rapidly came to usurp and incorporate 'policy making' and 'implementation', and to permeate the health policy discourse. Yet in the course of the ensuing years a number of analysts have voiced dissatisfaction with the dominance of targeting as a metaphor for policy – for example, Ilona Kickbusch, describing the epidemiological-rationalist approach characteristic of the late twentieth century, wrote: 'The wish for governability and order overshadowed the drive to establish a new territory and make history.'[7]

Increasingly it became evident that 'targeting' might prove too restrictive a means for our full purpose. Policy in pursuit of health is a socio-political exercise, and targeting is a purely technical conceit. Also, health policy begins with moral purpose, not data. And it is driven by our values. We required a more elaborate linguistic code adequately to express and explore the values embedded in evidence, policy, politics and the historical contingencies of particular societies.

In May 2003 an international workshop of health policy experts was held in Madrid, with the intention of considering the values that underpin policy making.[8] In my chairman's briefing for that meeting I wrote: 'The task that we have set for ourselves is to construct some sort of exploratory/evaluative instrument that can be applied to examples of health targeting . . . '[9] Armed with the thoughts of the participants in the Madrid conference, I attempted to outline such an instrument, and in May 2003 produced a first draft of the Framework. In the years since that meeting, and in the light of subsequent health policy workshops in Wales, Hungary, Spain and Scotland, the Framework has undergone a great deal of useful modification of detailed content, but its original structure and function have so far not been seriously challenged by those invited to experiment with its use, and remain intact.

The Madrid Framework[10] is imagined as a multi-dimensional space. Each dimension represents a salient force (equity, choice, democracy and so on) that acts on the creation and implementation of policy. I was seeking to describe a force field in which each group of concerns would pull in its own direction, so that policy and governance must perpetually adjust in order to find an equilibrium. This spatial imagery seemed appropriate because I wanted the Framework to represent a theoretical universe of health policy discourse.[11] However strained the metaphor, and it is strained, the dynamic imagery embraced the key notions of uncertainty and change, and was intended sharply to contrast with, and critique, the static imagery and rigid language of the dominantly fashionable 'targets', 'guidelines' and 'protocols'.

Initially the idea of a 'framework' came in for some criticism: was this not too prescriptive, rigid, concrete, constraining, a structure for our purpose? Why not present the issues, the so-called 'dimensions', as a checklist, an inventory, a lexicon? My contention was that 'framework' helps us to visualise not only the inventory of issues to be considered, but their relationships. When we speak of health, equity, choice and the rest, we employ 'lexical reasoning'. This allows us to explore their meanings in some fine detail. But lexical reason is less strong in helping us to see how these different, and often contradictory, elements relate to one another.

It is 'cartographic reason',[12] the ability to map, that allows us to see these spatial relationships, and to play with them. Maps trace the landscapes in which we live; they allow us, they compel us, to envisage location, destination, departure, arrival, and exploration. In his essay on the possibilities of inter-sectoral and inter-agency governance, Morton Warner (Chapter 10) describes the *spatial* relationships of the players, and offers us a diagram (page 123) that is actually a conceptual map. The Madrid Framework invites a coincidence of lexical and cartographic reason.

I began with an exhaustive list of the issues that had been raised at the Madrid conference, and in the wider literature on health policy. These I bundled into baskets of coherent value-laden qualities and concerns that seemed to belong together. They were composed to achieve maximum separation between the groups of related concepts, while acknowledging an irreducible degree of overlap. The brief descriptions of the 11 dimensions that follow, already the fruit of constructive conversations with very many stakeholders, are only indicative, and in no way comprehensive or definitive.[13]

1 **Health and wellbeing:** The protection and improvement of health is the *raison d'être* of all health policy, the ultimate goal of which is to enhance the capabilities of the citizen to live a full life. The WHO definition of health embraces physical, social, mental and spiritual wellbeing. Health policies are directed to determinants of health, risk factors for diseases, access to, and quality of, health services.

2 **Equity and fairness:** Inequalities in health, in the probabilities of disease, and in the quality of, and access to, services, are found within and between all societies. These are largely determined by social factors, income, age, ethnicity, education, housing and so on, such that the pursuit of health and social justice become inextricably entwined. Fairness relates also to such difficult concepts as merit and potential benefit.

3 **Choice:** What is deemed best for the population will only randomly be best for its sub-groups, or for the individual. Since personal choice is linked to the right to health, trade-offs have to be negotiated between the collective interest and the interests of individuals and particular groups. Choice and equity constitute one of the fundamental political fault lines in the landscape of health policy.

4 **Democracy:** In order to engender confidence in health policies, all stakeholders, and especially citizens and patients, need to be actively engaged. Access to health information and health literacy are crucial to such engagement. Health policies succeed in relation to the sense of solidarity and shared values that they foster.

5 **Stewardship:** Health is a vital public resource requiring investment by government. Traditionally governments were deemed to have three key duties: 'the defence of the realm', 'law and order', and 'the stability of the currency'. In the twenty-first century, a fourth duty, 'to protect and enhance health', emerges as of at least similar importance.

6 **Evidence:** Successful policies require good data comparable over time and locations. All data are socially constructed. It is therefore important to consider

not only the statistical, but also the ethical and political values embedded in evidence.

7 **Efficiency:** Government has a dual accountability: to protect and improve health; to ensure the optimal use of the public resources entrusted to it. Allocative efficiency is concerned both with the effectiveness of interventions and the priority accorded them. Operational efficiency is concerned with the optimal uses of resources to obtain the maximum benefit at the level of management. Efficiency in health policy is thus a matter of sound finance, sound science and sound ethics.

8 **Synergy:** Health policy and governance require cooperation between government agencies and a wide variety of other elements of civil society. When they interact so as to produce new ways of working, new functioning networks can be created, intractable problems can be redefined, and unanticipated solutions found.

9 **Sustainability:** Since most health policies are long-term exercises, provisions must be made to sustain political, organisational and individual motivations over the course of time, and of successive governments. This requires a fine balance between the benefits of stability and the creative potential of renewal.

10 **Interdependence:** Policy and services at both global and local levels must take account of concerns such as workforce mobility, the environment, international agreements – factors that transcend national boundaries. At every level there are biological, social and political interdependencies.

11 **Creativity:** Health policy and governance are not securely predictable and linear exercises. Successful policies and implementation require imagination, experimentation, innovation and flexibility.

In Chapters 3–13 these dimensions are considered, and their meanings expanded and challenged, by writers from a variety of perspectives and experiences.

In the two years since I first proposed them, the number of dimensions has varied between 10 and 13, and the names have been much argued over. For example, there were reservations about the adequacy of 'Democracy' as a title to capture all the complex concerns for public participation and social responsiveness. There were similar reservations about 'Stewardship', a reservation again given voice here by Constantino Sakellarides[14] (Chapter 7). Some complained that 'Human Dignity' seemed to be missing, or that 'Solidarity' should be considered apart from 'Equity and Fairness', and so on. However, it is not the particularity of the dimensions' titles that is important but the fact of gathering them together.

Michel Foucault[15] quotes an ancient Chinese encyclopaedia in which animals are divided into the following categories: (a) belonging to the Emperor, (b) embalmed, (c) tame, (d) sucking pigs, (e) sirens, (f) fabulous, (g) stray dogs, (h) included in the present classification, (i) frenzied, (j) innumerable, (k) drawn with a very fine camelhair brush, (l) etcetera, (m) having just broken the water pitcher, (n) that from a long way off look like flies. He comments on 'the stark impossibility of thinking *that*'. It is starkly impossible because we cannot imagine what the taxonomy was meant to accomplish. The only link that we can see between his creatures is that they appear together in the imagination of a long dead encyclopaedist. Our dimensions of health policy have a not dissimilar purpose. It is that they will appear *together*, that they will have interlinked meanings, resonances and relationships, in the imaginations of those who undertake a civilised discourse about health.

Words and values

In his poem *Burnt Norton* TS Eliot warns us:

> '. . . Words strain,
> Crack and sometimes break, under the burden,
> Under the tension, slip, slide, perish,
> Decay with imprecision, will not stay in place,
> Will not stay still.'[16]

So much rests on the ethical weight that we claim for the words we use.[17] A number of the essays in this book are written by colleagues whose native language is not English. They translate their thoughts into our contemporary lingua franca.[18] The danger, of which I became increasingly aware in the course of editing the chapters that follow, is that the overwhelming dominance of the English language in our times, although it appears to facilitate communication across societies and cultures, actually constitutes a threat. In translation, the full scope and richness of ideas, their most significant nuances and colorations, are easily bleached out. When we use statistics there is often an uneasy trade-off between reliability and validity. Similarly, when we use language, there is a compromise between reliable communication and valid meaning. The threat is the illusion of understanding, which, in particular, can distort our talk about values.

In their study of how people used the concept of values in Canadian health policy, Giacomini and her colleagues conclude that what really matters is not the exquisite definition of 'values' by academic ethicists, but the diverse ways in which the term 'values' is used by stakeholders in support of their health policies. They found that values were very broadly claimed – in relation to systems; ethical problems; relationships; goals; attitudes; feelings; responsibilities; rights; economic viability, and so on. The Humpty Dumpty approach.

Such a wide and indiscriminate use of 'value' might seem to do little more than signal our preferences and prejudices, or simply that the term 'value' is highly valued. Should we therefore strive to reserve it to distinguish something particularly profound, pervasive and binding? For example, in speaking of health policy, terms like fairness, honesty and human dignity seem evidently to represent deep human values, while others, also crucial in policy making, like evidence, efficiency and sustainability, seem somehow to be not so fundamental. They are necessary intentions, important means, but are they necessarily values?

In a monograph on the values inherent in the pursuit of science, Jacob Bronowski[19] identifies three: creativity, the habit of truth and the sense of human dignity. In a preface to this work he writes that he would add a fourth, one not generated by the practice of science. This he expresses as 'the values of tenderness, kindness, human intimacy and love'. Bronowski's quartet of values would seem capable of serving well most human endeavours, not least that with which we are concerned here. He also gives a most telling definition of values, when he concludes his essays with the following: 'The values by which we are to survive are not rules for just and unjust conduct, but are those deeper illuminations in whose light justice and injustice, good and evil, means and ends, are seen in fearful sharpness of outline.'

A culture is perhaps most precisely defined by its untranslatable words. In a recent collection of such words, the most powerful and the most complex examples proved to be those that refer to feelings.[20] These included *pohoda* – from the Czech, 'a pain-free, trouble-free state that we should all like to share'; *saudade* – from the Portuguese, 'a vague and constant desire for something that does not and probably cannot exist . . . an indolent dreaming wistfulness'; *bejaka* – from the Swedish, 'a welcome to all the vicissitudes that life may bring and an understanding and acceptance of people and things as they are'. Each of these words would require an essay to explore its roots, its feelings, its limits. The same is true of the words, much employed in this book, that represent values. Each of them will mean something finely nuanced, something utterly specific to the culture in which it is used; and something utterly specific to the individual citizen, to the mother of a five-year-old child who 'was not well'.

Values conflict. They point at one and the same time to our collectivity as human beings, how we act in relationship to one another, how we organise ourselves as societies, and to our individuality, how we defend our personal boundaries and freedoms. Rather than accepting any special pleading for this or that precept, in looking ethically to orient health policy, it may be more useful to think of value as signifying the ethical component of any and every aspect of policy making. In this sense the pursuit of equity and fairness is not *ipso facto* more or less ethically desirable than the pursuit of efficiency. Balancing the conflicting goods of these values would therefore become more explicit and acceptable because the judgement of policy makers would be seen to rest not on categorical grounds, but on contextual and contingent ones.

Many have posited that there is a set of values that are quintessentially European.[21] 'European' is often used in debate to signal concerns for equity, social fairness and solidarity, deriving from the expressed values of innovators like Rudolph Virchow and other European thinkers and health activists.[22] This somewhat romanticised concept of Europe is not to be pedantically defined by cartographic frontiers, but is infinitely extended by the minds of European thinkers, beyond the bourns of the continent. Will Hutton[23] claims that the European view is of a vigorous public realm, fundamental to the good society, and characterised by a belief in the social contract, in just capitalism, equity and qualified property rights. He describes the USA, with its emphasis on individual freedom and the safeguards of the market, as Europe's 'other'. Yet Hutton's European exceptionalism is perhaps misleading.

Norman Davies, in his panoramic history of Poland, points out that for much of its history Poland was not a nation state but an idea.[24] By the same token, Europe, whose dividing boundaries have been endlessly disputed, whose languages and cultures are diverse, was for much of its history most powerfully experienced as an idea, rather than as a particular geography or political constitution. While the concept of 'European values' remains useful and important, it refers not to an exclusive geopolitical, but to a commonly shared historical, culture, a long tradition of European thought about the public health and its function in the public arena.

The word solidarity, signifying unified interests, sympathies or aspirations, came into use, in this sort of European context, in the early 1980s. But originally it had a quite circumscribed meaning. It was the name of an independent trade union movement in Poland, registered in September 1980 and officially banned in October 1982. Where, now, are the boundaries of our solidarity? Graham Lister (Chapter 12) demonstrates how wide the concept of solidarity must become in a globalised world.

Jacob Bronowski[25] raises a fearful question about this. He relates hearing a popular dance tune of the day, played on a USA naval ship's loudspeakers. The tune was called 'Is you is or is you ain't ma baby?' Bronowski's memory shrinks to a pinpoint of unimaginable pain and expands into an exploding global connectedness when he tells us the circumstance. It is November 1945 and he is being driven in a military jeep along the harbour front of a ruined Nagasaki.

Values, policy and litanies

The expression of values often takes lyrical form. The notion of values as 'litanies' (in English the word is used bewilderingly to mean both a prayer, and a parody of prayer) directs our attention again to the elusiveness of real, as opposed to created, language. Giacomini *et al.*[26] note that '. . . almost all the Canadian health policy documents presented a list of a few *tenets countable by hand* with which to frame their reform proposals, such as "10 guiding principles", "9 vision statements", "7 major directions for change". Values also appear in *litanies* (e.g. "quality, access, efficiency, & accountability").'

A similar numerical escalation of intentions, and lyricism of cadence, is echoed in WHO policy '. . . *one* constant goal is to achieve full health potential for all people in the Region, with *two* main aims: to promote and protect people's health throughout their lives; and to reduce the incidence of the main diseases and injuries and alleviate the suffering they cause. *Three* basic values form its ethical foundation: health as a fundamental human right, equity in health and solidarity in action, and participation and accountability for continued health development. *Four* main strategies for action have been chosen to ensure that scientific, economic, social and political sustainability drive the implementation . . . '[27]

Julio Frenk (Chapter 14) employs a progression of mantras which constitute a hierarchy beginning with *four* ethical values – social inclusion, equality of opportunity, autonomy, and social responsibility – that are foundational. From these he derives *four* principles – citizenship, pluralism, solidarity, and the new universalism – that give social expression to the values. Finally he identifies *three* purposes – equality, quality and efficiency.

What is the function of these litanies? They serve in part as taxonomies, in part as mission statements, and in part as musical cadences that provide the health system with its mood music.

Policies and metaphors

The Madrid Framework, with its concept of the spatial dimensions of policy, is a metaphor. Familiarity with an extensive repertoire of metaphors appears to be helpful in the pursuit of productive discourse about health. Glouberman *et al.*[28] offer a number of metaphors for health policies. Some function as *levers* that exert predictable force and mechanical advantage; for example, regulations governing air and water quality. Others serve as *investments*, acknowledging the concepts of probability, risk, gain and loss; for example purchase of equipment or hospital building programmes. Some function as *seeds*, entailing the need to prepare the soil, to nurture growth, to prune; for example instituting experimental services. Each suggests quite contrasting approaches, timescales and expectations. The website of 'The Union of International Associations'[29] offers an abundant richness of organisational metaphors.

One of their telling examples is 'Knots and Basketry'. 'Knots are produced by interlacing one or more cords so that they lock together and resist forces acting to separate them.' They comment: 'Permanent social or conceptual structures are achieved by interlacing processes so that forces acting to separate them reinforce the mutual bonding. Complex structures are formed by multiple interlocking of functions . . . In achieving this self-reinforcement, elegant variations on the pattern may be favoured by particular cultures.' In the light of this, consider basketry as a metaphor to explain the dynamics of any political party. Consider basketry as a way of envisaging the interrelatedness, the tensions that bind closely together 'the interlacing cords' of the Madrid Framework's 11 dimensions.

Another of their metaphors is 'Flight'. 'True flight is produced by the simultaneous rotation of the left and right wings in a circle or figure-of-eight . . . This cycle produces the upward thrust required to overcome gravity and the forward thrust necessary to overcome drag.' They then suggest some social analogies: 'The structure of individual personalities or groups reflects their mode of movement in relation to public or peer group opinion . . . The complementary cycles produce the force necessary to counteract public or peer group opinion, enabling the group to rise to a more advantageous social position or move to a new position.'

Compare that statement, on the 'Governance through Metaphor Project' website, with Constantino Sakellarides' disquisition on policy as 'motion' (Chapter 7). He begins with a policy for improving road traffic flow in Bordeaux, and then explores the idea of circulation, of motion, by reference to holy pilgrimages, the fifteenth-century explorations of new worlds by Dias and Columbus in their fragile boats, the insights of Galileo and Newton, the dynamism of Rodin's art, and the playfulness of animated cartoons. Very soon we become aware that Sakellarides is offering us new ways of envisioning how we make policies, his metaphors taking us beyond the use of words to the very essence of movement and change.

Miquel Porta (Chapter 13) also takes us beyond words to consider a broad range of the senses – sight, smell, taste and touch – in a struggle to escape from past habits of thinking about health policy, and extend the reach of our imaginations. In all this it helps to remain conscious of the different metaphors we are using, the nature of their territories, and where, within their bourns, we may expect to travel and arrive. The purpose of the metaphors and allegories employed here by Sakellarides, Porta and others, is to remind us that policy makers, and those for whom policies are made, are at one and the same time rational, moral, sentient and emotional. Such metaphors create imaginary playgrounds within which we are able to experiment with the values that underpin everything that we attempt to do, to accustom ourselves to the priorities of others, and to come to an understanding with them.

The constructive conversationalist

Policies arise in the first instance from some initiating impetus, from new research findings, from epidemiological data monitoring trends, perceptions of needs, risks, threats, from evidence of public dissatisfaction with the status quo, the campaigns by special interest groups, political parties, the instant agendas of the media. For policy to ensue, these things must be talked about.

At some point the policy makers, groups of experts, health and social scientists, politicians and public servants, special interest representatives, public and corporate administrators, have to sit together and deliberate. This may occur at the highest levels, the WHO, the World Bank, the European Union, or the nation states, and at the most local levels, the smallest municipal districts or health authorities. What is the process of these deliberations? How is the initial impetus transformed into directives and then managerial plans for implementation? Derek Yach (Chapter 8) suggests that at the very highest global level of decision taking, the power of advocacy can overwhelm and override the evidence.

In recent years the aspiration has been that health policy be 'evidence based'. However policy is not the product of the data alone. It emerges from group interaction. In this, the light of evidence and reason is inevitably deflected through the prism of the values, preferences, emotions, intellect and personality of all the individuals who take part. The term conversation implies far more than 'speaking together'. The OED definition refers to 'having dealings with others', 'living together', and also to 'society' and 'intimacy'. The constructive conversationalist is a negotiator, an interpreter, and an explorer. How is 'constructive conversation' to take the place of partisan lobbying and special pleading? Or, if not to take its place – that may be asking too much of human nature – how is it to enable solidarity and moral efficiency in the choice of policies and in their ends?

Table 1.1 illustrates the different characteristics of committee process and the process of 'workshops' or 'think tanks'.[30]

Workshop members are either self-selected, or brought together on the basis of judgements about their personal fitness for, and commitment to, the task in hand.

Table 1.1

	Group work	*Committee work*
Characteristics	Social	Political
	Internal affiliation	External affiliation
	Process-oriented	Result-oriented
	Cooperative	Adversarial
Tasks	Explore differences	Decide intentions
	Define paradox	Reach agreement
Consequences	Focus on principles	Focus on actions
	Set limits to compromise	Generate rules
Dominant values	Beneficence	Non-maleficence
	Autonomy	Efficiency
	Advocacy	Justice
End points	Judgement	Agreement

Reproduced from Marinker (1994)[30] with permission from Blackwell Publishing.

They interact socially, in the sense that their personal values and prejudices are close to the surface of their deliberations, and legitimately so. Their commitment is to the group and its processes. For this reason their affiliations may be described as internal, and their mode cooperative.

Committee members are appointed by bureaucratic processes, to be representatives, or even delegates, of organisations or interests. They interact politically, and their personal values and prejudices, although inevitably in evidence, must always be subordinated to the committee's tasks, and to the agendas of the organisations and interests in whose name they attend. For this reason their affiliations may be described as external, and their mode adversarial.

Participants in workshops are encouraged to explore and define the paradoxes that abound, and to examine them in terms of the principles and values that individual members bring to the table. Consequently, the predominant values expressed are more likely to be the liberal and permissive ones of beneficence, choice and advocacy. The intention of the group's work is to produce judgement and reflection.

Committee members, when they encounter a paradox, are enjoined to decide between its conflictual elements, sometimes even to vote on them. Their job is to reach clear agreement, to take action and to generate rules. Consequently the predominant values expressed will be the more prudent and conservative ones of non-maleficence, efficiency and justice. The intention of the committee's work is to produce agreement and action.

The challenge is to reconcile the strengths of both approaches, and their mutual contradictions. Much of the literature on consensus in medicine refers to the function of ethics committees.[31] This is helpful, since what Handy[32] calls the management of paradox is little different from what medical ethicists have called the resolution of dilemmas. Jennings[33] urges us to think of consensus not as a thing, or a goal, but rather as an activity. He regrets the lack of a gerund form of the word (gerund: a form of a verb capable of being construed as a noun). In English the word would be 'consensing'. Jennings asserts that consensus enjoys moral weight in decision making only when it reflects 'a healthy community of open, inclusive moral discovery and growth'. But consensus speaks of compromise. Reflecting on the hard realities of policy making and implementation, Hans Stein (Chapter 16) remarks, 'If the choice you must make is between taking the left or the right road, to compromise by choosing the middle one won't get you anywhere, or at least not to the place that you originally had in mind.'

In an inescapable sense, a consensus must always be false. In the bargaining and the negotiations of policy making, some ideas succeed, others fail. More robust than consensus is the notion of keeping the differences in productive tension. Giovanni Moro (Chapter 5) says that policies '. . . must essentially be a matter of managing diversity'.

Constructive conversation will require something more open and flexible than the implied rules of the committee, the arena in which most health policy is made. Crucially, Per Carlsson and Peter Garpenby (Chapter 6) observe, 'Participants in the deliberative democracy model are expected to act without any predetermined opinions. The idea is that *the discussion itself*, and the arguments that are put forward, will contribute to reshaping preferences, and that following such discussion it should be possible to achieve a cooperation that includes the broad majority.'

We may need to invent new arenas for 'the discussion itself', for constructive conversation, new metaphors of discourse, much as Morgan[34] urges the invention of new metaphors for organisations. These, he suggests, will be the product of our ability to imagine them, a process that Morgan describes as 'imaginisation'.

Seven maxims

Committees are bound by conventions and rules – the rhythm of agendas, who speaks and when, how decisions are proposed, challenged, reached and minuted. There are no such generally recognised rules of engagement in the case of constructive conversation. I suggest that it might be helpful to adduce some maxims to guide us through the policy discourse, and offer the following list for critique, improvement and expansion.

1 **Search for the absent dimensions:** The Madrid Framework attempts to make explicit both the interconnectedness of, and the conflicts within and between, all of its dimensions. Discussions that habitually avoid one or other dimension may suggest an unconscious, or even a deliberate, avoidance by the policy makers. Any such persistent absence of issues may also suggest that the policy group lacks individuals with the relevant professional expertise or motivation, such that the balance of discussion in the group becomes *constitutionally* distorted.

2 **Resist 'stakeholder capture':** Discussions are inevitably driven by the professional or political or corporate imperatives of the participants. Constructive conversation requires the moderation of such self-interests or special pleadings, and the validity of the discussion may be tested by the degree to which participants are prepared to speak at variance from their expected partisanship.

3 **Expect the unanticipated:** Policies grow, evolve, adapt to changing circumstance, are blown off course by events, are capable of adapting to explore and exploit ecological niches in the health system. Uncertainty is the only certainty. There is no place for the constructive conversationalist in a discourse based on the fiction that every effect can be the precisely predicted product of a particular cause.

4 **Beware the claims of a common metric:** You cannot make quantitative comparison between custard and Tuesdays. Aristotle pictures choice as a quality-based selection among heterogeneous goods. Consequently, the following claims should be resisted. Firstly, the belief that in every situation of choice there is one value common to all the alternatives, and that this varies only in quantity. Secondly, the claim that in all alternatives, there is one and the same metric. Thirdly, that 'means' have values only in relation to the good consequences, the 'ends', that they produce. Fourthly, the myth of a common metric in all things belonging to the ultimate end – in our case to 'health' or 'equity', and so on.

5 **Distrust *de fide* claims of moral superiority:** Most of the dimensions imply ethical positions. These are often 'played' in debate as though 'equity' or 'choice' or 'evidence' and so on were the ace of trumps in a political card game. Such claims of *de fide* moral superiority are hard to resist, but they should be challenged.[35]

Daniels[36] compares a foundationalist with a relativist approach to discourse. In the former certain moral positions, values, are taken to be self-evident, fixed and unrevisable, because they derive from some absolute structures of value that reflect religious revelation or metaphysical theory. In health policy discourse the pursuit of equity or freedom of choice or quality of service are often presented in this way. Rawls[37] refers to these as 'fixed points'. Daniels argues for a relativist approach that he calls 'reflective equilibrium'. This 'consists in working back and forth among our considered judgments (some say our *intuitions*) about particular instances or cases . . . revising any of these elements wherever necessary in order to achieve an acceptable coherence among them.'

Whether we claim authority for our values from revelation or from reason, whether we believe them to derive from a universal reality or to be contingent on the insights of a particular moment in history, we argue for them on the basis that one is superior to another. Reflective equilibrium, constructive conversation, posits a dialogic, and not a dogmatic, resolution to the conflicts between the values implied in our policies.

6 **Shun easy consensus:** Consensus can be the lowest common denominator of agreement between the policy makers and stakeholders. The quest for this enfeebles robust debate and challenge. All the essays in this book reveal the complexities, the *intra*-dimensional conflicts within, and *inter*-dimensional conflicts between, such goods as 'health' or 'sustainability' or 'democracy'. Attempts to reach easy consensus by over-simplification of the real conflicts and paradoxes obscures the need for hard political choices. There is no consensus without loss. This should be faced and the cost counted.

7 **Consider your metaphors:** The various metaphors we use imply different ends, means and cultures. It's important to know in what metaphors we fashion our policies. If they seem inappropriate to the tasks, we can try to change them, to operate in alternative imaginations. In literature, mixing metaphors is deemed a vice; in constructive conversation about health, it can be a virtue.

Conclusion

Richard Rorty[38] resists the notion of foundationalist beliefs in a universal obligation on all humankind. Instead, he suggests that our sense of solidarity is grounded not in metaphysical absolutes, but in the particulars of how we have come to live in a liberal society. He holds that since our moral positions are contingent – on our histories and our contemporary situations – it does not help to try to express an *essence* of human solidarity (for example, with such collectives as 'all humankind' or 'all rational beings'). Rather, he believes that we express our liberal sentiments and aspirations more securely and more practically by 'reminding ourselves to keep trying to expand our sense of *us* as far as we can'. Rorty says that what is important is to separate out the question, 'Do you believe and desire what we believe and desire?' from the question, 'Are you suffering?' The former seeks to define the boundaries of our obligations. The latter invites answer from across all the frontiers of our partialities and our prejudices.

In November 2004 the UK government published its proposals to curtail smoking in enclosed public places. The political debate centred on the responsibilities of government. Many argued that in not making the ban absolute (a public house – the English 'pub' – that does not offer prepared food is likely to be exempt from the ban) the government was condemning many passive smokers (not least workers in the industry) to avoidable morbidity and premature mortality. Others argued that the ban was a substantial infringement of the individual's right to choose. Can the Madrid Framework help to illuminate the debate?

The impact of cigarette smoking on health is well established. In the UK it is estimated that smoking accounts for some 120 000 avoidable deaths per annum, and a massive burden of morbidity. Yet, because it is a major source of gratification to many citizens, particularly those in the lowest socioeconomic groups for whom so many sources of gratification may well be in poor supply, addiction to cigarette smoking remains widespread. The paradox is that, for these smokers, banning smoking in public places diminishes their sense of personal freedom and wellbeing, and their freedom of association – essential components of 'health' in the WHO's definition. This, despite the incontrovertible evidence of the shockingly destructive future cost of this gratification to them.

How should we judge the quality of constructive conversation about this policy? The expected avoidance of disease and premature mortality for those who would otherwise suffer as passive smokers is supported by the evidence. However, constructive conversationalists will recall Yach's warning (Chapter 8) that, 'Evidence is . . . selectively chosen for packaging in support of the political arguments.' Because all evidence is socially constructed, it presents not only the answers to the research questions posed, but also the agenda, the purposes, of the questioner. Those who argue from evidence must also take account both of the wider definition of health as freedom, and the implications of individual choice as a value. The freedom of the smoker (to prefer the immediate gratifications of smoking to the deferred gratification of a future without the burdens of heart and lung diseases) must be balanced by the freedom of others not to be damaged by the smoker's choice. Our choices perpetually impact on the choices of others, because, as Moro (Chapter 5), reminds us, there is 'need to correct the notion of citizens as pure, unrelated individuals, entities abstracted from their ties and the social fabric where they live'.

Not all 11 of the dimensions may be relevant to the conversation, but they should at least be considered. For example, any such legislation must be accompanied by the possibility of enforcement, and implementation will require a *synergy* between the policies of other government departments – those concerned with the licensing of premises, law and order, local government. What are the moral hazards for stewardship, for government, given the contribution to the public purse from the taxes on tobacco and alcohol, and the global economic dominance of these industries? Reference to the Madrid Framework can resolve none of the conflicts revealed. But it can set out the full field of discourse.

The essays that follow include examples of philosophical analysis, practical experience, visionary aspiration, and political credo. In the content of these essays, in their very differing reliance on research evidence and experience and belief, and above all in the authenticity of the writers' voices, is reflected that wide variety of approaches, opinions and prejudices that are mandatory for the rigour and vigour of constructive conversation.

Notes and references

1 Carroll L (1994) *Alice Through the Looking Glass*. Penguin Popular Classics, Harlow, Chapter 6.

2 At the 2003 Madrid conference on health policy and values, Ilona Kickbusch used the term 'constructive conversation'. I seized on this because I thought that it caught with fine precision what we were trying to achieve. Later, in the course of facilitating workshops in Wales, Hungary, Spain and Scotland, focused on the practical application of the Madrid Framework, 'constructive conversation' became the mantra for the way we talked about health and policy.

3 *See* Rosen RG (1974) *From Medical Police to Social Medicine*. Science History Publications, New York.

4 Rodwin VG (2001) Health in the City. In: M Marinker (ed) *Medicine and Humanity*. King's Fund Publishing, London.

5 Sen AK (1999) *Development As Freedom*. Knopf, New York.

6 World Health Organization (1978) *Health for All*. WHO, Geneva.

7 Kickbusch I (2002) Perspectives of health governance in the 20th Century. In: M Marinker (ed) *Health Targets in Europe: polity, progress and promise*. BMJ Books, London.

8 *Workshop on Health Targets in Europe: Values, Principles and Governance*, Madrid, May 8–9, 2003.

9 Note the persistent use of the politically correct term 'targeting', even when considering the underlying values of policy. The term 'evidence based' is now similarly part of our lingua franca, with consequent restrictions on what may be legitimately expressed. The words we use can turn against us, and take our thinking prisoner.

10 Marinker M (2005) The Madrid Framework. *Eurohealth*. 11(1): 2–5. Available from: www.euro.who.int/Document/obs/Eurohealth11_1.pdf.

11 In the course of wide consultation, the names and specific content of the dimensions have undergone iterative modifications. The number has also varied between 10 and 12. Finally I elected for *11* dimensions. It is only an amusing coincidence, and not a delusion of cosmic significance or *folie de grandeur*, that this is the approximate number of dimensions currently postulated by theoretical physicists to define the Universe.

12 Pickles J (2005) *A History of Spaces: cartographic reason, mapping and the geo-coded world*. Routledge, London. This is where I first came across this very useful term. I coined 'lexical reasoning' to complement it.

13 Neither the number nor the names of the dimensions are set in stone. If the Madrid Framework is to fulfil its purpose in supporting constructive conversation, these may well be modified to make it fit for particular purposes.

14 A classic problem of translation. 'Stewardship' is almost impossible to translate out of English, where its historic roots refer to the self-imposed duties of hereditary land owners to care for their estates and tied peasantries, and to ensure the continuing value of the estate for their heirs – hardly an attractive etymology for the twenty-first century obligations of democratic government. There is however another provenance which supports the use of 'Stewardship'. The OED records that in old Scottish usage the word 'policy' described the enclosed, planted, and partly embellished park or freehold possession lying around a country seat or gentleman's house.

15 Foucault M (1970) *The Order of Things*. Tavistock, London.

16 From 'Burnt Norton' in Eliot TS (1954) *Four Quartets*. Faber and Faber, London.

17 Susan Sontag (2001) Territorial imperatives. *The Guardian*. 16 June. 'We fret about words, we writers. Words mean. Words point. They are arrows. Arrows stuck in the rough hide of reality . . . And the more portentous, the more general the words, the more they also resemble rooms or tunnels. They can expand, or cave in . . .'

18 Marinker M (ed) (2002) *Health Targets in Europe: polity, progress and promise*. BMJ Books, London. 'It struck me that even when we think and speak in our own native tongues,

we are always translating. I came to suspect that it would be from these very approximations and ambiguities and ambivalences that we might reach a richer lingua franca . . .'

19 Bronowski J (1956) *Science and Human Values*. Penguin Books, London.
20 Moore CJ (2005) *In Other Words*. Oxford University Press, Oxford.
21 McKee M (2002) Values, beliefs and implications. In: M Marinker (ed) *Health Targets in Europe: polity, progress and promise*. BMJ Books, London.
22 Virchow R (1848) Die öffendliche Gesundheitsplege. *Medicinische Reform*. **5**: August 4. Virchow promoted the view that a democratic state should desire that all its citizens 'enjoy a state of well-being because it recognises that they all have equal rights.' He wrote that 'the state . . . must assist everyone so far that he (sic) will have the conditions necessary for a healthy existence.'
23 Hutton W (2002) *The World We're In*. Little, Brown, London.
24 Davies N (2005) *God's Playground: a history of Poland. Volume II*. Oxford University Press, Oxford.
25 Bronowski J (1956) *Science and Human Values*. Penguin Books, London.
26 Giacomini M, Hurley J, Gold I, Smith P and Abelson J (2004) The policy analysis of 'values talk': lessons from Canadian health reform. *Health Policy*. **67**: 15–24.
27 (1998) *HEALTH21* – the Health for All policy framework for the WHO European Region. WHO Regional Office for Europe, Copenhagen (European Health for All Series, No. 6).
28 Glouberman S (2001) *Towards a New Perspective on Health Policy: Canadian Policy Research Networks Study No. H/03*. Renouf Publishing Co, Ottawa.
29 Governance through Metaphor Project, on http://www.uia.org/metaphor/#pro.
30 Marinker M (1994) Evidence, paradox and consensus. In: M Marinker (ed) *Controversies in Health Policy*. BMJ Publications, London. I developed this model as a consequence of leading a number of expert think tanks in preparation for this publication.
31 Veatch RM and Moreno JD (1991) Consensus in panels and committees: conceptual and ethical issues. *J Med Phil*. **16**(4): 462.
32 Handy C (1994) *The Empty Raincoat*. Hutchinson, London.
33 Jennings B (1991) Possibilities of consensus: towards democratic discourse. *J Med Phil*. **16**(4): 462.
34 Morgan G (1986) *Images of Organisation*. Sage, London. Gareth Morgan suggests that we can understand organisations best if we think in metaphors.
35 'Conversation doesn't just reshuffle the cards: it creates new cards.' Zeldin T (1998) *Conversation*. Harvill, London.
36 Daniels N (2003) Reflective Equilibrium. The Stanford Encyclopedia of Philosophy. Summer 2003. www.plato.Stanford.edu/archives/sum2003/entries/reflective-equilibrium/
37 Rawls J (1999) *A Theory of Justice* (2e). Harvard University Press, Cambridge, MA.
38 Rorty R (1989) *Contingency, Irony and Solidarity*. Cambridge University Press, Cambridge.

Chapter 2

The value of values

Marc Danzon

In the 52 countries that comprise the WHO European Region, values are present in the preamble of almost every national health policy. However, they are not so visible in the core texts of these policies, in the parts that describe actions, resources, implementation and evaluation. Some sort of chasm seems to exist. On one side there are values, seen as inspirational, taken-for-granted, self-explanatory general statements. On the other side there is the reality of policy making in public health. The headline preambles and the detailed texts do not always link. It is easy to use values as a mantra rather than as an agenda.

The World Health Organization (WHO) Regional Office for Europe was confronted with this discrepancy when it began work on developing the 2005 update of the European Health for All policy framework, further referred to in this text as Health for All.[1] The process of preparing the update (2003–5) included a careful re-examination of the Health for All values, to render them more useful and relevant and thus encourage their practical implementation. Several important questions were raised:

- What role do values play in the Region's national health sectors?
- What are the values valid for the European health sector in the twenty-first century?
- Do these values also lie at the heart of policies formulated in other sectors – particularly the major policies dealing with national, social and economic development?
- How can these values be better understood; how can they be made more useful to policy makers?
- What kinds of mechanisms would contribute to the practical implementation of these values?

The Regional Office had sound reasons to ask these questions, and launched a broad exercise of reflection and analysis in order to answer them. The core Health for All values appear to be endorsed by the Region's Member States, and many governments referred to them explicitly in their national health policies. Yet this does not mean that these values are necessarily driving health systems. Also, while the ethical dimensions are easy to identify in health and health-related policies, they are 'rarely given a systematic scrutiny'.[2]

The approach was therefore to address these problems. The European Observatory of Health Systems and Policies made a systematic study of the health policies of all 52 Member States of the WHO European Region. Further, a think tank was created, bringing together experts with diverse professional backgrounds, with broad knowledge and experience in formulating, assessing and implementing health policies internationally, nationally and sub-nationally, all across the Region. Finally, a review was made of a wide range of available tools that might enable policy makers to assess whether values are present and respected in their national health policies.

The analysis revealed that, either directly or indirectly, many national policies referred to the core values described in the 1998 update of the European Health for All policy (HEALTH21). Indeed some of these values had been present in national health policy documents developed before that update. This suggests that the European Region shares a general ethical orientation.

However the Regional Office now wished to check whether these declared ethical commitments were in any way consistent with actual decisions taken and activities implemented. Was this measurable? In short, how to verify that the deeds matched the words? Although the work on the 2005 Health for All update revealed a general deficit of well developed methodologies capable of making such evaluations, at the empirical level some national experiences demonstrated a lack of consistency between stated values and actual practice. For instance, while most national health policy documents declare commitment to equity and solidarity, in practice equity is not progressing, and the gaps in health status and health gains between different social sub-groups are increasing. What's the value of a value, then, if evidence suggests that it is not respected in actions taken?

Raising these concerns does not mean denying the importance of values for European health policy making. Rather, it means that we are brave enough to ask the obvious question – 'Do we need values?'

Do we need values?

Modern science constantly brings people to new thresholds. The exploding progress in research and technologies offers significant benefits and health gains. At the same time, this progress raises some ethical problems. Improvement in health has no limits, but resources do have limits. In real life, not all advances can be made available to everyone who would benefit from them. 'Medicine . . . has no equity plan.'[3]

This means that policy makers always confront the need to make choices. And here is where values can be valuable. Policy makers can best justify their choices when they demonstrate, through their decisions, that they have respected and implemented the values cherished by their societies.

In reality, all health policies, and all other public policies, imply ethical assumptions. It is hard to imagine a health policy or a policy making procedure without them.[2] And because certain shared core values permeate all sectors of society, frameworks of common values are essential for any policy making process, and mark out the range of policy options that is politically acceptable.

The political context of values is very complex, not least because in today's rapidly changing and very diverse Europe, it is hardly feasible to reach a uniform understanding of some broad ethical notions. Values are subject to interpretations. No common definitions have yet been found that all – countries, and national and international stakeholders in health – would accept as accurate, acceptable and relevant. Another impediment for values-based governance is that values are only one among a range of factors influencing policy making. Policy makers have to make tough choices about which values to uphold and prioritise, and how much compromise is acceptable, when other salient factors, limited funds for instance, make compromise inevitable.

Nevertheless, countries need values and have become increasingly outspoken in stating this clearly. One of the most recent examples was the broad consultation on the European Union (EU) health policy, initiated in 2004 by the European Commission. In response to the Commission's call for reflection, a number of countries expressed concern that to consider health policy predominantly in economic terms could lead to the undermining of basic principles such as equity, neglecting the ethical issue of health as a human right. The message by member states to the Commission was clear. If EU health policy were to be too driven by market concerns, it could lose sight of the fact that health is not a standard market commodity, but also a goal and an end in itself.[4]

European countries gave similarly strong and plain messages to WHO. The Regional Office opened a broad consultation on a draft of the 2005 Health for All update in the first half of 2005. In their response, individual states clearly expressed a desire to preserve and sustain a core set of values. Many of them confirmed an interest in the values that comprise the heart of the European social consensus. During the consultation, and at the 55th session of the Regional Committee for Europe when countries adopted the 2005 Health for All update, they told the Regional Office that they were content to have the three core Health for All values – equity, solidarity and participation – reaffirmed.

Why do we need values?

Countries especially welcomed several findings of the 2005 Health for All update.[1] Based on this broad consensus, the following conclusions can more or less be confidently made.

- The core values of equity, solidarity and participation form the ethical fundament of health policies.
- At the international level, there is no need scrupulously and obsessively to redefine core values such as equity, solidarity, fairness, participation, even-handedness.
- In reality, values cannot be defined in a uniform manner that will reflect and resolve the wide diversity of the settings in which they are to be implemented; values are context-specific – culturally, historically, geographically, economically, and so on.
- Values, and the respect for them, form the basis of the legal human rights framework and the right to health, as stipulated in a number of international legally binding instruments and treaties.
- Values are therefore widely present in the international obligations that European countries have incurred in negotiating and adopting a variety of human rights instruments. When uncertain how to implement particular values or ensure respect for them, health policy makers do not need to start from scratch, or reinvent the wheel. Powerful instruments are available – the human rights treaties and conventions that the European states have already adopted.
- The values dominating the public health debate do not belong exclusively to the health sector; most often, they are ethical norms, standards and aspirations that are held to be respected across all sectors, by the society at large.

- In periods of profound reforms of the health sector, values are essential and irreplaceable. They comprise a compass for orientation that can help policy makers retain a focus on what their societies believe is right and fair, at times when they are obliged to introduce what are often very painful and unpopular, but necessary, changes. This is true not only for countries in the turmoil of transition, but also for all countries that are committed to reforming their health systems.
- Respect for values and for human rights is a means of empowering the public health sector both to lead and to meet the challenge of stewardship.
- To do this, public health policy makers need to have clear evidence of the benefits of adherence to commonly shared values. They also need to have at their disposal a range of tools for putting values into action.

Health for All? Yes, for all

Equity is a core Health for All value.[5] There was a period when WHO was seen as somewhat idealistic and ideological in encouraging countries to consider that everyone has the right to reach their full health potential. But today the notion and language of equity are regaining currency, and are stronger than ever – for national policy makers, for researchers, for the international community.[6] From WHO's perspective, this is welcome because these values have always been at the heart of the Organization's policy making and at the core of the Health for All movement in particular.

Nor is WHO alone in its 'for all' aspiration. It is highly indicative of what is valuable in Europe, that this 'for all' agenda, in a number of guises, appears in the statements of a wide range of national and international actors.[7] The decision to adopt a programme of community action in the field of public health for 2003–8 postulated that the programme was to contribute to tackling inequalities in health. In July 2004, the European Commissioner for Health and Consumer Protection said that the 'overarching goal of EU health policy can be concisely expressed as a pursuit of good Health for All.'[8] In June 2005, the Council of the European Union took this notion further, calling on the EU member states to 'pay special attention to the access to affordable . . . treatment for all in need'.[9] It also declared, as a guiding principle for sustainable development, 'the respect for fundamental human rights, including . . . equal opportunities for all; promotion and protection of fundamental human rights, solidarity within and between generations, involvement of citizens in decision-making'. The Council clearly highlighted social equity and cohesion as key policy objectives. Another major partner of WHO, the Council of Europe, strongly subscribes to these same values.[10] National governments do so too. When launching a new national health strategy in 2001, one European health minister (of Ireland) said that the concern for equity is a national value and that everyone is encouraged to have a say.[11] Another European country (the United Kingdom) made tackling health inequalities its core programme for action, and chose this as one of the core topics for the EU during the period of its presidency.[12]

It is amazing how persistent we – health policy makers, actors or visionaries – are in our ambition to bring health gains to all. Reality confronts and frustrates us all the time, and yet we continue, even though it is a fact of life that no matter how much we wish and try to do so, we cannot bring what we feel is right to all who need it.

The distribution of wellbeing and health is uneven. Researchers systematically point to the discrepancy between commitment to health as a human right, and the realisation of this right. Disparities grow between health outcomes for the well-to-do and the poor.[13] Social and economic inequalities are reflected epidemiologically in the disproportionate burden of diseases,[3] and there is evidence that social disparities in health outcomes are widening, not narrowing.[14,15] At the national level, debates continue. Does a country want a healthcare system that offers greater equity of access so as to ensure that everybody's needs are met, or should the distribution of healthcare be left to the market?[16]

Internationally as well, there is consistent and convincing evidence of the problem of achieving health equity. The Organisation for Economic Co-operation and Development (OECD) draws attention to income-related inequality in the use of medical care.[17] The World Bank's report 2006[18] points to inequality as a key barrier to global development. It is very relevant that the report interprets equity in exactly the same way as WHO – not as equality of health *outcome* but as equality of health *opportunity*, irrespective of race, caste, gender, inherited social and economic privileges. Lastly, individual widely renowned thinkers and politicians point to the urgency of the need to address health inequalities. They state that the magnitude of suffering, disease and premature death in the world today is caused by social factors and widening inequalities, and conclude that if the major health determinants are social, so must be the remedies.[19,20]

In summary, there is a wide commitment to the values of equity, solidarity, fairness and participation. But they are not always clearly reflected in practice. Why?

Health systems

Increasingly, shortcomings in health systems are seen as one possible explanation of why values are not fully reflected in the way services are delivered to all members of society. Inevitably, the way a health system works reflects the ethical choices made. This is true for all four functions of health systems – provision of services, financing, resource generation, and stewardship and governance. Of these, the biggest challenge to solidarity and equity lies in how a health system is financed.

In a system based on the Health for All values, budgets should be drawn up to reflect the relative contributions of the various budget items to health improvement. For example, a policy that favours sophisticated, high-technology investment should make sure that all population groups can benefit equitably. All decisions about allocation of resources involve setting priorities that inevitably express values. Clarifying how values affect both the process and the content of health policy decisions is therefore essential. Some researchers pose uneasy and challenging questions – for example, is the economic evaluation of health systems and health funding in touch with society's values?[21]

For a national health system to be consistent with the Health for All vision and values, it should have the following important features, all of which are clearly linked to values.

- *Universal availability*. There should be enough functioning health and public health facilities, goods and services to meet the needs of everyone in the country.
- *Universal accessibility*. The need for accessibility applies to every element of the health sector, but is particularly critical for primary care. Access has an economical dimension (affordability), a geographical dimension (physical accessibility), an ethical and human rights dimension (accessibility to all population groups equally, without discrimination) and a communications dimension (accessibility of information).
- *Universal acceptability*. All health facilities, goods and services, including communication and information, should be culturally appropriate and respectful of cultural differences and traditions.
- *Quality improvement*. The benefits of the continuous improvement and upgrading of health services should be evenly distributed among all social groups and not merely available to people who can pay for it. Quality improvement programmes should specify the expected resulting health gain. For instance, adopting procedures that ensure patient safety is one efficient way to boost quality. The benefits of quality improvement include better health, improved relations between the general public and health professionals, and a decrease in costly failures in patient treatment.

In the European Region, health systems can be described as having three essential goals – health gain, fairness and responsiveness. All three are in harmony with the Health for All ethical framework. In reality, however, these goals are not always met – 'Health systems are consistently inequitable, providing more and higher quality services to the well-off, who need them less, than to the poor, who are unable to obtain them.'[22] Evidence shows that, in the absence of a concerted effort to ensure that health systems reach disadvantaged groups more effectively, such inequalities are likely to continue. Values may be used to test, evaluate and improve the way health systems function, and this is most useful if carried out by individual countries. For all these reasons putting values at the centre of health systems is crucial.

Checking the performance of health systems against commonly shared values proves to be useful especially today, when national policy makers often receive conflicting views on the most efficient way to strengthen them. The views conflict because of the sensitivity of the issues. A government may be willing to distribute money in an equitable and fair manner to everyone in need, but how can it do so when resources are extremely tight?

Overall, the health systems message from different national and international health stakeholders is pretty consistent. For example, the Gastein Health Declaration 2003 clearly calls for affordable, accessible healthcare[23] – the same characteristics seen as essential by Health for All and WHO. In June 2005, the Council of the European Union called on the EU Member States to work continuously on developing and maintaining a sustainable, affordable and accessible healthcare system as a basis for all prevention, treatment and care, and in this context to pay special attention to ensuring access to affordable health services.[9]

Values and targets

Even when we talk the common language of values, we do not always agree about the best ways to express and realise them. Although there may be a broad consensus about what is important, sometimes we disagree on how exactly to proceed, for example on how to design and measure progress. In Europe, the great diversity of settings, views and experiences is a given in all debate.

Many argue that we do not need to take values into account because we already have a proven and useful approach to policy making – health targets. Health targets have a solid, serious history in Europe. At the heart of the Madrid Framework there lies a publication called 'Health targets in Europe'.[24] In the Gastein Declaration 2004 to the European Parliament, the Madrid Framework is recommended for all health systems. Setting targets is described as 'an incentive to shape the future'.

Thirty-eight European health targets were adopted by WHO as far back as 1984, as the core of the European Health for All, and the 1998 update suggests 21 targets.[25] Target-setting was actually the traditional approach in Health for All policy formulation across the WHO European Region. Recently, however, a new consensus has been building. Establishing common targets for all countries in the Region can often be artificial, unfair or simply uninspiring. They do not necessarily take account of significant differences in Member States' population, health and economic development. Analysis of the HEALTH21 targets in 40 national Health for All policies reveals the following interesting points.

- Countries prefer concrete, technical targets. For instance, three targets appear in three-quarters of the policies – improving mental health; healthier living; reducing harm from alcohol, drugs and tobacco.
- In contrast, broadly formulated, vague and general targets seem to be of little interest. For instance, three targets appear in less than a quarter of the policies – solidarity for health in Europe; mobilising partners for health; policies and strategies for Health for All.
- Countries systematically reformulate and adjust the regional targets to reflect their individual needs and circumstances.
- Some national policies also introduce health targets not yet covered by Health for All, reflecting particular national and sub-national priorities.

The message is clear. Setting targets can be an important exercise at the national, and sometimes at the sub-national, level. Targeting can provide guidance, enhance implementation, and can be an excellent means for a country to articulate its degree of ambition. And when all stakeholders are involved, the formulation of national health targets can help ensure their joint ownership of health policy.

Implement, monitor, evaluate, plan for the future

Acknowledging the different choices that could be made does not mean underestimating the role that values play in European policy making. In fact, quite the opposite, it means that values are both useful and valuable, provided always that their implementation is verified, measured and monitored. Such a vision is not entirely new. In developing it, the Madrid Framework and Health for All have points of consensus.

As stated in a letter of October 2004, from M Marinker to D Byrne,[26] the European Commissioner for Health and Consumer Protection, the aim of the Madrid Framework is described as follows – 'to develop a flexible, robust and practical tool with increasingly wide international applicability'. As for Health for All, before 2000 it was mainly oriented towards *outcomes* as a means of protecting and improving health. Recently, the *process* of reaching these outcomes has become equally important and interesting for the Regional Office. How to support countries with the process? For the Regional Office, this comes down to helping them implement what they state they want to achieve. Policy makers need instruments at hand.

That's why the 2005 Health for All update took a pragmatic approach towards values. It proposes a toolbox, a variety of instruments, methods, actions and techniques that health ministers can use when designing and implementing Health for All policies. The examples correspond to four generic questions.

- How can policy makers establish a national framework for ethical governance?
- How can they incorporate up-to-date evidence into their health policies?
- How can they assess the implementation of values?
- How can they make policies more effective in improving health?

To be able to promote equity and other values across social groups, generations, genders and countries, however, policy makers need to understand the under-lying trends in their societies. This is a new challenge for public health. Health trends must be continuously observed, monitored, checked and evaluated, with seriousness and professionalism. Evaluations are needed so that we are able to compare policy in action with the original policy intent. If we find out that they diverge, it is our responsibility to find the cause and to assess the implications. Only thus can we meet the challenge to forecast, to plan for the future. The need for evaluation in public health is one area of quick, vast new development and change.

How do we talk about values?

Another domain is the tone, the way we speak about ethical issues. There has been a visible and exciting change in the style, the language and the approach with which the international community talks about values in health policy. From being somewhat instructive and prescriptive, it has moved to what the Madrid Framework describes as *constructive conversation*.[27] Previously tending to be monologic and patronising, international health stakeholders have now moved to a communications style of dialogue and partnership. We have all become more receptive, more modest, less 'preachy' and more respectful of the right of individual countries to formulate their own health imperatives, values and targets. We also seem to be more willing to be flexible in whatever we give as recommendations. It is a Region-wide common process of change, marked on the surface by the new tone and language, but revealing a deeper transformation in attitudes, towards greater openness and interaction.

Examples are abundant. The European Commission took this approach as early as 2000, when it called for the creation of a European Health Forum – one of its new mechanisms to involve in the debate not only policy makers, but all relevant groups in societies, in an open forum of consultation, exchange of views and experience.[28] The Madrid Framework describes itself as not intending to be a gold standard, but rather an evolving reference of values – to boost the European cooperation in establishing common values that can be embraced and implemented at all levels.[25]

The Regional Office has also evolved. A lot of time has passed since 1984, when WHO adopted the first set of Health For All targets for the European Region. One analyst said of its approach, 'WHO operated at the time in the only way it knew.'[24] Since then, WHO has learned much. The main lesson was summarised in a comment given by a country in its deliberation on the 2005 Health for All update that this consultative approach is really welcome. The Region is not anymore in a situation where one common normative European strategy could capture the realities of the fast-changing Region. The 2005 update takes Health for All Europe another step forward. It is offered not as a users' manual, but as one possible architecture for a health policy.[29] It is already adopted and the work continues.

WHO Europe has committed itself to an open-ended Health For All process, a process that will be continually enriched by a variety of national experiences and perspectives, and by the continuing input and work of the Regional Office. The consultation with countries has already generated some intriguing proposals that will be taken up, including the following:

- to explore further the financial dimension of implementing Health for All policies in the Member States;
- to scrutinise precisely how ethical, values-based governance relates to health system functioning;
- to study the impact of health determinants on sectors other than health;
- to monitor systematically the use and applicability of the Health for All concept of ethical governance in individual countries;
- to develop concrete tools for comparative analysis of Health for All policies in relation to the implementation of the core values;
- to explore the connections between the Health for All policy framework and the core policies of other key international stakeholders in public health;
- to develop benchmarks for the progressive implementation of Health for All;
- to develop a broad Health for All communications platform at the regional, national and sub-national levels.

Most of these are about how to position values in the reality of policy making. No matter what different health actors choose to call it – constructive conversation, open-ended process, joint reflection, health forum – the underlying approach is the same: openness, ability to listen and adjust, transparency, sharing. The international dimension of this process is seen by all as interaction and cross-fertilisation, creating opportunities for the exchange of views and experiences. Countries expect the Regional Office to set the stage and stimulate such an open-ended process, in cooperation with its key partner organisations in the domain of health. However, it is individual countries themselves that will find the best ways to implement values, to make sure that the functioning of health systems reflects respect for them; in essence, to transport values from the wishful preambles into the main texts of national public health policies and programmes.

Putting frameworks in the frame

Can we see the forest, not only the trees?

Finally, an observation about an intriguing and increasingly common phenomenon: the international community has displayed an amazing tendency to call everything 'a framework'. This goes to the root of a problem with major implications. How can we frame all the proposed frameworks? How can a national policy maker find a meaningful way to deal with the growing number of cross-cutting issues, generic concerns that are supposed to be reflected in each and every policy action? Examples are alarmingly numerous.

In 1993, the European Commission set out a '*framework* for action in the field of public health' and eight action programmes for the period 1996–2001 were adopted within this framework. In 2000, in its proposal for adopting the 2001–6 programme of the Community action in the field of public health, the Commission said this programme would be successful and possible only in the new public health *framework*.[28,30,31] Two very recent publications of the World Bank and of WHO describe the *Millennium Development Goals* (MDGs) as the core *framework* for measuring progress. The MDGs are seen to provide an overarching framework for development efforts, and benchmarks against which to measure success.[32] DGs set quantifiable and ambitious targets against which to measure progress.[33]

Next comes the *poverty framework*. As part of their efforts to reach the MDGs, countries worldwide are designing and implementing poverty reduction strategies. These strategies have a strong health component. To make it even more difficult to see the whole forest for the trees, the *human-rights based approach* lies also at the core of the international efforts for better health: human rights can make powerful contributions in improving health outcomes.[34] The right to health has a normative substance, obligations associated with it and a range of measures are required for its implementation.[35] WHO was quick in linking human rights to the poverty framework, moving fast in providing health policy makers with tools for designing, implementing and monitoring a poverty reduction strategy through a human-rights based approach.[36]

On top of that, the central role of good health was recently explored in the *framework* of macroeconomic development and growth. *Human development* approaches have evolved rapidly, adding further to the complexity of all the frameworks. Originally, social and economic development was seen only through the prism of the outcome of development efforts.[37] How these outcomes were achieved was not the centre of attention. However, since the start of the new century it is widely recognised that the ways and means of achieving human development are no less important than their outcomes. Human rights are one such means. Those populations whose development is at stake should have their rights respected and realised. Thus, in 2000, UNDP noted that human development and human rights are two approaches 'harmonious enough to be able to complement each other and diverse enough to enrich each other'.[38] That is, these two *frameworks* also overlap.

Even broader issues frame the picture. Leading politicians in Europe declare that '*global security*, not just common humanity, demands that we renew the vigour with which we address poverty, the environment and disease. In 2005, the world must remind itself of the goals set in the Millennium Declaration and why they were set . . . Crucially, we must focus on better ways of achieving them . . . it will be propelled forwards by the ever-greater awareness of global interdependence.'[39]

To put it bluntly, everything of value is interdependent, so everything of true value is being labelled and promoted to countries as a *framework* – Health for All, the Commission's public health strategy, the MDGs, human development, human rights, poverty reduction, security. What else? Gender? Health systems? Socioeconomic determinants of health? The 11 dimensions of the Madrid Framework? Health targets? The list continues . . . All these and many more are equally crucial frameworks for policies, decisions and actions. How can we orient ourselves in this patchwork of frameworks? How can we make a meaningful link between them all? A useful way may be to see how health comes into the picture.

Health seems to be universally recognised as the hard currency of modern times. Health is at the heart of the MDGs. Recognition of health is central to the global agenda of reducing poverty, as well as an important measure of human wellbeing. Health generates wealth;[23] health should be considered as an investment . . . not a cost (European Commission); health is a cause of progress (United Nations); good health drives economic growth (United Nations Development Programme, World Bank); investing long-term means to be able to bridge the health gaps and tackle inequalities (current UK EU presidency).

Health governance is good governance. This is what the 2005 Health for All update calls ethical, values-based governance. It implies a willingness to search for the best solution in a rational rather than in an ideological way. In this situation it is crucially important to be open and honest about the values on which your system and your judgements are based. It also implies a provision for future generations, which in essence is about the value of solidarity both within and between generations.[9,39]

In the end, in order to grasp the complexity of the issue, we need to go back to the basics, to the simplest and most obvious questions about health policy in Europe. One such key question was posed in 2002 with some passion: 'Who will carry the flame? And how?'[24]

Maybe it is not for one international or national body to carry the flame alone. Because our common shared values are themselves the flame. Maybe these values are that common denominator of all international frameworks and efforts. If this is the case, health policy makers can draw strength from values, can be persistent in their commitment to ethical, values-based governance, and not allow fatigue to overwhelm them, or desperation, because they do not see sufficient results, and quickly enough, from the enormous efforts they make.

As long as we share the same values and are able to talk openly and honestly about how to bring them into the reality of everyday policy making, the passion for and commitment to them will endure.

References

1 WHO Regional Office for Europe (2005) *The Health for All Policy Framework for the WHO European Region: 2005 update*. WHO Regional Office for Europe, Copenhagen (document EUR/RC55/8). Available from: www.euro.who.int/Document/RC55/edoc08.pdf.

2 Churchill LR (2002) What ethics can contribute to health policy. In: N Danis, C Clancy

and LR Churchill (eds) *Ethical Dimensions of Health Policy*. Oxford University Press, Oxford.

3 Farmer P, Furin J and Katz J (2004) Global health equity. *Lancet*. **363**(9423).

4 Byrne D (2004) *Enabling Good Health For All. Reflection paper*. European Commission, Brussels. Available from: http://europa.eu.int/comm/health/ph_overview/ strategy.

5 Ritsatakis A, Barnes R, Dekker E *et al*. (eds) (2000) *Exploring Health Policy Development in Europe*. Copenhagen: WHO Regional Office for Europe; 2000 (WHO Regional Publications, European Series, No 86). Available from: www.euro.who.int/Information Sources/Publications/Catalogue/20010911_37.

6 Barnard K (ed) (2003) *The Future of Health – the Health of the Future: Fourth European Consultation on Future Trends*. Nuffield Trust, London.

7 Decision No. 1786/2002/EC of the European Council and of the Council of 23 September 2002 adopting a Programme of Community action in the field of public health (2003–8). *Official Journal* 2002;L271:1–12.

8 Byrne D (2005) Enabling good health for all – the future of health in Europe. Speech/ 04/367 [online] [cited 2005 Oct 5]. Available from: http://europa.eu.int/rapid/press ReleasesAction.do?reference=SPEECH/04/367&format=HTML&aged=0&language= EN&guiLanguage=en.

9 Presidency Conclusions, 16–17 June 2005. Council of the European Union, Brussels (10255/05).

10 Council of Europe (1998) *The Human Rights, Ethical and Moral Dimensions of Health Care: 120 case studies*. Council of Europe, Strasbourg.

11 Department of Health and Children, Ireland (2001) *Quality and Fairness: a health system for you – health strategy*. Stationery Office, Dublin. Available from: www.dohc.ie/ publications/quality_and_fairness.html.

12 Department of Health (2003) *Tackling Health Inequalities: a programme for action*. Department of Health, London. Available from: www.dh.gov.uk/PublicationsAnd Statistics/Publications/PublicationsPolicyAndGuidance/PublicationsPolicyAnd Guidance Article/fs/en?CONTENT_ID=4008268&chk=Ad%2BpLD.

13 World Health Organization (1998) *The World Health Report 1998 – life in the 21st century: a vision for all*. World Health Organization, Geneva. Available from: www.who.int/whr/ 1998/en/index.html.

14 Dyer O (2005) Disparities in health widen between rich and poor in England. *BMJ*. **331**: 419.

15 Menke R, Streich W, Rössler G and Brandt H (2003) *Health Inequalities in Europe and the Situation of Disadvantaged Groups: report on socio-economic differences in health indicators in Europe*. Netherlands National Institute of Public Health, Bilthoven.

16 Deeming C (2004) Choice and equity: lessons from long term care. *BMJ*. **328**: 1389–90.

17 van Doorslaer E, Masseria C and OECD Health Equity Research Group Members (2004) *Income Related Inequality in the Use of Medical Care in 21 OECD Countries*. OECD, Paris. (OECD Health Working Papers.) Available from: www.oecd.org/dataoecd.

18 World Bank (2005) *World Development Report 2006: equity and development*. World Bank, Washington, DC. Available from: http://web.worldbank.org/WBSITE/EXTERNAL/ EXTDEC/EXTRESEARCH/EXTWDRS/EXTWDR2006/0,,menuPK:477658~pagePK: 64167702~piPK:64167676~theSitePK:477642,00.html.

19 Lee J-W (2005) Public health is a social issue. *Lancet*. **365**(9464).

20 Marmot M (2005) Social determinants of health inequalities. *Lancet*. **365**: 1099–104.

21 Coast J (2004) Is economic evaluation in touch with society's health values? *BMJ*. **329**: 1233.

22 Gwatkin D, Bhuiya A and Victora C (2004) Making health systems more equitable. *Lancet*. **364**: 1273–80.

23 International Forum Gastein (2003) *Gastein Health Declaration 2003*. International Forum Gastein, Bad Hofgastein.

24 Marinker M (2002) *Health Targets in Europe: polity, progress and promise*. BMJ Books, London.

25 WHO Regional Office for Europe (1998) *HEALTH21 – the Health for All policy framework for the WHO European Region*. WHO Regional Office for Europe, Copenhagen. (European Health for All Series, No. 6.) Available from: www.who.dk/document/health21/wa540ga199heeng.pdf.

26 Marinker M (2004) *The Madrid Framework: twelve dimensions of health targets in Europe*. Letter to Hon. D Byrne, Commissioner for Health and Consumer Protection, 15 October 2004.

27 Marinker M (2005) The Madrid Framework. *Eurohealth*. 11(1): 2–5. Available from: www.euro.who.int/Document/obs/Eurohealth11_1.pdf.

28 New European Community health strategy [online] (2000) [cited October 5 2005]. Available from: http://europa.eu.int/scadplus/leg/en/cha/c11563.htm.

29 *Health for All: the policy framework for the WHO European Regions*. 2005 update. WHO Regional Office for Europe, Copenhagen. (Fact sheet EURO/12/05.) Available from: www.euro.who.int/document/mediacentre/fs1205e.pdf.

30 Directorate-General for Health and Consumer Protection (2003) *A Programme of Community Action in the Field of Public Health (2003–2008)* [online] [cited 2005 Oct 5]. Available from: http://europa.eu.int/comm/health/ph_programme/programme_en.htm.

31 World Bank (2005) *Millennium Development Goals: progress and prospects in Europe and central Asia*. World Bank, Washington, DC.

32 World Health Organization (2005) *Health in the Millennium Development Goals*. World Health Organization, Geneva. Available from: www.who.int/mdg/publications/mdg_report/en/.

33 World Health Organization (2005) *Human Rights, Health and Poverty Reduction Strategies*. World Health Organization, Geneva (Health and Human Rights Publication Series, No. 5). Available from: www.who.int/hhr/news/en/HRHPRS.pdf.

34 Committee on Economic, Social and Cultural Rights (2000) *The Right to the Highest Attainable Standard of Health: substantive issues arising in the implementation of the International Covenant on Economic, Social and Cultural Rights*. Committee on Economic, Social and Cultural Rights, Geneva. (E/C.12/2000/4, General Comment No. 14.) Available from: http://cesr.org/generalcomment14.

35 Organisation for Economic Co-operation and Development and World Health Organization (2002) *Poverty and Health*. World Health Organization, Geneva; OECD, Paris (DAC Guidelines and Reference Series). Available from: http://whqlibdoc.who.int/publications/2003/9241562366.pdf.

36 Jonsson U (2003) *Human Rights Approach to Development Programming*. UNICEF, Nairobi.

37 UNDP (2000) *Human Development Report 2000*. Oxford University Press, Oxford.

38 Solana J (2005) Jointly does it. In: D Franklin (ed.) *The World in 2005*. The Economist, London.

39 Gunning-Scheppers L (2004) *Governance and Health Targeting – experiences and future potential*. University of Amsterdam, Amsterdam.

Chapter 3

Health and wellbeing

Ilona Kickbusch

Health is a highly dynamic force which has shaped modern societies. After a long period in which health was thought of very much in relation to medicine's perceptions of disease, we are at a point in time where our view of health is being redefined – increasingly and persistently both by the market and by citizens. Health, it seems, is everywhere and we are caught up in a debate of what this ubiquity means.[1] Is it a new tyranny or a means to greater self-determination? Is better health a personal responsibility, or should there be significant action by the public sector to ensure health, including a restriction on goods and services that endanger health? Is health a private good or a joint responsibility of all citizens? How much health security should we expect from the state and how much can really be provided?

In the national political arenas, declarations about the importance of health, public health, health promotion and disease prevention abound, but are usually uttered in connection with a determined call to citizens to show more individual responsibility and to live healthier lifestyles. It is too tempting to reduce the spread of chronic diseases to a victim-blaming strategy with echoes of nineteenth century punitive attitudes to the causes of ill-health: those that become ill have only themselves to blame for smoking, over-eating or having sex with the wrong person. This type of argument ignores 150 years of European public policy experience. It neglects the commitment to address the conditions, the knowledge and the skills which enable people to live healthy lives, individually and collectively; it fails to address such factors as social inequalities, child poverty, tobacco control, the labelling of food products, sex education in schools. And above all it fails to have a positive vision of health and its contribution to society. There are very few countries that can claim to have a *health* policy deserving of the name, and only two countries in Europe – England and Sweden – have a minister dedicated to public health. Indeed, only one country – Sweden – has a health policy that focuses on inequality, and addresses the determinants of health.

A European opportunity

But this neglect by nation states could prove to be a window of opportunity for the European Union and for active European citizenship. The European Commission, through its work on public health, aims, 'together with the Member States, to protect and promote the health of European people. The Commission strives to improve public health in the European Union, to prevent human illness and diseases and to obviate sources of danger to human health . . . For the Commission, health is a key priority. That is why the Commission has developed a more coordinated approach to European health policy: a high level of human health protection should be assured in setting out all Community policies' (from the Commission's public health programme website).[2]

The Commission was able to develop its work in public health precisely because European member states had begun to neglect their public health systems and saw no danger in giving the Commission the latitude to deal with this rather vague and undefined area of health to which they did not in fact accord very much importance. Their main concern was that the Commission would not interfere with the countries' healthcare *systems*. This shortsightedness on the part of nation states gave the Commission the opportunity systematically to strengthen its activities in public health, particularly in the past decade, for example through the establishment of a European Centre for Disease Prevention and Control (ECDC), an Executive Agency for its Public Health Programme in 2005, and strong legislative action on tobacco control through a number of Commission decisions and directives. Indeed, the more that health becomes a trans-national issue, the more health becomes a market, the more it becomes a concern of citizen's action groups at the European level, the more the Commission is challenged to provide public health strategies that concern Europe as a whole and that fit well with global health strategies.

Compared to its relevance and its potential, public health policy is still relatively weak within the Union's overall responsibilities. Indeed, other EU policies frequently contradict public health policies, despite the declared intention of the public health programme to '. . . promote health and prevent disease through addressing health determinants across all policies and activities'. A clear case in point is European agricultural policy. In view of the public health challenges that Europe faces in terms of health determinants and chronic and infectious diseases, all of which transcend the borders of the nation states and require trans-national responses, the time is ripe for a significant European effort that focuses on health in a new way, and gains the support of the European public. One attempt by the European Commission to do so is the proposed new joint programme that combines public health and consumer protection.[2]

Yet an even more critical argument for a strong public health policy at the European level is social citizenship. Major differences in health status and health services exist within and between countries in the European Union, particularly since the recent inclusion of new member states. Addressing them will be a challenge that goes to the core of what it means to be a European. Why should a Swede live longer than a Hungarian? Why should a European who is materially poor have poorer health and shorter life expectancy than someone who is better off? While there are many active patient organisations and groups that advocate on specific health issues, there is not yet a strong citizen's movement that advocates according the same rights to health to all citizens throughout the Union. Evidence shows that smoking kills; why, then, can some European countries still disregard this fact to the detriment of the health and lives of their citizens? Why is there an approach to standardisation in the European internal market, yet no standard for what European citizens can expect from their governments in terms of public health, disease prevention, health protection and promotion? Why is health not seen as being as critical to the future of Europe as is competitiveness? Indeed, why is health not recognised as a driving force of competitiveness in knowledge and information societies?

A key problem lies in the fact that, in the context of most European debates, health is usually understood as a distinct and narrowly defined organisational and policy sector, i.e. the healthcare system or the public health system. It is not regarded as a guiding value of European policy making, as a key *raison d'être* for a European Union that wants to move beyond being a common market to a union that promotes the common good for Europeans. It would seem that in order to move forward, the European Union would need to discuss *health* in different terms – to frame a health agenda in a manner that the European public understands, that European media will adopt, that policy makers can relate to, and that non-governmental groups can advocate in order to strengthen health protection and promotion and overall wellbeing. In a union of European peoples, health and wellbeing would then play a central role and constitute a core value.

New frames and mindsets

Framing '. . . refers to how messages are encoded with meaning so that they can be efficiently interpreted in relationship to existing beliefs or ideas'. Frames convey meaning and can help uphold consistent biases. For example, in terms of economics Amos Tversky and Daniel Kahneman[3] have shown that framing can affect the choices one makes, so much so that several of the classic axioms of rational choice do not hold. Much depends on how the problem is presented. Similar insights come from Erving Goffman's work[4] in sociology; Gregory Bateson's work in anthropology shows that cognitive models, or mind frames, influence action.[5] Their insights are particularly applied in strategic communication approaches such as media framing and agenda setting.

It is therefore worthwhile considering how, in recent years, a number of new frames have emerged that can provide a useful entry point for a new European debate on health. These frames consider health as:

- an intrinsic value and human right;
- fairness and social justice;
- an overarching policy goal which addresses social determinants;
- a trans-national public good.

These frames obviously overlap. They represent different entry points to a common key concept – other frames also exist such as health as a resource[6,7] or health as an investment.[8] Each relates to specific reference and advocacy groups. Alkire and Chen[9] argue that a rights-based approach ('fulfilling our obligations so others are dignified') and an equity approach ('achieving a fairer distribution of health capabilities') differ from one that is utilitarian ('maximising aggregate subjective happiness') or humanitarian ('acting virtuously towards those in need'). However, in real life these approaches are not so easily differentiated, and health advocates from various schools of thought do not always clearly elucidate their platforms – thereby ensuring that they appeal to a wider audience and so generate more agreement. Such frames also appear in other configurations, for example in the dimensions of the Madrid Framework[10] – which is itself, as indeed is this book, an exercise in framing.

Health as a value and a human right

Health is a value worth striving for in itself, as well as a factor that contributes significantly to other values, like equity, dignity, solidarity and diversity, that are relevant to the 'European social model'. Amartya Sen[11] emphasises that health is not only a means of reaching other individual or societal goals, but also is an end of political and societal activity in itself. This clarifies the *intrinsic* value of health. Various types of human capability (such as the capability to avoid preventable morbidity and premature mortality, or to be literate and numerate) are considered by Sen both as ends in themselves, and as key means to the achievement of other intrinsically valued ends, such as political freedoms and the capability to participate actively in life and in trade and production. It is the expansion of these human capabilities that are the real freedoms of life, and the ultimate end of public policy. Health therefore, has both a constitutive and an instrumental value – and frequently the two are difficult to disentangle, as they complement one another. Indeed it is a characteristic of the 'European social model' that social citizenship is intricately linked to political citizenship.

In many countries, the commitment to a certain system of protecting and improving health is seen as a value in itself. The Canadian report 'Medicare: A Value Worth Keeping'[12] asserts: 'Canada's healthcare system is one of this country's foremost social accomplishments, a core value that helps define our national identity.' Sorrell claims that, 'the NHS functions in the UK not only as a source of medical treatment, but as a prime medium of national solidarity and national identity.'[13,14] At this level, health and the health system as values are 'part of the cultural fabric that allows people to engage each other with language, develop their institutions, maintain the social order necessary for survival and prosperity, play social roles, and assume personal identities'.[15] This indeed seems a critical function of health in terms of the 'European social model' and European citizenship.

As inequities in health become more and more obvious, the notion of health as a human right is gaining new support.[16] The human right to health was codified as such in the Declaration of Human Rights in 1948, and appears in the constitution of the WHO. This raises the issue of the interface between European values and what has been termed *universal values*. Nigel Dower points out, 'If citizens are increasingly motivated by global concerns then cosmopolitan goals enter domestic policy in that way and people can be effective global citizens by being effective globally oriented citizens of their own states.'[17] In particular, this would imply a common notion of social justice and a system of international law where the right to health constitutes a legal claim. It is very relevant to the European Union, in terms of access rights to health of third country nationals within Europe, as well as with European positions taken in the global health arena. One critical such arena is women's rights and reproductive health.

Health as fairness and social justice

From the very beginning of modernity, health has been at the centre of debates on inequity, initially within the context of the nation state, and today as a key dimension of globalisation. Health governance debates are in their essence predominantly about social justice, about inclusion and exclusion – even if they are presented as fiscal debates. The value of equity commonly arises in relation to access to, utilisation of or financing of health services, and also with regard to health outcomes and health status. Two main forms of health equity can be identified: vertical equity (preferential treatment for those with greater health needs) and horizontal equity (equal treatment for equivalent needs). *Inequalities* that are unfair, or arise from social injustices, and are also avoidable are considered *inequities*. Fairness, in this context, is used to describe the unacceptable disparities in health.[18]

Health inequities arise from unequal access to the determinants of health, such as education, housing, employment, and from the unequal distribution of resources and power relating to gender, race and ethnicity, and from unequal access to healthcare. This, of course, has been at the historical roots of the public health movement and is the basis for the significant action on health inequalities that is now underway, with a focus on the social determinants of health. The WHO Commission on the Social Determinants of Health describes its goal as 'to lay the foundations of health equity to be a shared global goal, and for an understanding that acting on that goal demands action on the underlying causes of ill health'.[19]

A shift to a model of policy and intervention based on equity and the social determinants of health will require policies that acknowledge the *structural* causes of health problems, and the constant tension between the goals of different policy sectors.

The strong correlation between the socioeconomic position of people and their life expectancy has been firmly established by research.[20] Not all Europeans have the same chance of remaining healthy. The WHO Health for All database clearly shows significant differences in health expectancy between social groups and between countries.[21] As Europe has grown richer it has also become more unequal. This again reinforces the critical function that health plays in terms of the European social model and European citizenship, and the need for citizens' movements to demand European action, policies and funding mechanisms, in order to attempt to close the gaps.

Health as an overarching goal in all policies

Good health in Europe has historically been linked to good governance. Today this means two things: firstly, governing the health sector to ensure universal and equitable access, as well as quality of outcome; secondly, governing across sectors to address the determinants of health and enable healthy choices.

Several advances have been made in this direction. The European Commission, for example, has determined that all its policies should be judged on their potential impact on health.[22] Commissioner David Byrne embarked on an effort to make health central to all EU policies,[23] and the EU presidency of Finland in 2006 will follow up on this theme of 'health across policy sectors'.[24] The UK presidency in 2005 selected the theme of health inequalities,[25] and the Commission has created a European working group on the social determinants of health.[26]

The new Swedish Public Health Policy, adopted in 2003, aims to create more equity in health. It was the result of a ten-year process in policy making. In the 1980s, a parliamentary commission was asked to develop a strategy for equality of good health, focusing on the structural determinants of health. The main objectives included, but were not limited to, economic and social security, secure and favourable conditions during childhood and adolescence, participation and influence in society, healthier working life and increased physical activity. Many ministries and governmental agencies have become involved in the implementation of Swedish Health Policy, because of its focus on the determinants of health. Policy makers in Sweden have concluded that economic policy (redistribution between income groups, age groups and regions), social welfare policy (accessibility of basic social services), labour policy (employment rate), secure conditions for early child development (quality of schools and daycare), environmental policy, food and agricultural policy (food subsidies), and alcohol policy (reducing the supply) are all integral to the aim of creating equity in health in Sweden.[27]

Political resistance to the foundations of such a new Public Health Policy is in large part due to differences in values. The Swedish National Institute of Health in Sweden asserts, 'There is strong popular opinion for defending and developing the social welfare. On the other hand there are strong opposing forces, especially on the international level.'[28] The underlying issue in this case is expressed well by T McMichael and R Beaglehole: 'Tension persists between the philosophy of neo-liberalism, emphasizing self-interest of market-based economies, and the philosophy of social justice that sees collective responsibility and benefit as the prime social goal. The practice of public health, with its underlying community and population perspective, sits more comfortably with the latter philosophy.'[29]

Health as a trans-national public good

Whether a good is considered public or private within a society is a political decision. In the 'European social model' health clearly constitutes a public good and end in itself – a view that is increasingly under attack. In her groundbreaking work on global public goods Inge Kaul[30] reinforces this point: 'The privateness or publicness of a good is rarely an innate property. In most instances, it is a policy choice – our policy choice – to make a good more or less public or private.' Indeed in Europe, from the eighteenth century on, claims for access to health and access to citizenship increasingly converge and become a driving force of social and political movements. The growing understanding that health and disease could be influenced through clearly described and circumscribed interventions by the nation state made the sanitary revolution part of the big reform project of the first wave of European modernity. Health or disease were not just a personal choice, they became a political choice.

The discussion on health as a global public good has also given new impetus to the discussion of health as a public good at other levels of governance. The public good concept implies that health cannot be reduced to a commodity and needs political will and a 'public push'. It must be supported by a governance infrastructure with public financing mechanisms. In this sense, health is also a *public value*. Public values are 'concerned with *State intervention to promote morally desirable ends'*.[31] They extend beyond both individual preferences and the private realm and, in terms of health, increasingly expand from considerations of medical care provision to the provision of the social determinants of health. Wickham[14] adds another dimension to this from a European perspective. He observes that in Europe the state is also the guarantor of two very European concepts: social cohesion (also explicitly mentioned in the Lisbon Agenda);[32] and social inclusion. Inclusive health systems – for example migrant-friendly hospitals – play more than just a medical role, they reflect societal values. 'In the short term the health sector may be one of the promising points of entry for policies and interventions to tackle health disparities, to prevent impoverishment due to healthcare expenses, and to prevent the decline in social position of those with chronic diseases' (WHO priorities for research to take forward the health equity policy agenda 2004).[33]

In the literature on health, at national and international levels, there is a renaissance of Geoffrey Rose's public health dictum – 'The primary determinants of disease are mainly economic and social; therefore its remedies must also be economic and social.'[34] This concept forms the foundation of a new and broader public health field and expands it into a wide arena of economic and social rights, including a new empowerment of citizens, consumers and patients. As such it reflects a combination of social, economic and political rights which has been typical of the historical development of good health in Europe.

The concept of health as a public good and a public value is clearly under threat from economic developments, such as the growth of the private healthcare market, from social trends such as increasing individualisation, and from the view that health is an expenditure that our rich societies can no longer afford as a joint social effort. In consequence, European societies must debate the value they assign to health – as a right of citizenship, as an individualised private product and responsibility, and as an ultimate value.[34]

Future European dialogue on health

The four frames introduced above provide a set of references for a European dialogue on health: understanding health as an intrinsic value in itself as well as a human right; seeing it as a basic contribution to fairness and social justice within a European context; ensuring that health is part of a range of policies that address determinants of health; and relating European health to global developments through an understanding of health as a global public good.

The 'European social model' is not a vague idea – it can only be understood in the context of citizenship, which means in the context of rights. Different concepts of citizenship can further help clarify European values in relation to health. According to Ralf Dahrendorf, European citizenship lies between *theoretical/soft citizenship* (such as feeling part of a community, having common goals and values) and *practical/strong citizenship*, which encompasses real rights (such as voting, fair trials, expression and association). *Active citizenship*, frequently mentioned in citizenship literature, refers to citizens who actively participate in political and social discourse. Historically, national citizenship has been constructed through social participation. Active citizenship in the EU means that citizens defend human, political, economic and social rights – including the right to health and healthcare.[33] Finally, *social citizenship* is relevant to the European context because it constitutes the core idea of a welfare state. Social rights are granted based on citizenship, not performance in the market.[35]

In European history, health has been linked to changing concepts of citizenship. In the eighteenth century it was linked to the individual moral responsibility of the man of property. In the nineteenth century it changed radically to a collective good which became part of the rallying cry of the disenfranchised – the poor, the working class, women. In consequence it moved out of the realm of the charity of the church and philanthropic organisations, and into the realm of rights and social justice.[1,14]

Health can again become a positive force of European citizenship. For this to happen there needs to be a health debate with many stakeholders, in order to clarify the role and value of health in the European Union. This debate will need to include dialogue with many other sectors – building on the dialogue initiated by David Byrne,[23] and on mechanisms such as the European Health Forum.[35] Such dialogue is crucial for a European civil society.

A comparative value study of European health documents would probably reveal, just as the Canadian study[15] did, that European health policy makers have very different understandings of the 'value' of health. It would be crucial, however, to create the political space to discuss the common health core of the European social model, and for this discussion to be with the citizens, and not only between heads of state. This can help take values out of the realm of moral speculation and into the realm of rights at all levels of governance. Only as rights can values become instrumental in European public policy making.[36] Health needs to be recognised as a key dimension of social citizenship in a Europe committed to the wellbeing of its citizens, now and in the future.

Europe has the potential to be a global leader in shaping policies that promote health in the twenty-first century. The social Europe of the future requires a focus on a European identity which is inextricably linked to the concept of health rights and social citizenship in health. Health can and must play a major role in the establishment of citizenship, identity and allegiance to the modern European Union (EU), just as it did historically to the nation state. Health is an area that very concretely affects people's wellbeing and feelings of security. Indeed a strong commitment of the European Union to health could be seen as a concrete expression of the potential that lies in its commitment to wellbeing and social justice. Health needs to move into the centre of EU policy making, especially in relation to citizens' needs and rights.

Such a concept of citizenship also accepts a commitment to global solidarity. Europe needs to apply the lessons learned in the historical development of public health in Europe to its global responsibilities. A strong European voice in global health is presently lacking; it could make a major difference in moving forward an agenda for more equity in health in an interdependent world.

References

1 Kickbusch I (2006) Health governance: the health society. In: I Kickbusch. *Health and Modernity: the theoretical foundations of health promotion.* Palgrave, London.
2 http://europa.eu.int/comm/health/overall_mission_en.htm.
3 Tversky A and Kahnemann D (1981) The framing of decisions and the psychology of choice. *Science.* **211**: 453–8.
4 Goffman E (1974) *Frame Analysis: an essay on the organization of experience.* Harper and Row, London.
5 Bateson G (1985) *Mind and Nature: a necessary unity.* Bantam, New York.
6 Breslow L (1999) From disease prevention to health promotion. *JAMA.* **281**(11): 1030–3.
7 World Health Organization (WHO) (1986) Ottawa Charter for Health Promotion. *Health Promotion.*1: iii–v. www.euro.who.int/AboutWHO/Policy/20010827_2 (accessed 3 August 2005).
8 UN Millennium Project (2005) *Investing in Development: a practical plan to achieve the Millennium Development Goals.* Earthscan, London.

9 Alkire S and Chen L (2004) Global health and moral values. *The Lancet.* **364.**

10 Marinker M (2005) The Madrid Framework. *Eurohealth.* 11(1): 2–5.

11 Sen A (1999) *Development as Freedom.* Knopf, New York.

12 Health Action Lobby (1992) *Medicare: a value worth keeping.* Canadian Association of Social Workers, Ottawa.

13 Sorrell T (2003) Health care provision and public morality: an ethics perspective. In: A Oliver (ed) *Equity in Health and Healthcare: views from ethics, economics and political science.* The Nuffield Trust, London.

14 Wickham J (2000) *The End of the European Social Model: before it began.* Available from: www.ictu.ie/html/publications/ictu/Essay2.pdf.

15 Giacomini M, Hurley J, Gold I, Smith P and Abelson J (2001) *'Values' in Canadian Health Policy Analysis: what are we talking about?* Canadian Health Services Research Foundation, Toronto, Ontario.

16 De Feyter K (2005) *Human Rights: social justice in the age of the market.* Zed Books, London.

17 Dower N (2003) *An Introduction to Global Citizenship.* Edinburgh University Press, Edinburgh.

18 Evans T, Whitehead M, Diderichsen F, Bhuiya A and Wirth M (eds) (2001) *Challenging Inequities in Health: from ethics to action.* Oxford University Press, New York.

19 www.who.int/social_determinants/en/.

20 Marmot MG and Wilkinson R (eds) (1999) *Social Determinants of Health.* Oxford University Press, Oxford.

21 www.euro.who.int/hfadb.

22 OECD Health Project (2004) *Towards High Performing Health Systems.* OECD, Paris.

23 Byrne D (2004) *Enabling Good Health for All. A reflection process for a new EU Health Strategy.* 15 July 2004. Available from: http://europa.eu.int/comm/health/ph_overview/Documents/byrne_reflection_en.pdf.

24 www.valtioneuvosto.fi/vn/liston/base.lsp?r=90650&k=en&old=716.

25 UK Presidency Tackling Health Inequalities Summit. October 2005 www.dh.gov.uk/PolicyAndGuidance/International/EuropeanUnion/EUPresidency2005/EUPresidencyArticle/fs/en?CONTENT_ID=4119613&chk=Xa2sOh.

26 http://europa.eu.int/comm/health/ph_determinants/socio_economics/socio_economics_en.htm.

27 Hogstedt C, Lundgren B, Moberg H *et al.* (2004) The Swedish Public Health Policy and the National Institute of Public Health. *Scandinavian Journal of Public Health.* **December** (Supplement 64).

28 Agren G (2004) The New Swedish Public Health Policy as a Tool to Improve Equity in Health. Swedish National Institute of Public Health, Powerpoint Presentation.

29 McMichael T and Beaglehole R (2003) The global context for public health. In: R Beaglehole (ed) *Global Public Health: a new era.* Oxford University Press, Oxford.

30 Kaul I and Faust M (2001) Global public goods and health: taking the agenda forward. *Bulletin of the World Health Organization.* **79:** 2.

31 Staley K (2001) *Voices, Values and Health: involving the public in moral decisions.* King's Fund, London.

32 Lisbon Strategy, Available from: http://newropeans-magazine.org/index.php?option=com_content&task=view&id=1836&Itemid=227.

33 (2005) *Bulletin of the World Health Organization.* December. **83**(12): 948–53.

34 Citizenship and Identity. From: El sitio web de la historia del siglo XX. Retrieved on 29 September 2004: www.historiasiglo20.org.

35 Esping-Andersen G (1990) *The Three Worlds of Welfare Capitalism.* Princeton University Press, Princeton.

36 Habermas J (1992) Citizenship and national identity: some reflections on the future of Europe. *Praxis International.* **12**(1): 1–19.

Note

This chapter is based in part on a paper prepared by Ilona Kickbusch for the 7th European Health Forum Gastein 2004 on 'Values, principles and objectives of health policy in Europe', which can also be found in: Kickbusch I (2005) The need for common values, principles and objectives for health policy in a changing Europe, in: Svenson P-G (ed) *International Hospital Federation Reference Book*. Pro Book Publishing, London.

Chapter 4

Equity and justice

Jennifer Prah Ruger

Research over several decades has identified social inequalities in health, both between and within countries.[1-3] This research has prompted some countries to pursue strategies to reduce socioeconomic inequalities in health,[4-7] although these initiatives have not been without controversy.[8-11] Such efforts have fuelled the debate over the relative contributions of health determinants and how to weight and direct public policies that affect health.[12-17] The debate centres on the tension between the need to account for the impact of health determinants outside the healthcare system (social determinants of health) and the need to balance health as an objective with other valuable social ends (in other policy domains).

Alongside this practical debate exists a parallel debate at the philosophical level:[18-23] one that will in many ways inform the policy choices that societies make to improve the health of their populations. The implications of theories of justice (e.g. fair and equitable treatment of people) for social determinants of health has thus become an important topic of philosophical inquiry, although little work has been done in this area.[19-21] Although a survey of the main issues relating to the fairness of social inequalities in health has been provided elsewhere,[19,21-23] this essay focuses more specifically on the application of John Rawls' theory of justice to the social determinants of health and then proposes an alternative philosophical framework, rooted in Amartya Sen's capability approach and Aristotle's political theory, for thinking about such inequalities.

Justice as fairness

An important starting point for a philosophical discussion of the social determinants of health is the application of John Rawls' theory of justice to such determinants.[18,21] In *A theory of justice*, Rawls[24] argued that justice requires the fair distribution of primary goods and that rational people behind a 'veil of ignorance' about their personal circumstances would choose principles of justice that maximise the minimum level of primary goods. Primary goods are allocated to individuals on the basis of 'fair equality of opportunity', due to the disadvantages that these individuals have accrued through the 'natural lottery' and the 'social lottery' of life.[24]

In applying Rawls' theory to the social determinants of health, Norman Daniels and colleagues[18,25] argue that justice requires flattening 'socioeconomic inequalities in a robust way, assuring far more than a decent minimum'. From this point of view, 'a society complying with these principles of justice would probably flatten the socioeconomic gradient even more than we see in most egalitarian welfare states of northern Europe'.[18] The implications, they argue, are that, 'we should view health inequalities that derive from social determinants as unjust unless the determinants are distributed in conformity with these robust principles.'[18] From a policy perspective, therefore, governments should pursue social strategies (to reduce health inequalities) by implementing policies 'aimed at equalizing individual life opportunities, such as investment in basic education, affordable housing, income security and other forms of antipoverty policy'.[25] Daniels and colleagues give at least five examples of social policies that might improve health by reducing socioeconomic disparities: investment in early childhood development, nutrition programmes, improvements in the quality of the work environment, reductions in income inequality, and greater political fairness.[25]

Although there is much to applaud in a Rawlsian analysis of the social determinants of health, this approach has not been spared criticism. Some critics are concerned that these policy prescriptions are too far-reaching without sufficient evidence of their effect on population health.[26] Francis Kamm[27] notes, for example, that policy proposals related to social inequality and health must compare the health gained by economic growth associated with social inequality with the health that would be gained from complete social equality. These types of comparisons are necessary to fully understand the net effects of policy measures.[27] Barbara Starfield[16] adds that although 'income redistribution may go a long way to improve health', there also has to be 'simultaneous attention to changing other social and health policies . . . There is no simple solution to reducing systematic health inequalities.'[16] Ezekiel Emanuel[28] and Ted Marmor[15] have made similar points, and have added concerns about the political and policy problems associated with the strategy of eliminating all socioeconomic inequalities.

Sudhir Anand and Fabienne Peter[20] offer a critique that underscores the importance of taking into account health differentials between and within multiple groups (e.g. between African-American and white men with the same income levels) – not just average health across socioeconomic groups. They also expressed concern that attention to health inequalities is indirect (e.g. a 'side effect') in the analysis of Daniels and others, and highlight the problem in using Rawls' original theory to come up with the premise that 'inequalities in health are unjust if, and only if, they are the result of unjust social arrangements'.[20] Ezekiel Emanuel and Emmanuela Gakidou and colleagues independently reiterated this critique, expressing concern with the idea of justifying improvements in social justice based primarily on their impact on health inequalities.[28,29] They also underscore how complex the relation is between socioeconomic status and health inequalities and the need for further study.[29]

Anand and Peter go on to argue that there is a tension in using different aspects of Rawlsian justice because such views might conflict in their policy recommendations and might therefore be redundant. In a sense, Daniels and colleagues are still treating socioeconomic and health inequalities as independent spheres of justice,[30] but they provide little guidance when accounts of social and economic justice conflict with accounts of justice with respect to health.[30] For example, 'economic inequalities permitted by Rawls's Difference Principle may cause health inequalities that are condemned by the account of health equity'.[30] Justice and health needs a philosophical framework for assessing trade-offs between health inequity and other inequities. It is insufficient to assume that 'health is the by-product of justice'.[31]

At a more fundamental level, Amartya Sen,[32–34] and more recently Michael Marmot,[35] have expressed concerns with the Rawlsian focus on means rather than ends because it does not take account of human diversity. The Rawlsian approach is problematic, they argue, because resources and means cannot be good in their own right – they have no intrinsic value (they cannot be the object of social activity), they are good only insofar as they promote human functioning.[32–34] As Sen notes, 'if the object is to concentrate on the individual's real opportunity to pursue her objectives (as Rawls explicitly recommends), then account would have to be taken not only of the primary goods the persons respectively hold, but also of the relevant personal characteristics that govern the *conversion* of primary goods into the person's ability to promote her ends. For example, a person who is disabled may have a larger basket of primary goods and yet have less chance to lead a normal life (or to pursue her objectives) than an able-bodied person with a smaller basket of primary goods.'[34] Ensuring possession of primary goods, therefore, might not address inequalities in health; that reduction of socioeconomic inequality will necessarily lead to reductions in health inequalities should not be assumed.[35,36] It therefore cannot be said that it is necessarily the case that 'health is the by-product of justice', since this 'oversimplifies the demands of health equity vis-à-vis the extensive requirements of social justice'.[36] This critique throws light on the distinction between a 'resource-orientation' (Rawlsian) and a 'results-orientation' (capability) in public policy. Thus, although a focus on fair distribution of primary goods and equal opportunity is a useful way of elevating the importance of the social determinants of health, this view has limitations, especially in acknowledging the intrinsic value of health and other capabilities in analysing the relative effectiveness of resources on health and health inequalities, and in understanding public policy more broadly.[37,38]

A capability perspective

By contrast with Rawls' theory and other well known philosophies, Amartya Sen developed the capability approach.[32–34] This philosophical framework, with roots in Aristotle's political theory,[39–43] applies to the social determinants of health,[37,38] but it is more 'people-centred' and 'agency-oriented' in its philosophical basis and more nuanced in its practical application. This view sees the expansion of human capabilities – the real freedoms that people have – as the ultimate end of public policy. As such, it values health intrinsically and more directly than non-intrinsic or solely instrumental social goods such as income or healthcare.[37,38] In this context, different kinds of capabilities (e.g. the capability to avoid preventable morbidity and premature mortality, or to be literate and numerate) are regarded both as ends in themselves and instrumentally important for the achievement of other (also intrinsically valued) ends (e.g. economic facilities (such as the capability for participation in trade and production) and political freedoms). For example, the degree to which individuals have the capability actively to participate in their work, social and political life, to be well educated, or to be secure in their economic facilities, are ends in themselves, but they may also be related to individuals' capability for health functioning since the lack of those capabilities could be harmful to health – as Michael Marmot and colleagues' work suggests.[1–3,44,45] Thus, such social determinants of health have both constitutive and instrumental value, and they serve not only to contribute to the 'general capability of a person to live more freely, but they also serve to complement one another', as stated by Sen.[34]

Indeed, often such freedoms as economic facilities, social opportunities (e.g. capability to avoid premature mortality and to be well educated), political freedoms (e.g. capability for self-determination), and protective security (e.g. capability to avoid economic vulnerability) will supplement one another and 'strengthen their joint importance'.[34] For example, better education for women reduces child mortality directly through a woman's expanded ability and desire to obtain, understand and act on health-related information, but also indirectly by increasing her respect and empowerment in intrafamilial and extrafamilial decision making. Lower child mortality rates, in turn, help reduce birth rates, reinforcing the influence of better education on fertility. As Sen notes, 'different kinds of freedom inter-relate with one another, and freedom of one type may greatly help in advancing freedom of other types'.[34] Conversely, the coupling of disadvantages can exacerbate an individual's overall freedom, for example, a disabled person might have difficulty both in earning a decent income and in converting more income into capabilities.[34] Income inequality assessment alone, therefore, cannot tell us how well such a person is living.

The capability perspective is also an agency-oriented view. It emphasises the importance of human agency – i.e. people's ability to live a life they value. It underscores that agency is essential for both individual and collective action and is critical for changing policy, norms and social commitments. Reducing social inequalities in health therefore requires more than 'flattening the socioeconomic gradient', it requires improvement of the conditions under which individuals are free to choose healthier life strategies and conditions for themselves and for future generations.[37,46] A capability perspective emphasises the empowerment of individuals to be active agents of change in their own terms – both at the individual and collective level.[37,46] Agency is important for public policy because it supports individuals' participation in economic, social, and political actions and enables individuals to make decisions as active agents of change. This view contrasts with the perspective that individuals are passive recipients of medical care or even income redistribution decisions or other public policy programmes. An agency-centred view promotes individuals' ability to understand and 'shape their own destiny and help each other'.[34]

A broad and multifaceted approach

A capability approach to the social determinants of health thus recognises the importance of addressing health needs on multiple fronts, in multiple domains of policy that affect all determinants of health (not just socioeconomic inequalities). It emphasises the integration of public policies into a comprehensive set of health improvement strategies delivered through a plurality of institutions. Information about the factors and processes that can improve health (and reduce health inequalities) should form the basis of policies designed to avert health problems. According to Sen, such policies may address a number of different influences, such as 'individually inherited proneness to disease, individual characteristics of disability, epidemiological hazards of particular regions, the influence of climate variations'.[36] Public policies should focus on making 'simultaneous progress on different fronts, including different institutions, which reinforce each other'.[34] This 'integrated and multifaceted'[34] approach supports the idea that society is obligated to reduce inequalities in the capability for functioning (including health functioning), and it recognises the 'respective roles and complementarities' of different kinds of capabilities.[34] However, this approach extends this reach with caution; recognising that considerable work is to be done to better understand the relative impacts of various policy domains (including politics)[8,47] and their interrelationships before embarking on major social changes.[36] This approach is also cautious about extending the traditional boundaries of health policy to include all policy domains that affect health and about assuming that social and economic policy reforms will be associated with health improvement in a linear way (e.g. the relation between income and health could be variable and depend on a number of factors such as age, gender, job status, location, and environment).[36] As Michael Marmot[48] notes, the idea of abolishing hierarchies altogether, and making everyone exactly the same, does not seem promising for public policy. So before abolishing hierarchies, we need to understand the precise factors that influence health, including the underlying political structure. We must then determine how to weight different social objectives, once we have this information. The capability perspective thus rejects a narrow and compartmentalised view of inequality (e.g. focus on income distribution)[8] and the search for a 'single all-purpose remedy'[34] for reducing health inequalities. Several distinctions are relevant to this viewpoint.

First, such an approach necessitates improving the assessment of other (non-health sector) policy domains, such as employment policy, by using health indicators as well as traditional indicators (e.g. employment rates). For example, in terms of economic policy, a capability approach would be concerned not only with whether a person's annual income falls below society's average, but with the extent to which that person's income level affects his or her health. This suggests that analysis of mortality and morbidity data can be used as an additional indicator in evaluating economic and social arrangements, to take into account the effect of these policies on health. In developing countries, in particular, economic arrangements have been found to be critical for preventing death and avoiding disease and disability. For example, one study of famine and under-nourishment found that starvation results when a large proportion of the population loses the means of obtaining food and that this loss results from three economic factors: unemployment; a fall in the purchasing power of wages; and a shift in the exchange rate between goods and services sold and food bought.[49] Policy recommendations to prevent famines and reduce starvation would then, according to these results, incorporate improvements in these three economic factors (non-health sector domains) and information about the effects of these factors should necessarily 'form the basis of policies designed to avoid famine and relieve hunger'.[49] Thus, the more conventional ways of measuring the effectiveness of economic and social policies can be enhanced by indicators of a population's health that illuminate important aspects of social inequality, help understand the relation between these factors and health, and identify policies to address these disparities. Adding such measures to the existing array of policy indicators might improve assessment of all policies that affect health, while maintaining the strengths of other public policy domains.

Second, information about the factors and processes that can improve health should form the basis of policies designed to avert health problems. However, the traditional boundaries of health policy should not be extended to include all policy domains that affect health, such as employment policy. Employment policy may be a useful way of thinking about health policy, but is not a substitute. For instance, employment indicators are not necessarily valid for assessing health policies because a person who is unemployed but wealthy does not necessarily incur the same morbidity and mortality risks as an unemployed person with no financial support. Moreover, an employed person might have a high degree of stress or lack of control, which could precipitate illness. Thus, employment status alone should not be identified with health policy in a linear way; the crucial information is the extent to which it affects a person's health.

Third, although health policy and other policies must remain separate, it is important not to assume that they are independent, especially in developing countries. Thus, while health policy and other public policies affecting health are related, it is important to keep the concepts of health policy and other policies distinct, without assuming them to be independent of each other. So, before giving substantially greater weight to broader socioeconomic policies than to health policies, we need to understand the precise mechanisms through which various factors influence health. We must then determine how to weight different social objectives, once we have this information. In light of existing information on social determinants of health, it would be unwise to prescribe sweeping policies, such as completely flattening of socioeconomic inequalities, in an effort to improve health. Such prescriptions blur, rather than clarify, the means and ends of health policy, hindering evaluations of the impact of public policies on health.

Fourth, such an approach to public policy would also likely entail what could be called horizontal and vertical integration, respectively. The horizontal dimension integrates policies across disease-specific programmes to create a comprehensive package of complementary interventions to improve health. In North America, western Europe, Australia, Brazil, Senegal, Thailand and Uganda, for example, the spread of HIV/AIDS has been slowed through multiple prevention strategies, including: health education; behaviour modification; social, economic and political environments that allow individuals to protect themselves against infection; condom promotion; HIV counselling and testing; blood safety; reduction in mother-to-child transmission; needle-exchange programmes; and treatments for sexually transmitted infections.[46,50] Such an integrated set of strategies has also been more effective for controlling tobacco use in a number of countries than narrower approaches.[51] Successful efforts have included simultaneous bans on advertising and promotion and on sales to children; mandatory health warnings; smoke-free environments; higher taxes on tobacco products; investment in health education; and smoking prevention and cessation programmes.[51]

The vertical dimension integrates domains of public policy that build upon each other. For example, better education, especially for women, makes individuals more likely to protect themselves from contracting sexually transmittable diseases including HIV/AIDS.[46,52] And improved economic, cultural and social conditions for women – through, for example, real employment, political and civil opportunities that empower them within the family and in their relationships with men – enhance the effectiveness of HIV/AIDS prevention and treatment programmes because such freedoms enable women to choose safer life strategies for themselves and their children.[46] Improving a woman's agency and education, thus, can improve the health of herself and her family, which in turn can improve overall health in a developing country.[46]

Fifth, the capability perspective also recognises the importance of a many-sided approach that addresses the functions of plural institutions, including nongovernmental actors and market forces to achieve public policy objectives. This contrasts with a predominant focus on government action and intervention (e.g. on the governmental redistribution system), important as that is. For example, government agencies can widely distribute health information, while market-based approaches can expand employment opportunities for women and nongovernmental organisations can provide aid and technical assistance in the health sector. The movement in global health toward better public–private partnerships reflects this view, but such efforts should be more closely linked with specific health improvement efforts and broader development activities.[52]

Conclusion

It is important to reflect on the richness of the Rawlsian approach to social justice generally and to the social determinants of health more specifically. Such efforts have advanced our thinking about health equity and its determinants. Despite its many strengths, however, the Rawlsian approach has limitations; an alternative approach to health and its determinants (within and outside the health sector) is found in Sen's capability approach. This approach takes human capabilities and freedoms as the real ends of public policy and calls for an integrated and multifaceted approach to health improvement that involves multiple institutions making simultaneous progress on various fronts.[53] Although this more comprehensive approach[54] may seem less deterministic, its more nuanced application calls for institutional arrangements to support greater freedoms for all persons so that people can 'help themselves', 'support each other', and 'influence the world'.[34]

Acknowledgements

Thanks are due to Amartya Sen, Sudhir Anand, Michael Marmot, and participants in the workshop on Rights, Dignity and Inequality at Trinity College, Cambridge, UK, for helpful comments. Thanks are also due to the Washington University School of Medicine and Centre for Health Policy for support. Jennifer Prah Ruger is supported in part by a Career Development Award (grant 1K01DA016358-01) from the US National Institutes of Health.

References

1 Marmot MG (2001) Inequalities in health. *N Engl J Med*. **345**: 134–6.
2 Amick BC, Levine S, Tarlov AR and Chapman D (eds) (1995) *Society and Health*. Oxford University Press, New York.
3 Marmot MG (1998) Improvement of social environment to improve health. *Lancet*. **351**: 57–60.
4 Acheson D (1998) *Independent Inquiry into Inequalities in Health Report*. Stationery Office, London.

5 (1999) *Reducing Health Inequalities: an action report.* Stationery Office, London.
6 Mackenbach JP and Stronks K (2002) A strategy for tackling health inequalities in the Netherlands. *BMJ.* **325**: 1029–32.
7 Black D, Morris JN, Smith C and Townsend P (1999) Better benefits for health: plan to implement the central recommendation of the Acheson report. *BMJ.* **318**: 724–7.
8 Horton R (2002) What the UK government is (not) doing about health inequalities. *Lancet.* **360**: 186.
9 Smith GD, Morris JN and Shaw M (1998) The independent inquiry into inequalities in health is welcome, but its recommendations are too cautious and vague. *BMJ.* **317**: 1465–6.
10 Evans PG, Barer ML and Marmor TR (eds) (1994) *Why Are Some People Healthy and Others Not?* Aldine de Gruyer, New York.
11 Macintyre S (2000) Prevention and the reduction of health inequalities. *BMJ.* **320**: 1399–400.
12 Leon DA, Walt G and Gilson L (2001) International perspectives on health inequalities and policy. *BMJ.* **322**: 591–4.
13 Deaton A (2002) Policy implications of the gradient of health and wealth: an economist asks, would redistributing income improve population health? *Health Affairs.* **21**: 13–30.
14 Martikainen P, Valkonen T. Inequalities in health: policies to reduce income inequalities are unlikely to eradicate inequalities in mortality. *BMJ.* 1999; **319**: 319.
15 Marmor T (2000) Policy options. *Boston Review.* **25**. Available from: http://boston review.net/BR25.1/marmor.html (accessed 6 February 2004).
16 Starfield B (2000) First contact. *Boston Review.* **25**. Available from: http://bostonreview. net/BR25.1/starfield.html (accessed 6 February 2004).
17 Woolhandler S and Himmelstein D (2000) Lost in translation. *Boston Review.* **25**. Available from: http://bostonreview.net/BR25.1/ woolhandler.html (accessed 6 February 2004).
18 Daniels N (2002) Justice, health, and health care. In: R Rhodes, MP Battin and A Silvers (eds) *Medicine and Social Justice: essays on the distribution of health care.* Oxford University Press, New York.
19 Evans T, Whitehead M, Diderichsen F, Bhuiya A and Wirth M (eds) (2001) *Challenging Inequities in Health: from ethics to action.* Oxford University Press, London.
20 Anand S and Peter F (2000) Equal opportunity. *Boston Review.* **25**. Available from: http://bostonreview.net/BR25.1/anand.html (accessed 6 February 2004).
21 Peter F and Evans T (2001) Ethical dimensions of health equity. In: T Evans, M Whitehead, F Diderichsen, A Bhuiya and M Wirth (eds) *Challenging Inequities in Health: from ethics to action.* Oxford University Press, London.
22 Macinko JA and Starfield B (2002) Annotated bibliography on equity in health, 1980–2001. *Int J Equity Health.* **1**: 1–20.
23 Braveman P and Gruskin S (2003) Defining equity in health. *J Epidemiol Community Health.* **57**: 254–8.
24 Rawls J (1971) *A Theory of Justice.* Harvard University Press, Cambridge, MA.
25 Daniels N, Kennedy B and Kawachi I (2000) Justice is good for our health: how greater economic equality would promote public health. *Boston Review.* **25**. Available from: http://bostonreview.net/ BR25.1/daniels.html (accessed 6 February 2004).
26 Angell M (2000) Pockets of poverty. *Boston Review.* **25**. Available from: http:// bostonreview.net/BR25.1/angell.html (accessed 6 February 2004).
27 Kamm FM (2001) Health and equality of opportunity. *Am J Bioeth.* **1**: 17–19.
28 Emanuel EJ (2000) Political problems. *Boston Review.* **25**. Available from: http:// bostonreview.net/BR25.1/emanuel.html (accessed 6 February 2004).
29 Gakidou E, Frenk J, Murray C (2000). A health agenda. *Boston Review.* **25**. Available from: http://bostonreview.net/BR25.1/ frenk.html (accessed 6 February 2004).

30 Brock D (2000) Broadening the bioethics agenda. *Kennedy Inst Ethics J.* **10**: 21–38.

31 Daniels N, Kennedy B and Kawachi I (2000) *Is Inequality Bad for Our Health?* Beacon Press, Boston, MA.

32 Sen AK (1985) *Commodities and Capabilities*. North-Holland, Amsterdam.

33 Sen AK (1992) *Inequality Re-examined*. Harvard University Press, Cambridge, MA.

34 Sen AK (1999) *Development as Freedom*. Knopf, New York.

35 Marmot MG (2000) Do inequalities matter? *Boston Review.* **25**. Available from: http://bostonreview.net/BR25.1/marmot.html (accessed 6 February 2004).

36 Sen AK (2000) Foreword. In: J Cohen and Rogers (eds) *Is Inequality Bad for Our Health?* Beacon Press, Boston, MA.

37 Ruger JP (1998) Aristotelian justice and health policy: capability and incompletely theorized agreements. PhD thesis. Harvard University, Cambridge, MA.

38 Ruger JP (2003) Health and development. *Lancet.* **362**: 678.

39 Aristotle (Welldon JEC, translator) (1987) *The Nicomachean Ethics*. Prometheus Books, Amherst, NY.

40 Nussbaum MC (1990) Nature, function, and capability: Aristotle on political distribution. In: H von Gunther Patzig. *Aristoteles Politik*. Vandenhoeck and Ruprecht, Gottingen.

41 Nussbaum MC (1998) The good as discipline, the good as freedom. In: DA Crocker and T Linden (eds) *The Ethics of Consumption and Global Stewardship*. Rowman and Littlefield, Lanham, MD.

42 Nussbaum MC (1992) Human functioning and social justice: in defense of Aristotelian essentialism. *Polit Theory.* **20**: 202–46.

43 Aristotle (Lord C, translator) (1984) *The Politics*. University of Chicago Press, Chicago, IL.

44 Marmot MG, Shipley MJ and Rose G (1984) Inequalities in death: specific explanation of a general pattern. *Lancet.* **1**: 1003–6.

45 Marmot MG, Smith GD, Stansfeld S *et al.* (1991) Health inequalities among British civil servants: the Whitehall II study. *Lancet.* **337**: 1387–93.

46 Ruger JP (2004) Combating HIV/AIDS in developing countries. *BMJ.* **329**: 121–2.

47 Ruger JP (2005) Democracy and health. *QJM.* **98**: 299–304.

48 Kreisler H (2002) Redefining public health: epidemiology and social stratification. Sir Michael Marmot Interview: conversations with history, 18 March 2002. Institute of International Studies, UC Berkeley. Available from: http://globetrotter.berkeley.edu/people2/ Marmot/marmot-con1.html (accessed 6 February 2004).

49 Sen AK (1993) The economics of life and death. *Scientific American.* **268**: 40–7.

50 United Nations. *Preventing HIV/AIDS*. Available from: http://www.unaids.org/en/other/functionalities/ViewDocument.asp?href=http%3a%2f%2fgva-doc-owl%2fWEB content%2fDocuments%2fpub%2fPublications%2fFact-Sheets02%2fFS_prevention_en%26%2346%3b.pdf (accessed 6 February 2004).

51 Ruger JP (2005) Global tobacco control: an integrated approach to global health policy. *Development.* **48**(2): 65–9.

52 Ruger JP (2005) Changing role of the World Bank in global health. *American Journal of Public Health.* **95**(1): 60–70.

53 Ruger JP (in press) Toward a theory of a right to health: capability and incompletely theorized agreements. *Yale Journal of Law and Humanities.*

54 Ruger JP (in press) Health, capability and justice: toward a new paradigm of health policy law and ethics. *Cornell Journal of Law and Public Policy.*

Note

Chapter 5

Choice

Giovanni Moro

Choices

The concept of choice has a long history in Western culture. In philosophy, from Aristotle onwards, choice has been conceptualised as the meeting place of the intellect and the will, the place where the intellect and the will interact in a variety of ways. In ethics, choice is the crucial point of the exercise of freedom and responsibility. In politics, it is a necessary condition of democracy and a basic element of sovereignty. These different understandings of choice are highly relevant. When we come to consider choice as a component of a framework of values in health policy, however, we have also to consider some more concrete concerns, such as the illness and the social situation of patients, the role of doctors, market dynamics and public policy directives. These many considerations indicate how multifaceted is the idea of choice. The attempt to clarify what we mean when we speak about choice in healthcare is a task as complex as dealing with the history of ideas in the philosophical realm.

Semantics does not help us to clarify the matter. According the dictionary,[1] choice means both an act and a possibility: the act of choosing between two or more possibilities, and the right or possibility of choosing. In other words, choosing is both about the choice of a possibility, and the possibility of a choice.

Looking at choice as part of a discourse on values in health policy, as defined in the Madrid Framework,[2] an even more complex picture emerges. In the context of such a framework choice can be intended to signify any of the following:

- a value or a worthwhile tool to put some (intrinsic or extrinsic) values into practice;[3]
- a requirement or an outcome;
- an individual or a social and collective matter;
- a market matter or one of public policy.

Furthermore, and specifically in relation to healthcare, choice can be observed *prima facie* as:

- a matter of healthcare or a matter of health policy, i.e. of treatments or of services;
- referring to individuals either as patients or as consumers;
- referring to very different objects of choice, such as surgery, hospitals, medicines, etc.;
- involving one or more patients, doctors, governments, companies and other stakeholders.

In the last decades, in addition to the foregoing characteristics, some unexpected and increasingly widespread facts affecting choice have emerged:

- patients suffering from serious or rare diseases are independently accessing information about their conditions, and are therefore able to challenge the doctors' diagnosis or treatment;
- people are able to buy medicines directly on the Internet, thereby bypassing the doctors' prescriptions, national regulations in respect of medicines, and the officially recognised suppliers of medicines;
- there are citizens' and patients" organisations that offer counselling;
- doctors are refusing to make a choice between different treatments, so leaving the choice to patients, who consequently have often to deal with differences of opinion between the doctors themselves;
- the choices that doctors make are increasingly disregarded by patients;
- within the constraints of current legislation, pharmaceutical companies seek to deliver information about their medicines directly to the public.

In the past the traditional view has been that patients accept that decisions are taken by fully responsible, and not to be questioned, doctors; that relevant information is reserved to experts; that the state, representing the whole community, designs and implements policies of general scope; that citizens' organisations are engaged mainly in charity, assistance to patients being confined to non-medical matters; that pharmaceutical companies adopt a very low profile in their public relations and lobbying activities. What the new developments indicate is that (no matter whether we see them as positive or negative) they go well beyond the traditional view of choice-related matters in healthcare.

This being the case, the attempt to clarify what we mean when we speak of choice in healthcare and health systems cannot be confined to a preamble in this chapter. It becomes its main purpose.

The citizens

My field of observation and reflection is delineated by the following statements:

- choice is about citizens;
- by citizens I mean to include the notions of consumers, patients, users, caregivers and so on;
- choosing can be defined as the practice, by citizens, of a relevant role in selecting both treatments and services;
- this role is not superseded by, but is rather interrelated with, those of other relevant actors in healthcare, for example doctors;
- choice as a practice is conditional (positively or negatively) on a number of external factors, so that choices regarding healthcare are substantially inter-related with health policy;
- dealing with choice in health policy, therefore, implies considering those factors that can affect the choices of citizens, or that can be affected by them.

These statements, which are empirical and not value-driven, are nevertheless consistent with the vision of citizens' choice as a value. This latter vision is well expressed by the European Charter of Patients' Rights:[4]

Each individual has the right to freely choose from among different treatment procedures and providers on the basis of adequate information.

The patient has the right to decide which diagnostic investigations and therapies to undergo, and which primary care doctor, specialist or hospital to consult. Health services have the duty to guarantee this right, providing patients with information on the various centres and doctors able to provide a certain treatment, and on the results of their activities. They must remove any obstacle that limits the exercise of this right.

A patient who does not have trust in his or her doctor has the right to choose another one.

Of course recognising choice as a *value* makes sense in the case of citizens. For other actors engaged in health – from governments to doctors – choice, though of the utmost importance, is best understood not as a value, as such, but primarily as a duty, a function, and so on.

The last methodological warning I want to give is that I will deal with this issue from a European perspective, and in particular on the basis of the Active Citizenship Network's research and policy activities on patients' rights. It is not only a matter of competence. Rather, it must be said that the issue of patients' choice is in a sense at the core of ongoing dynamics of health systems in the European Union – and is thus emerging as a relevant heuristic tool. That said, in what follows I will try to show and discuss some of the conditions and constraints on choice as a citizens' value.

The Janus-faced paradox of citizens' choice

My discussion on choice now moves from the realm of ideas to that of concrete reality, checking what choice means for the citizen's daily dealings with health systems. I will use some of the results from the Active Citizenship Network's Report on the implementation of the European Charter of Patients' Rights.[5]

The research gave information on the state of patients' rights by identifying phenomena that can be considered *indicators of attention* towards those rights; and it reflected an approach to healthcare issues based on the point of view and the condition of citizens, patients or users of health facilities. Its findings, therefore, are especially valuable for the purpose of this chapter.

From the ACN survey, attention to the right to free choice was accorded one of the lowest rankings by the health authorities, as Table 5.1 shows. In all the countries surveyed, it was reported that there was a requirement for specific authorisation in order to get some treatments. In 8 out of the 13 comparable countries, there were differential fees in the public and private hospitals, and supplementary insurance coverage for only some hospitals. There was also some evidence of incentives being given to seek treatment in private hospitals, and of indigent patients being restricted to seek treatment only in certain designated hospitals. According to key witnesses, in more than half of the countries surveyed new measures were adopted over the past year, further to restrict the possibility of citizens to choose their healthcare services.

In addition to this picture, the research adds much information regarding the

Table 5.1 General classification of patients' rights according to the degree of attention

Degree of attention	Right	Score
High	Access – physical	26
	Complain	26
	Privacy	25
	Information	24
	Safety	24
Medium	Personalised treatment	22
	Quality	21
	Innovation	20
	Avoid pain	20
Low	Free choice	19
	Compensation	19
	Prevention	18
	Consent	18
	Access – care	17
	Time	16

Score: min 9, max 27, average 21
Active Citizenship Network, 2005

situation of other, choice-related, patient rights, namely the rights to access, to information and to consent. All these rights can be considered as factors affecting the actual possibility for citizens to make choices about their health; factors such as barriers to access to services, lack of information, the habit of 'uninformed consent', all limit free and responsible choice.

Regarding the right of *access* to health services, the survey identified the following as the most common problems: the lack of public insurance coverage for services considered essential by the public; administrative and/or economic obstacles in accessing services; the impossibility in some European countries of getting access to medicines that are available in others. Specific examples, where the right to guaranteed equal access of health services without discriminating was not respected, were reported in more than half of the surveyed countries.

As regards the right to *information*, the least available relates to hospital waiting lists for diagnostic tests and surgery; to complaints received from the public; to data for benchmarking; and, most frequently mentioned, to data on outcomes (patient satisfaction, clinical performance measures, etc.).

As for the right to *consent*, it must be pointed out that, while forms to obtain the patient's consent are widespread, in only some of the European countries were they used when patients underwent invasive diagnostic tests and surgical operations. Usually they were reserved only for use in the course of clinical research. Furthermore, while all the consent forms contained information on the nature of the procedure, only in two cases did they include information on risks and benefits, and in no case were existing alternative treatments mentioned.

Despite any limitations of the research, these data tell us something very interesting and really very concerning: in current health policies, the term 'choice' seems to carry highly ambiguous and contradictory meanings.

On the one hand, the availability of free, responsible choices by citizens is generally considered of crucial importance in making health systems perform more efficiently and effectively. Reforms aimed at establishing markets, or quasi-markets, are actually based on the supposition that citizens, choosing the most appropriate and effective services and professionals, will create the conditions for fair competition on quality, and compel healthcare stakeholders to improve their performances and avoid waste.

On the other, however, those who make health policies, and those who implement them, appear to attempt to make it as difficult as possible for the citizen or patient to exercise choice. Our research data revealed that this second task – making choice as difficult as possible – is achieved in the main by the following three strategies:

- creating bureaucratic barriers;
- hiding information;
- rationing services.

In other words, on one hand citizens' choice is required for the sake of sustaining well functioning health systems, and on the other hand it is hindered for the very same reason (usually in the name of financial sustainability).

But this is just one face of the paradox. It also has another face, which makes it even more interesting and concerning.

Obviously citizens cannot be invited to make choices outside their competence to choose. Also, in such cases, they should be helped to choose with the support of competent advice and fully available information. It is the role of health systems actors to perform these functions, to provide information, advice and counsel. However, citizens are very often left alone to choose between alternatives of which they are not aware, on the basis of information that they do not have. This is the second face of the paradox.

Such (un)informed consent is a clear indicator of this: citizens are called upon to choose, usually without information, in terms of risks, benefits and existing alternatives. Further, according to an Active Citizenship Network's research on citizens' organisations in 26 'New Europe' countries,[6] almost everywhere citizens' healthcare organisations are engaged in providing health information, and in the education of patients and public. In almost half of these countries advice services and call centres are provided by citizens' organisations, and in more than one in four countries, they provide medical counselling and training of professionals and patients. All of these activities would not need to be undertaken were health systems and their actors operating effectively.

The second face of the Paradox of Citizens' Choice, therefore, can be expressed as follows:

> While there are some choices that citizens cannot make, or make alone, those who should make, or facilitate, such choices seem to offload their responsibility back onto the citizens themselves.

The two faces of the Paradox of Citizens' Choice can be combined as follows:

> When citizens wish to make choices, they are not enabled to do so; when they wish to be advised or supported in making choices, they are left to their own devices.

It is well known that contradictions are innate in public policies, so we should not be too surprised by this situation. This, however, should not make us less concerned. Rather it should spur us to take a further step: to try to identify more factors related to the Paradox of Citizens' Choice that might be accommodated by more pertinent public policy.

Information, competence, trust

The Paradox of Citizens' Choice is linked to a number of factors of various kinds – cognitive and operational; economic, social, cultural and political; global and domestic; specifically focused on health, and more general factors. Of course, it is impossible to identify all of them. However, the purpose of this book is to encourage constructive conversation. Therefore, in line with the purpose of this book, I will stress some of the more pertinent elements that contribute to creating the paradox of choice, according to which citizens' choice is both a winning strategy and a deadly danger, both necessary and impossible. It should be added that a policy on choice in health should, in any case, cope with these factors.

The Paradox of Citizens' Choice refers to a general cultural pattern. In relation to governments interacting with civic organisations, this has been called the *Dr Jekyll–Mr Hyde Syndrome*: citizens are at one and the same time considered and managed by governments both as a resource and as a threat.[7] This syndrome, which implies in turn an over- and an underestimation of the role of citizens in public life, is deeply rooted not only in political and administrative culture, but also in that of private actors, including companies, professionals and experts. With reference to welfare systems, and especially to health systems, it is translated in the double-headed statement that citizens are the very purpose of health systems, and at the same time their highest, unbearable, cost. Health, wellbeing, the safety of citizens are the very *raison d'être* of health systems, of policy, and for professionals. Therefore, one element of the paradox is that this priority is contradicted by other views and practices (especially in the name of financial constraints). And this is precisely the starting point of the European Charter of Patients' Rights.

To this general paradigm, three specific factors that feed the paradox can be added. They are the existing informational asymmetries in health, uncertainty about the competence of citizens, and a lack of trust in the sources of information.

The *first*, and probably best known or most recognised, factor is *informational asymmetry*, something that happens 'when the producer does not supply the amount of information that maximizes the difference between the reduction in dead-weight loss and the cost of providing information'.[8] What is to be stressed here is that, in the case of healthcare goods, only a small proportion of them are *search goods*, that is, goods whose characteristics can be determined by consumers with certainty prior to purchase. Rather, for the most part, they are either *experience* or *post-experience goods*: that is, either goods for which consumers can determine their characteristics only after purchase, or goods for which it is difficult for consumers to determine quality even after they have begun consumption.[9] Obviously, while in the case of *search goods* informational asymmetry is negligible, the last two types of goods imply a significant degree of informational asymmetry.

The *second* factor is the issue of *citizens' competence* in healthcare. What is commonly agreed is that:

- citizens have experiences related to their possible or actual illnesses;
- they have perceptions related to the services they receive (this is the basis of consumer satisfaction surveys);
- they have highly subjective opinions about how things should work.

In other words, citizens' competence is usually considered as something belonging to the realm of subjectivity, meaning that citizens can manage feelings and opinions, but not information. For these reasons, they are usually supposed not to be able to make choices, but rather to constitute the targets of public action and professional performance. Of course, citizens are not, and cannot be, changed into doctors or experts in health economics.

Nevertheless, on the basis of their own experiences, of 'social technology transfer', and of deposits of memory of collective actors, they produce and use limited but reliable information both on healthcare and services.[10]

The Paradox of Citizens' Choice seems to interact with the foregoing as follows. The ability of citizens to make choices is denied in those instances where they are clearly competent to choose, and this ability is expected and required in those instances where they are not. In both cases, even though accepted in theory, in practice the autonomous subjectivity of citizens is denied.

In primary markets, informational asymmetries can be reduced by informative advertising and warranties on the sellers' side; and in secondary markets, by the intervention of private third parties, such as certification or auditing services, and professionals.[11] This leads us to consider a *third* factor, *trust*. All possible measures aimed at reducing informational asymmetries can be effective and successful insofar as those who carry them out are trusted by the public. A source of information can be highly competent and honest, but if it is not trusted, those concerned will not be confident of its advice. The problem is that trust and confidence are among the scantest common goods in contemporary societies, and this affects daily face-to-face relations (triggering a vicious circle with social capital).[12] It also affects the public arena, bringing into question the reliability both of political actors (such as political parties) and other public and private actors (such as companies, the media and public administration itself).[13] Obviously, this is not at all foreign to the concerns of healthcare and health policy. Distrust in medical doctors is a well known phenomenon, as well as suspicion of the motives of companies engaged in healthcare. This worrying situation, by the way, does not seem to be taken seriously into account in the EU debate about proposals for direct-to-consumer information on medicines by pharmaceutical companies. And distrust extends to citizens themselves, who are usually distrusted, for example, when they try to communicate information on their diseases.

In the field of healthcare there are therefore three factors that seem to worsen rather than resolve the Paradox of Citizens' Choice. Citizens, when they make choices about healthcare, are faced with significant informational asymmetries. In some cases citizens are not in fact competent to make choices, and these are precisely the situations where citizens are called to take decisions by themselves, replacing other actors who should but do not exercise their responsibilities. Patients have no trust in those sources of information that could reduce these asymmetries; and they themselves are not trusted.

These three factors are, without doubt, of the utmost importance. Any discussion about choice in healthcare from the citizens' point of view has to cope with them. They cannot be ignored. However, rather than foreclosing further constructive conversation on this matter, I want now to attempt an exercise of 'looking differently' at the problem.

Looking differently

Looking with different eyes at the Paradox of Citizens' Choice, and at its related factors, we could envisage an approach to choice capable both of reinforcing knowledge, and becoming a reference for designing a policy aimed at empowering citizens as choice actors on health issues, putting them in a position properly to exercise this role.

First of all, although it might seem an obvious point, no one can replace citizens in making choices on health-related issues. The temptation to replace citizens may have, and has had, quite varying, even opposite, inspirations and motivations – for example, a left-wing enlightenment or a right-wing paternalism; authoritarian state planning or consumer orientation. The substitution of the citizen's right of choice is, in any case, nothing but a shortcut. In turn, the right and duty of citizens to make choices cannot release other actors from the task of exercising their own choices, whether they are governments, professionals or companies. The weight of these choices cannot be offloaded onto citizens. In other words what this means is that healthcare policy must be managed in a governance framework, which at one and the same time calls for clear divisions of labour, and cooperation among the actors.[14]

Another factor to be taken into account is that, in present welfare systems, various dimensions of health are often overlapping and not easy to distinguish from one another – in particular, for example, the distinction between healthcare and health policy. The first includes treatments and drugs; the second quality and cost of structures and services. Choices made in one dimension have effects in, and are influenced by, choices made in the other, and vice versa. Something like a 'clear-cut' choice is difficult to find in practice. The public discourse on citizens' choice should be based on what actually happens, rather than on what should happen, and does not.

Linked to this commitment to reality, another element has to be considered. This is the need to revise the notion of the citizen as a pure, unrelated individual, an entity abstracted from his/her ties and the social fabric where he/she lives. When we deal with the choices of individuals, we are in fact speaking about persons who are parts of a number of networks, have multiple interests and concerns, have family and neighbourhood links, have independent access to health information through the media and the Internet. The individual who makes choices is thus both complex and interrelated, and these choices are influenced or supported by a number of factors and actors that may render the individual more expert or, on the contrary, less expert, confused and uncertain. None of this is can be clearly understood if we only look on people as islands. This understanding of the relatedness of the individual is not at all incompatible with the newly recognised value of the patients' experience and evidence. Finally and importantly, all this makes clear that citizens (and patients) are neither autonomous nor artless; both these views are in fact myths. We need to go beyond myths.

It should be recalled that citizens are also self-organised, acting collectively to protect rights and pursue common goods, from advocacy to the delivery of services. Community-based, voluntary, consumer, and patients' organisations are some of the forms taken by citizens who have a new attitude to the exercise of power and responsibility in the public arena.[15] With reference to choice, and to the factors highlighted in the previous paragraph, they play a relevant role in:

- informing, advising and assisting patients, both on medical and non-medical issues;
- advocating and bargaining on choices with public authorities and other stakeholders;
- 'lending trust'[16] to public and private actors, helping to ensure their reliability as sources of information;
- auditing, monitoring and reporting on health actors' behaviours, so functioning as third parties in relation to informational asymmetries;
- pushing medical doctors and other actors (such as pharmaceutical companies) to be fully responsible in choosing and delivering information;
- giving priority to individual differences, in the delivery of services, and emphasising the ability to tailor, or adapt, the service to the users' needs;
- taking part in managing conflicts between alternative competing needs, especially in situations of scarcity.

The role of citizens' organisations must not be overestimated. But neither should it be underestimated. According to all available data from surveys, pretty much everywhere such organisations are at the top in rankings of social trust.

None of this resolves the Paradox of Citizens' Choice, and I have not aimed to do so here. Rather, these observations reveal that matters are much more complex than is usually considered, and so may be of some worth in attempting to manage the ensuing problems.

Memo for a policy

In concluding, I return to the Madrid Framework, the point of reference of this book. As to policy on choice the Framework highlights two main issues. The first is the potential conflict between those choices made with regard to collectivities, if not to whole populations, and those made with regard to the needs of individuals and specific groups. The second is that, since choice in health policy implies the gain of 'something' but not of 'everything', the resulting menu of choices must be 'transparent' and challengeable by citizens. Both these elements pose real and serious problems that deserve the highest level of our attention.

In a sense, these two considerations – the conflict between the individual and the group, the possibility of obtaining some goods but not others – characterise not only health policy, but policy making in general. The typical problem for public policy (and for politics) is precisely how to make choices that look at problems in a rounded way – by attempting to reduce the gap between the specific needs and conditions of people, as well as taking into account cultural, religious, social, economic and other differences; and by adopting the minimum standard for a democracy, that policy choices are made transparent, so that people, especially those directly involved and affected, are able to question them.

In another sense, however, these statements are insufficient and more is required. Firstly, in contemporary societies, 'the interest of the whole population' is very difficult to identify because of the existence of multiple identities and networks, and the overlapping of interests. As we have seen, the individual is not as 'individual' as the traditional representation of society suggests. So, the problem of making policy choices is to define the general interest, not by deducing them from some *a priori* scheme, but by starting from an acknowledgement of the many differences in a society. Things, therefore, are much more complex than is suggested by the task of managing the divide between general and special interests. A policy on choice in health (and in welfare in general) must essentially be a matter of managing diversity.

Secondly, it seems to me that, following the way in which I have defined and argued for citizens' choices in this chapter, these must be part of the general process of policy making, and neither over- nor underestimated. In this sense, a new democratic standard should clarify and establish that citizens must have a say and a role in defining the menu itself. It is not enough to be given the opportunity to question it *after* it has been defined. Consultation policies, involving individuals as well as organisations increasingly now at local, national and trans-national levels,[17] though at the moment absolutely insufficient, nevertheless go in this direction.

Thirdly, it is necessary to avoid any risk of policy *bricolage*, and recognise that conflict cannot be eliminated by policy making. On the contrary, conflict is one of its constitutive elements. A without-conflict definition or implementation of a policy simply does not exist, either in principle or practice. What is important, from this point of view, is rather to make sure that citizens can participate in policy conflicts on an equal basis, recalling that citizens' positions are often those closest to common concerns.

Fourthly, it is far too reductive to consider choice as something that happens only at the moment of the definition of a policy (i.e. the idea of a unique and definitive macro-decision). Throughout the whole policy making cycle a number of choices (macro and micro) are being made. As we have seen, several choices to the detriment of citizens' and patients' rights have been made in European countries, particularly in the implementation of policy, which could possibly have been identified and avoided with the active participation of citizens' organisations. The problem, thus, is how to ensure that citizens' choices are taken into consideration as a relevant part of the policy making process, and recognised as a distinguishing and value-added element. This should be the concern not only of citizens' organisations, but also of governments, policy makers, experts, and the whole policy community.

Fifthly and lastly, a policy on choice should have as its final aim the empowerment of citizens as choice owners, in two senses. The first is that citizens must be provided with enabling know-how and skills on choice-related issues, and helped to feel themselves really able to exercise their own rights and powers on choice. The second is that citizens can demand of all health actors, and impose on them, that they take responsibility for, and are held accountable for, their own choices.

References

1 *Oxford Advanced Learner's Dictionary of Current English* (1993) Oxford University Press, Oxford.
2 Marinker M (2005) The Madrid Framework. *Eurohealth.* 11(1): 2–5. Available from: www.euro.who.int/Document/obs/Eurohealth11_1.pdf.
3 Dunn WN (1981) *Public Policy Analysis: an introduction.* Prentice Hall, Englewood Cliffs, NJ.
4 Active Citizenship Network (ACN) (2002) *European Charter of Patient Rights.* Paper presented in Brussels on 15 November 2002. See also: Kickbusch I (2004) *The Need for Common Values, Principles and Objectives for Health Policy in a Changing Europe.* Paper presented at the European Health Forum Gastein 2004.
5 Lamanna A, Moro G and Ross M (eds) (2005) *Citizens' Report on the Implementation of the European Charter of Patients' Rights.* Working paper February 2005. ACN, Rome. The first stage, reported in 2005, was carried out in 2003–4 in the 15 'old EU' countries. In all but two of them the results were comparable.
6 Active Citizenship Network (ACN) (2004) *Public Institutions Interacting with Citizens' Organizations. A Survey on Public Policies Regarding Civic Activism in Europe.* Paper. ACN, Rome.
7 Id.
8 Weimer DL and Vining AR (1992) *Policy Analysis: concepts and practice.* Prentice Hall, Englewood Cliffs, NJ. See also: Shmanske S (1996) Information Asymmetries in Health Services. The market can cope. *The Independent Review.* 1(2) (Fall 1996): 191–200.
9 Weimer DL and Vining AR (1992) *Policy Analysis: concepts and practice.* Prentice Hall, Englewood Cliffs, NJ.
10 Moro G (2002) *Involving the Citizen in the Debate on the Selection and Prioritising of Health Targets and their Implementation.* Paper presented at the Conference on 'Health Targets in Europe: polity, progress and promise'. London, 7 June 2002. See also: Wildavsky A (1993) Citizens as analysts. In: A Wildavsky. *Speaking Truth to Power.* Transaction Publishers, New Brunswick. See also: Marinker M (ed) (2002) *Health Targets in Europe: polity, progress and promise.* BMJ Books, London.
11 Weimer DL and Vining AR (1992) *Policy Analysis: concepts and practice.* Prentice Hall, Englewood Cliffs, NJ.
12 Cf. Putnam RD (1993) *La tradizione civica nelle regioni italiane* (Making Democracy Work). Mondadori, Milano; ID (2000) *Bowling Alone. The Collapse and Revival of American Community.* Simon & Schuster, New York; Sztompka P (1999) *Trust: A Sociological Theory.* Cambridge University Press, Cambridge.
13 Cf. Schmitter PC, Trechsel AH (eds) (2004) *The Future of Democracy in Europe: trends, analyses and reforms.* Council of Europe Publishing, Strasbourg; Zadek S (2004) *The Civil Corporation: the new economy of corporate citizenship.* Earthscan, London and Stirling.
14 Moro G (2002) The citizen side of governance. *The Journal of Corporate Citizenship.* 7(Autumn): 18–30.
15 Active Citizenship Network (ACN) (2004) *Public Institutions Interacting with Citizens' Organizations. a survey on public policies regarding civic activism in Europe.* ACN, Rome. See also: Petrangolini T (2002) *Salute e diritti dei cittadini. Cosa sapere e cosa fare* (Health and Rights. What to know and what to do). Editori Riuniti, Roma.
16 Zadek S (2004) *The Civil Corporation: the new economy of corporate citizenship.* Earthscan, London and Stirling.
17 See, for example, European Commission (2002) *Towards a Reinforced Culture of Consultation and Dialogue: general principles and minimum standards for consultation of interested parties by the Commission.* COM(2002) 704; OECD (2001) *Citizens as Partners: OECD Handbook on Information, Consultation and Public Participation in Policy-Making.* Paris, OECD.

Chapter 6

Democracy

Per Carlsson and Peter Garpenby

Who is against democracy?

For most people in Europe, democracy is a concept that stands for inalienable values like other concepts such as freedom, equality, human dignity, respect for human rights – and good health. These basic values have played a vital role in the construction of healthcare and other parts of welfare systems. They often appear in political manifestos and legislation, but sometimes they are neglected, or fail to be implemented, in practical policy making.

Democracy in terms of healthcare refers to citizens' potential to exercise power over the content and scope of the healthcare system, and to the exercise of power over their own situations when they end up as a patient or as a user in some other way. Can democracy work in relation to healthcare? Since we lack a uniform definition of democracy and its applications in different contexts, it is not easy to answer this key question.

We can, however, say that healthcare is in the midst of a cultural revolution. Respect for the individual patient's human dignity, in terms of autonomy and integrity, has gradually increased, but there is need for more. Examples of injustices in the access of adequate care are attracting increasing attention. The need for criteria of *need* for care, contrasted with *demand* for care, is increasingly accepted. Why then have these self-evident values proven to be so difficult to realise in practice? One explanation is that, in real life, there are many conflicts between values that cannot be resolved in a manner that simultaneously gives equal weight to them all. For this reason, people, politicians, representatives of care-providing professions, tend to focus on one issue at a time, which means that certain values have to give way to others.

The self-determination of patients in healthcare was discussed extensively throughout the 1990s, and politicians in many countries took action to strengthen the position of patients in the system. As a result, 'patient rights' have been laid down in laws and manifestos, for example in the UK as early as 1991, when the 'Patients' Charter' was introduced by a Conservative government. When a Labour government took office in 1997, it instigated a review of the Charter, and a report was produced later that year. The Charter was abandoned as part of changes to the NHS implemented in the year 2000 under the new 10-year NHS plan. We interpret this as a shift away from regarding the patient foremost as a consumer with individual rights, to a citizen with both rights and obligations, and acting in partnership with the providers of healthcare.

In practice, much remains to be done. A recent European survey shows significant variations between European countries in reported levels of involvement. Results indicate that many European patients want a more autonomous role in healthcare decision making.[1] What does this imply for democracy in health policy? Democracy is something much more complex than a political mechanism for satisfying individual self-interest. And we note that while there is much activity in support of patient involvement in clinical decisions, analogous initiatives to enhance *citizens'* involvement in health policy are rare.

There are considerable differences between European countries in the operation of democratic processes in relation to healthcare. Some countries, for example the United Kingdom, the Netherlands and Norway, tend to a more centralised system of government. In Sweden, the services are decentralised. There is a relatively strong element of representative democracy, with thousands of local politicians engaged in healthcare policy making. Despite this, questions about the actual power of politicians over healthcare, and their legitimacy to make difficult decisions, is gaining in importance.

In times of economic expansion, during the 1960s and 1970s, when decisions were being taken to increase the budget for the public sector, representative democracy worked relatively well. But in recent years, with economic development no longer supporting continuing expansion of the public sector, democracy appears to be working less satisfactorily. One reason for this may be that in Sweden, the County Councils that control healthcare are relatively large and are currently in the process of being combined into ever larger administrations, each with a population of more than a million.

These proposed enlargements are a response to the new health technologies that will transform the ways in which care can be provided to the population. But what are the implications of such large administrations and populations for the democratic process? Will citizens be able to feel fully involved? This confronts us with a classic clash between two values – efficiency and democracy.

Who has sufficient legitimacy to make a difficult decision?

Irrespective of the healthcare system, policy makers in Europe face a number of challenges that place new demands on *how* decisions are made, and on politicians' ability to conduct a dialogue with citizens. Health, and access to good healthcare, are increasingly seen as a right in modern society. According to a survey conducted among the Swedish population in 2000, 39% responded that healthcare was the single most important political issue for them,[2] and received the highest percentage of all responses. However, the individual's right to good healthcare can conflict with the interests and needs of other citizens. Since resources in the public sector are limited, it must follow that the right of any one person to obtain the best possible care will come into direct conflict with the rights of others. If we are to balance the demands and wishes of all individuals in society, the majority must share a number of values – such as solidarity, justice and altruism.

During the second half of the twentieth century, thanks to good economic growth, it was possible to expand the public sector, which roughly kept pace with the cost of advances in modern medicine and the growing demands from the population. Technological progress contributed, or seemed to contribute, to continuous improvements in public health, and this motivated continuous expansion. We can now see indications that this trend is over. The connection between medical progress and health improvement is no longer perceived to be so clear. In many countries the ability to expand welfare services by means of tax increases seems to have reached its limit. In old welfare countries like Sweden, politicians have been forced to introduce cutbacks in benefits.

The health technology field continues to progress, but currently it seems that new technologies such as genetic engineering contribute primarily to improvements in diagnosis rather than treatment. With the tremendous development in imaging techniques the accuracy of diagnosis improves greatly. But we are left with the impression that physicians are becoming better at diagnosis, rather than the treatment of diseases. This overtaking of treatment by diagnosis often leads to cost increases that do not correspond to improved health. The dramatic increase in the media coverage of health matters, with promising reports of future technologies, combined with critical reports on shortcomings in health services, kindle expectations on the one hand and dissatisfaction with the system on the other. A growing gap between public expectations and what can actually be done can, in the long run, lead to a lessening of trust in those who are responsible – the politicians.

Nonetheless, in Sweden, trust in healthcare as a social institution remains high. In 2000, 65% of people responded that they had 'great' or 'rather great' trust in the healthcare system.[2] The scores were significantly lower for the democratically elected institutions – like the Swedish parliament and government, and the EU parliament. As regards trust reposed in different professional categories, physicians are at the top of the list and politicians are at the bottom. These results may have implications for the design of healthcare policies. How much room for action do we have? How should the necessary decisions be made? Will it be possible to change this trend of distrust in political institutions? Is it a real problem that public confidence in the political institutions of a democracy is lower than in the institutions concerned with implementing public policies?

We do not believe that the problem of a growing deficit of trust will disappear. Rather, we hold that health policy makers should be helped to understand the context in which they are acting, and to be more sensitive to what people want. It is not sufficient to listen only to the voices of the majority. The voices of the minorities must also be heard, and their right to equality of care defended.

If politicians are to be able to make unpopular but necessary decisions, they will have to create a legitimacy of their own. Generally speaking, all structural changes in healthcare systems face the risk of being perceived as negative. All limits on public services lead to general dissatisfaction, and specific dissatisfaction among special interest groups. To gain acceptance for difficult policy decisions, those actors with an 'outside perspective', those who sporadically come into contact with healthcare as patients or as patients' relatives, must have sufficient trust in the actors with an 'inside perspective', those whose job it is to lead and operate the service. Today the level of such trust in healthcare policy makers is low. How can we better understand this?

It is clear that citizens and the different actors in healthcare perceive the problems very differently. While there are reports in the media of more effective treatments that achieve more cures, better symptom relief, and so on, other reports present a contrasting picture of citizens who doubt if healthcare will be available to them when they get sick, and feel increasingly driven to seek alternative remedies. These perceptions are all challenges for the provision of healthcare as we know it. A few of these, with direct implications for the democratic component in the system, are listed below.

- Greater transparency in the provision of information reveals that there are differences in practice and health within and between countries.
- Medical progress produces new pharmaceuticals and other medical technologies that tend to be substantially expensive, in part because of the need to cover the costs of their R&D.
- With the growing number of elderly in the population, and changes in the panorama of disease, the need for healthcare increases.
- There are growing demands on healthcare because of growing public and individual expectations.

Does greater transparency lead to less confidence?

Healthcare involves a number of paradoxes that contribute to difficulties in creating clear-cut and straightforward policies. If citizens are to have confidence in these, they must be based on, and reflect, popular views about such basic values as equality, quality and accessibility. This requires that citizens, patients and their families, are involved in decision making in some way. This means involvement in the direction that health policy is to take, the distribution of resources, and decisions concerning individual patients.

One condition for such a real involvement in the decision making process is greater access to relevant information on how healthcare services actually work, on resources, processes and outcomes. We can already see the beginning of such a trend in many countries. Because of greater transparency on the part of government agencies, directors and administrators, because of the desire of physicians and other care providers to report what they do, and because of improved information systems that describe how healthcare actually performs, there is increasing evidence of real differences in the supply, quality and outcome of care. While there is reason to believe that these differences in health and style of practice have always existed, they have been largely hidden. As recently as the early 1980s, health service researchers such as Wennberg and others attracted great attention when they demonstrated not only great health and practice variations between countries, but also between small geographical areas in the same country.[3]

Smoothing out significant differences is not only a matter of the distribution of resources, but also of service policies concerning performance. Data on quality of care have, over time, become important considerations in health service policy, as in the UK where politicians have struggled with the Resource Allocation Working Party (RAWP) formulae, which attempt to model 'need' in allocating resources to the different parts of the National Health Service.[4]

Publication of outcome data, however, is not uncontroversial.

When pursuing a policy with the aim of smoothing differences, politicians must act to increase the transparency of health service policies to the general public by encouraging care providers to better and standardised documentation on their services. This, however, conflicts with the traditional autonomy of health professionals, and, when flaws come to light, runs the risk of causing a crisis in confidence. Every report on malpractice or negligence means that a problem, having been identified, can be attended to, and so can lead to improvements in the service. Yet at the same time this can lead to an erosion of public confidence in the service.

Erroneous information can be disseminated because of flaws in basic data, and unnecessary misunderstandings can arise because the interpretation of these data can be far from simple. In Sweden, since the late 1980s, the national government, together with County Councils and the medical profession, have established quality registries.[5] Today there are about 50 of them. A number have been in existence for more than 15 years, but their content remains relatively unknown to the general public, or indeed to healthcare policy makers! However, reporting has gradually become more accessible and specific: it is now possible to see the results for much smaller service units than heretofore. This reporting of results for individual hospitals, rather than for large geographic areas, has proven to be a major step.

Healthcare services in all countries have probably become significantly more transparent to the general public in past decades, and policy makers are relatively in agreement on continuing along this path. However, this transparency causes problems both for health professionals and for politicians.

Medical innovations: a driving force not easy to handle

On a weekly basis we are informed by the press, radio and TV about new advances in medicine. Other reports signal variations in clinical practice between different areas. For the individual citizen, politicians and other decision makers, it can be difficult to judge the relevance of such reports. This raises many questions in the public mind about priority-setting. In addition, some new medical technologies, for example pharmaceuticals, are supported by strong economic interests and are therefore advantaged over other useful technologies that lack such support.[6] It can also be difficult to determine whether or not a new technology is compatible with prevailing values. An all too hasty or extensive introduction of new health technologies can court risks.

Many attempts have been made to control the development and dissemination of medical technology. Most initiatives have been unsuccessful. The primary reason is that the decision making processes are complex, that prediction can be difficult, and that the bureaucratic systems seem relatively slow, old-fashioned or inadequate. Previous attempts in many countries to determine the need for computer tomography are one example of this difficulty with technology assessment.

By the same token, there may be reasons to slow down the dissemination of certain technologies, while others may need speeding up. The introduction of technologies presented for rapid dissemination should be stringently examined for scientific evidence on patient benefit, risks and cost-effectiveness. The introduction of laparoscopic cholecystectomy 15 years ago is one example of rapid diffusion, where the health and financial costs and benefits are still a matter of debate. When there is good evidence of positive benefit, and a reasonable cost-effectiveness, it is not so much a matter of uncertainty about the value of the technology, as of reallocating funds within the frame of a finite budget.

The expansion of coronary artery surgery in the 1980s required considerable political initiatives in order to fit the resulting technological development into the existing health service organisation. Another example, from the late 1990s, was the introduction of new, expensive pharmaceuticals for the treatment of rheumatoid arthritis, which required a reallocation of resources across traditional clinical borders.

It is obvious that technological changes play a major role in the development of health systems. Furthermore, the use of technology is affected by a number of factors in addition to its effectiveness and cost-effectiveness. Pressure groups and special interests must be balanced by a democratic government that seeks to safeguard the common good by using appropriate control measures. One that has certain advantages in this context is control by dissemination of knowledge. Concepts such as evidence based medicine (EBM) and transparency in priority-setting are important in this respect. In particular, EBM has had a major impact in many European countries, not just on medical practice, but on health service policies, such as the best possible scientific data being employed in explicit decision making. To support this approach, an attempt is being made to bridge the knowledge gap between experts and laypersons. In many countries there is a system for health technology assessments in which national agencies produce scientific evidence. SBU in Sweden and NICE in the UK are well known examples, and to an increasing extent citizens are being involved in making an input into these evaluation processes.

Better health demands more healthcare

The EU Commission has estimated that from 2005 to 2030 the number of people over 65 years will rise by 52% – to about 40 million. At the same time those in the age group 15–64 years will decrease by 7% – to about 20 million.[7] According to the Commission, in order to offset this loss of working-age people, we will need an overall employment rate of more than 70%. These predicted demographic changes will have major implications for all parts of society, and will put extreme pressure on welfare systems, not least in relation to the care of the elderly.

Citizens have growing expectations about the state of their own health and the function of health services. In a modern society, easy access to all forms of service is a high priority. But strong interest groups such as the large pharmaceuticals companies, using their enormous marketing power, can distort the balance of health goods available in the health system. This can threaten such basic values as effectiveness and efficiency. The inability of policy makers to act firmly to guard against this can create a permanent situation of implicit rationing which can seem arbitrary and unfair, such that confidence in publicly funded health services can be eroded.

Openness in priority-setting – an advance on democracy?

It will probably be necessary to test more transparent and systematic processes for priority-setting and rationing. This has been on the political agenda in some countries throughout the 1990s, but has proven complicated to achieve in practice.[8] In 1997 the Swedish parliament decided on an ethical platform for priority-setting in healthcare. Since then not much has happened in practical policy making, and many questions remain to be answered:[9]

- How can greater fairness be achieved in practice?
- Which aspects have been given fair priority?
- Who is to make this sort of decision?
- How can politicians and care providers be involved?
- What sort of material evidence is needed to form the basis for decisions?
- How transparent can decisions be?
- How can the general public be involved?

In Sweden the topic of priority-setting has attracted many actors in recent years but it is still an issue, which tends to cause disturbance in political circles. A number of regional and local health authorities and national bodies are in the process of developing systematic and transparent approaches. The ranking of services, within broad disease groups, and made by the medical profession, is one of the first steps towards such greater transparency. In 2003, the Östergötland County Council drew up a list of 'low-priority services' which would not be included in its provisions and would have to be funded by the patients themselves. Despite preparations for this move, which had been ongoing for several years in line with the Swedish parliament's decision, the reactions of the media, the general public and among central government politicians were strongly averse.[10] The entire process bore testimony to a lack of trust in the political allocation of public goods. How can we understand this paradox? Why is the general public so reluctant to accept this sort of democratic process, and at the same time unwilling openly to discuss priority-setting in healthcare?

Will the social trap shut without trust?

In all countries healthcare is rationed, and for the most part decisions about rationing are made by health professionals. This new resolve to make this rationing more open, and to involve the representatives of the public – the politicians – causes new problems.

Based on the theory of social capital and its wider implications, the Swedish political scientist Bo Rothstein[11] has attempted to disentangle the problem of trust in democratic societies. He claims that it is obvious to most people that a society benefits from a functioning legal system, a financial system, and a social insurance system that cares for the elderly and the sick. Effective cooperation in pursuit of mutual aims, however, requires a large degree of confidence both in others and in democratic institutions. If a member of society cannot trust the other members of that society, then it becomes rational to act egotistically, even though, in the long run, such action leads to poorer outcomes for the society at large. What is good for me is not necessarily good for everybody else, and vice versa. Without trust there is the risk that we all lose, in other words that 'the social trap shuts'.[12]

Solidarity in the welfare state is conditional. That is to say, it is based on the trust reposed by members of society that its institutions will function fairly and in the common interest. In such circumstances, political actors as well as individuals can be motivated by what both parties perceive to be fair, by what they perceive to be their own good, and by the desire that their own good correspond with what they perceive to be morally correct. How can this state be achieved?

There are a number of rival theories in responding to this question. A central premise of these theories is the creation and maintenance of social capital.

According to the Swedish Commission on the State of Democracy[13] there are a number of conditions that should be fulfilled in order to achieve a democratic form of government. One is that there must be plenty of social capital or civic virtue, mutual respect and trust that is maintained in the family, in the workplace, in kindergarten and at school, in civil society, and naturally in politics. The Commission was influenced by the theory of social capital as developed by the American political scientist Robert Putnam. Putman claims that social capital can be traced to the basic conditions of civic society, and that it can be measured by the extent to which people have a rich associational life (participation in voluntary organisations) which in turn, and in the long run, creates a climate for good government.[14]

A competing theory for explaining political confidence, a better concept than trust, according to Hardin,[15] is based on the empirical finding that people have a strong understanding of procedural fairness in a legal context, and that they value the opportunity to make their voices heard.[16] If people perceive injustices in *judicial* institutions, this will have a negative impact on their perception of *political* institutions. Similarly, Ostrom emphasises the significance of institutions: according to institutional theory, confidence is created on the basis of how institutions act, and how individuals assess these actions. Ostrom maintains that perceptions of decision making processes play a decisive role in individuals' view of what is in their best interest, and in their ability to think collectively.[17]

Based on short-term selfishness, individuals may be motivated to act egotistically. However, placed in a situation in which they must debate publicly, and morally defend their positions, social norms then play a decisive role in resolving the problem of 'social traps'. Ostrom argues that many decisions made in a democracy deal with matters that are common to everyone in society. Goods that cannot be limited in a natural way, for example natural resources or social welfare provisions, risk being overused, and short-term benefits for one individual can mean that everyone loses in the long term.

For this reason, politicians must encourage users to set up their own regulatory systems, and themselves take the responsibility of seeing to it that regulations are followed. This is practised in Sweden by means of far-reaching decentralisation of decision making, and independent local governments. In healthcare services, a major part of the allocation of resources has, in addition, been handed over to professional groups who are expected to act unselfishly for the common good.

According to Rothstein, Ostrom's studies support the hypothesis that there is a connection between trust and deliberative democracy. Participants in the deliberative democracy model are expected to act without any predetermined opinions. The idea is that the *discussion itself,* and the arguments that are put forward, will contribute to reshaping preferences, and that following such discussion it should be possible to achieve a cooperation that includes the broad majority.[11] If we translate this into the problematic situation of healthcare services, a successful policy must be formulated by institutions perceived to have a high degree of legitimacy by both the healthcare organisations and the citizenry.

How are health policy makers to win this political legitimacy? In a survey study from six European countries, Newton shows that social trust is based on information acquired mainly from personal experience.[18] People tend to act on the assumption of a public norm – that healthcare decisions are fair, and that the care provided will be of high quality. However, they have then to test this assumption, to see how far they can trust the healthcare services. Hence, personal experience becomes more important in creating public and personal trust than the publication of political manifestos.

How can we interpret the prevalence of low confidence in political systems? Is it due to lack of interest by the public in the common issues? Is it a reflection of increasing egoism on the part of citizens? Is it that citizens no longer trust the ability of politicians? It appears that none of these explanations holds true. In fact many studies indicate a growing interest in politics. However people are turning their backs on traditional forms, and instead choose to work politically in temporary single-issue parties.[19] In line with this trend, Sweden has seen the formation of several local political parties dealing solely with issues of healthcare. According to Rothstein[11] this increase in individualism is not necessarily indicative of egoism and selfish values, or of a decrease in social solidarity. The data point in the opposite direction. More people have more social contacts than was previously the case. He argues that impartial institutions create social capital, rather than, as had been commonly held, that it is the social capital in society that creates the possibility of a well functioning democracy.

The institutions of the democratic state are not limited to parliamentary representation. Not least in the health sector there are numerous other public institutions concerned with the implementation of policies. Healthcare institutions, not only in a tax-financed system but also in social insurance systems, can be regarded as part of a democratic continuum. Particularly in the case of healthcare services, for most citizens direct contact with providers of care is more common than contact with representative political institutions (national or local governments). Very few Swedish citizens know how a County Council is democratically governed, and most have little personal experience of influencing their democratically elected politicians on the content of health services. But nearly everyone has personal experience of healthcare as a patient, or a family member of a patient. For this reason, it is not difficult to understand why confidence in health services as an organisation can be very high, while confidence in health services at the political level, and in politicians as actors, can be low. This lack of perceived legitimacy in political decisions may therefore have its basis not only in dissatisfaction with any decisions actually made and perceived as unfair, but in the public's ignorance of how healthcare policies are made, and of how the decision making process actually works.

Is there a way forward?

We identify five potential strategies for creating trust in democratic decision making related to health.

1   In civic society, by increasing the social capital at a meta level, for example by encouraging people to become engaged in voluntary organisations. This can be regarded as a long-term strategy to increase confidence in democratic government (see, for example, Putnam[14]).
2   At the political level, by increasing deliberative democracy through establishing an *a priori* dialogue with citizens concerning the basic values governing healthcare (see, for example, Callahan[20]).
3   At the political level, by focusing on procedural justice in single issues (see

Daniels and Sabin[21]). This strategy focuses on transparency, reason-giving and measures for appeals in the decision making process.

4 At the provider level, by focusing on fair treatment of clients in their contacts with healthcare providers, and encouraging patients to take part in decision making about their own care. Healthcare professionals can play a key role in strengthening patient empowerment and shared decision making.

5 At the provider level, by focusing on the openness of healthcare activities and on transparency about quality and outcomes, and by increasing citizens' choice, for example the ability to choose their preferred providers.

We do not have enough evidence to suggest any one particular strategy, and it is important to be aware of the potential conflicts between them. We believe that in most countries combinations of such strategies will appear, but in the end policy makers will have to make choices between them.

As there are no simple solutions, we argue for a relatively unprejudiced approach. Our standpoint is that if citizens are to have confidence in public health systems, decision making will need to reflect social values. For this to happen all stakeholders – citizens, patients and their agents – will need to be actively involved in some way. A key question is of course what that way is to be. What are the different ways forward? Are citizens to become more involved in decisions about the provision of healthcare at the political level, or, at the individual level, about their own care as patients? Are citizens to become more actively involved in the allocation of resources, or in the evaluation of the results of the care system, or in both?

Our own limited experience indicates that it is hard to engage the general public in an overall discussion about difficult choices related to health and healthcare. This view is supported by evidence on the difficulties of engaging citizens on a regular basis in the running of government.[22] Consequently, our assumption is that the creation of political and provider institutions that can be regarded as legitimate and fair is the primary goal.

We believe that people are not only interested in the final result of their personal contacts with public institutions, but are also interested in whether or not the process will lead to results that can be considered as fair, for example whether they were treated with respect and dignity, while at the same time being treated as one among others in relation to the prevailing regulations and practice. According to Rothstein[11] the collective memory can play an important part in this. The availability of social capital in a society is a function of the design of its political institutions, as is the perceived degree of universalism in the institutions guaranteeing impartiality, objectivity and equal treatment.

It is interesting to note the conflict between a universal principle of fairness at an overall level, and the ethical principles that the health professional is expected to follow, in providing first and foremost for the individual patient, and then for the needs of particular categories of patients. We have found that there is enough evidence for us to advocate strategies of procedural justice in the quest for democratic institutions with a high degree of legitimacy.

The 'accountability for reasonableness' proposed by Daniels and Sabin[21] is such a framework for a fair and legitimate procedure for priority-setting in healthcare. Their standpoint is that people are not able to agree on abstract ethical principles. Instead, they believe that it is possible to provide procedures that people generally find fair and legitimate. They argue that four conditions have to be fulfilled in order to achieve acceptance.

1 **Relevance:** The rationales (evidence, positive arguments and principles) must be considered relevant for priority-setting decisions by fair-minded people.
2 **Publicity:** The basis for priority-setting decisions must be public.
3 **Appeals:** There must be mechanisms for challenging decisions and revising them in light of new evidence and arguments.
4 **Enforcement:** There must be either voluntary or public regulation of decision making processes to ensure that the first three conditions are met.

This framework has had an impact on efforts in many places and has been used for analysing efforts to increase fairness in healthcare. It represents a type of deliberative approach, but it is not clear to what extent the general public should be involved in the decision making process. It has already had some influence on Swedish policy making in healthcare (for example, in the process used by the Pharmaceutical Benefit Board, LFN) and it has been used in Canada as an analytic model for evaluation of priority-setting in several projects (see, for example, Reeleder *et al.*[23]).

Conclusions

For most people in Europe democracy is an inalienable value, and has played as vital a role in the construction of health and healthcare as it has in other parts of the welfare system. Nonetheless there is much uncertainty still about how democracy should be practised in relation to healthcare. In many countries, healthcare and other public welfare systems are now facing great challenges. The pressure on these systems may contribute to an escalating frustration and a deteriorating confidence among the public. Policy makers are forced to employ priority-setting and rationing while enjoying only limited legitimacy among public. The part to be played by democracy in enhancing the citizen's potential to exercise power over the content and scope of healthcare remains a key challenge for all policy makers in Europe. Although there are many suggested approaches aimed at improving the degree of democracy, there is not enough evidence to recommend any one single strategy. Rather, it is important to be open-minded, critical and constructive.

One way forward is a combination of several strategies, but we acknowledge the potential conflicts between them. In a democratic society there will always be an element of tension, a gap between the pursuit of the overall good of society and that of the individual citizen. The key for the future democratic governance of healthcare is to close that gap as far as possible. We strongly recommend more systematic development and interdisciplinary research.

References

1 Coulter A and Jenkinson C (2005) European patients' views on the responsiveness of health systems and healthcare providers. *Eur J Public Health.* **Jun 23.**
2 Holmberg S and Weibull L (eds) *Land du välsingnade? SOM – undersökningen 2000, SOM rapport 26.* SOM institutet, Göteborgs universitet.
3 Wennberg JE and Gittelsohn A (1982) Variations in medical care among small areas. *Sci Am.* **246:** 120–34.

4 Carr-Hill R, Jamison JQ, O'Reilly D, Stevenson MR, Reid J and Merriman B (2000) Risk adjustment for hospital use using social security data: cross sectional small area analysis. *BMJ.* **324**: 390–2.
5 Garpenby P and Carlsson P (1994) The role of national quality registers in the Swedish health service. *Health Policy.* **29**: 183–95.
6 European Commission (2005) Employment, Social Affairs and Equal Opportunities. Available from: http://europa.eu.int/comm./employment_social/news/2005/mar/demog_gp_en.html.
7 Sennfält K (2005) *Economic Studies of Health Technology Changes.* Linköping University Medical Dissertations No. 889. Linköping University, Linköping.
8 Ham C and Robert G (eds) (2003) *Reasonable Rationing: international experience of priority setting in health care.* Open University Press, Maidenhead.
9 Bäckman B, Carlsson P and Andersson A (2005) *A More Transparent Priority Setting Process in Sweden – does it make sense?* Submitted for publication.
10 Bäckman B, Carlsson P and Lindroth K (2005) *A More Transparent Priority-setting Process in Sweden – reactions in mass media.* Manuscript.
11 Rothstein B (2005) *Social Traps and the Problem of Trust.* Cambridge University Press, Cambridge.
12 Platt J (1973) Social traps. *American Psychologist.* **28**: 641–51.
13 *Sustainable Democracy.* Swedish Official Government Reports, SOU 2000:1.
14 Putman R (2000). *Bowling Alone: the collapse and revival of the American community.* Simon & Schuster, New York.
15 Hardin R (2000) The public trust. In: SS Pharr and RD Putnam (eds) *Disaffected Democracies: what's troubling the trilateral countries.* Princeton University Press, Princeton, NJ.
16 Tyler T (2002) *Trust in the Law: encouraging public cooperation with police and courts.* Russel Sage Foundation, New York.
17 Ostrom E (1990) *Governing the Commons: the evolution of institutions for collective action.* Cambridge University Press, NY.
18 Newton K (2002) *Who Trusts?: The origins of social trusts in six European Nations.* Department of Political Science, University of Southampton, Southampton.
19 Petterson O (ed) (2001) *Demokratirådets Rapport 2000: Demokrati utan partier?* SNS Förlag, Stockholm.
20 Callahan D (1990) *What Kind of Life: the limits of medical progress.* Simon and Schuster, New York.
21 Daniels N and Sabin J (2002) *Setting Limits Fairly: can we learn to share medical resources?* Oxford University Press, Oxford.
22 Hibbing JR and Theiss-Morse E (2002) *Stealth Democracy: Americans' beliefs about how government should work.* Cambridge University Press, Cambridge.
23 Reeleder D, Martin DK, Keresztes C and Singer PA (2005) What do hospital decision-makers in Ontario, Canada, have to say about the fairness of priority setting in their institutions? *BMC Health Services Research.* **5**: 8.

Chapter 7

Stewardship

Constantino T Sakellarides

'Stewardship' is the name of the fifth dimension of the Madrid Framework, hence it is the given title of this chapter. However, I believe stewardship to be too limited and limiting a concept to convey the full purposes of 'health governance in a network society' – the subject of this essay and the chapter title I would have preferred.

A world of life and motion

Almost three decades ago an ingenious team of traffic experts in Bordeaux pioneered a road traffic management system called 'Gertrude'. The team seemed to have something like the following underlying philosophy – 'life is movement; movement is life'. Their main professional obsession was with traffic bottlenecks. These slow down and interrupt circulation in city arteries, increase tension and impatience, decrease air quality, reduce working and leisure hours, and turn everyone's time schedule into a futile exercise.

Their purpose in inventing Gertrude was to keep things moving by relentlessly regulating traffic flow throughout the urban maze. Late at night, when traffic was light, while still faithful to their belief in the virtues of movement, they would calm the traffic in certain sections of the city, so as to save the citizens from the disturbance of noisy nights. Motion needs its ups and downs.

For them, movement meant mainly connectivity. They were attempting to bring different points in space and time into close proximity. Also, these flow engineers had a feeling for the quality of life. Their experience had made it clear that quality of life was in fact their core business.

Since medieval times, pilgrimages moved believers towards holy places. Travelling to Finisterre (which means 'the end of land') on their way to Santiago, their voyage towards sunset was in fact the allegory of a life. This was a time to revisit one's own life path in a new light, and then move on.

Motion propelled austere gothic art into the renaissance – it steered the earlier Florentine harmony into the distress of 'mannerism', expressed in terms of its provocative use of colour and unusual contortions in its composition, before settling into the 'baroque' new harmony. Later styles, like the 'baroque' returned to far more harmonious forms. Meanwhile by moving tiny and fragile sailing boats through immense, distant oceans, Dias, Gama, Cabral or Columbus became the first great globalisers. Old diseases and new medicinal herbs travelled with them.

From our perspective today, early science was about understanding movement in key domains of knowledge. By comprehending the circulation of blood in the body, Harvey contributed considerably to the development of modern medicine; insisting that the earth moves around the sun allowed Galileo to discover fundamental principles about our universe, as did Newton in revealing the laws governing the falling of objects. In eighteenth-century London, a centre of maritime trade, there was great concern to learn how to navigate precisely by measuring longitude, a concern of the government at Westminster, of Greenwich astronomers, and of a man of science in the Royal Society. A prize of £20 000 (a huge sum at that time) was instituted by the 1714 Longitude Act 'for such person or persons as shall discover the Longitude'. It turned out that it was necessary to invent a time measurement machine based on sustained quasi-perfect motion – Harrison's Chronometer – to arrive at a quite precise ascertainment of longitude at sea.

Rodin's vitalism is expressed in the dynamics of his sculptures. Brancusi's egg-shaped volumes can be seen as symbolising both the life potential inscribed in embryonic matter, and the ability to move effectively through inner intimae, darker corridors towards brighter prospects, a world of life and motion.

The impulse of motion turned drawings into animated cartoons and photographs into movies. But beyond motion, what creates the notion of 'the story' is the way images and sounds become interconnected.

Current philosophers, trying to know the universe and fathom its meanings, look for theories that can bring together movement on the unimaginably large scale (the expansion of the universe that followed the 'Big Bang') with motion in the very smallest, most intimate particles of matter (the insights of quantum physics). In this, they defy our more intuitive preconceptions about the unchanging nature of time and space, what had been the most fundamental underpinnings of our understanding of both life and motion.

Biology too has been transformed in our times, and has evolved from the understanding of life to giving us the ability to change it profoundly – genomics, cloning and stem cells are largely about dynamics of life, influenced and moved by humans.

The so-called information age also has its mysteries. The number of transistors in computer microchips has been doubling every four years since the 1980s, and is expected to continue to do so throughout the next decade.[1] Explanations for this peculiar trend are not evident. But the trend has far reaching consequences. Information storage and management capacity are the technological backbone of connectivity and motion in the emergent network society.

In fact, a number of interrelated pathways, where different sorts of flow occur, can be identified in our advanced post-industrial societies.

Firstly, information is everywhere. Information is an extraordinarily uncommon kind of resource – it expands with use, as it moves from one person to the next. And as it circulates, the likelihood that it will became internalised as knowledge is enhanced. This knowledge is then translated into actions, and these in turn then generate more information, expanding knowledge and changing the way people act. Knowledge/action networks become the prime paths of influence in the network society.

Secondly, consider simple daily living. It is made up of multiple encounters. Some become frequent and regular, and create tight and strong ties. This comes about by building confidence, by inviting reciprocity and inculcating trust – trust perceived as 'a state of positive expectations about each other's motives, in situations entailing risks'. These attributes tend to expand communication and produce the desire for even more encounters. Some of these encounters are lighter, less regular or frequent, and also at a greater distance. However, because weak ties are much more numerous than our strong ones, they tend to be more useful in disseminating innovation and values.[2] 'The network society is where we live. It's not a society comprised by isolated cyber-navigators and telecommunication robots.'[3]

Finally, imagine navigating in a virtual universe. Favourite ports for regular visits are charted, some clustering into tight communities of practice, knowledge or interest. Others remain as part of a large array of more episodic encounters. As navigation proceeds, in documenting our thoughts, or glimpsing the unexpected, a single, surprising, extraordinary encounter may set our minds travelling in completely new directions.

Enter a seamless world shared by many and owned by everyone, where we can move freely from today's challenges to yesterday's memories, from local action to global concerns, from intellectual abstractions to tangible realities.

Stillness in essence

While the pace of change in the network society is overwhelming, from science and technology to communication and lifestyles, an unsuspected stillness in essence glooms over health systems. Particularly in the last two decades, European health systems, insofar as they have attempted equitably and significantly to affect health gain, to develop more efficient and effective health services, to respond to healthcare needs, and to improve social justice in health financing, have fallen far short of even relatively modest expectations.

Significant changes in health systems took place under the following historical circumstances. Firstly, by the late nineteenth century, the economic and the social tensions of the industrial revolution had given rise to new forms of social protection. Secondly, in the mid-1990s, a post-World War II spirit of social generosity favoured stronger and more comprehensive public policies. These remain fundamental historical landmarks in the development of European health systems.

Bismarckian social insurance reforms included the financing of access to healthcare, and were an important expression of a social contract for sustainable development. Trade, enhanced by the industrial revolution, gave new impetus to public health as sanitary protection and to health education.

Duncan represented a new kind of full-time public health officer. He worked in Liverpool in the mid-nineteenth century, a city concerned with the effect of diseases on the wellbeing of its inhabitants, the health of its trade and the safety of its port operations in a rapidly industrialising world. In Germany, Virchow's observations on the social determinants of health and disease pioneered the notion of 'social medicine'.

Beveridge-type reforms in Europe – focusing on state health budgets – had two important consequences. They contributed to the transition from a framework of social protection (financing access to the existing healthcare supply) to a public policy on looking for organisational solutions best able to contribute to health policy objectives. At the same time, they were also instrumental in bringing together the 'bits and pieces' scattered around an expanding health domain into a more comprehensive whole.

A number of salient landmarks in health policy development can be identified in the late 1970s and throughout the 1980s. Primary healthcare principles,[4] adopted more than 25 years ago, very visibly redirected health systems into paying more attention to common health concerns, rather than to the more rare and serious medical conditions.

European health targets from 1983 to 2005,[5] a key element of WHO's European 'Health for All' strategy, were conceived as an expression of a new kind of social contract for health. The target approach has expanded into many different sectors of governance as an alternative, or a complement, to more normative traditions. The 1986 Ottawa Charter on Health Promotion[6] played an important role in advocating the notion that, as a central aim of health governance, people should be helped to acquire the knowledge and skills to promote their own health, and in more supportive environments.

People, not services, were to be the drivers of health promotion.

However, in spite of these developments, there seems to be some sort of pause, a failure of impetus, in progressing towards more effective health governance. There is a considerable gap between conceptual and technical progress, on one hand, and the ability of health policies to steer changes in European health systems appropriate to the twenty-first century, on the other.

The political discourse of health reform, and the profusion of organisational and managerial initiatives in heath policy and services, seem to have little influence on local health landscapes. These are moved by other influences than those coming from health policies.

A number of theoretical frameworks attempt to contribute to a better understanding of these evident limitations in managing health systems change. The study of structured resistance to change, or path dependence in the process of change, merits increased attention. As long as 30 years ago, Alford's structural interest theory[7] stated that 'institutions are organized to serve the more powerful interests in society'. More recent developments in the area of the new institutionalism, and particularly in that of historical institutionalism, are of great relevance to health policy: '[With] conflict between rival groups for scarce resources, institutions develop to favour some groups and demobilize others – this institutional organization of the economy is the predominant factor in structuring the outcome of group conflict, with the state serving as a non neutral broker of competing interests.'[8]

If culture can be seen as a sort of first order institution, where others are embedded, the opportunities for, and constraints on, the evolution of health systems can then be seen as integral parts of the dynamics of cultural change.[9] In this context, there is understandable interest in searching for 'change engines' in health systems.[10] Some emphasise the role of social actors in contrast to the role of institutions: 'Social change is predominantly affected by collective actors . . . there are three main sources of social power resources (SPR) – ownership, knowledge and political support. The distribution of SPR across political organizations is the main driver of policy.'[9,11]

Those who study human development pay special attention to the convergence, or critical conjunctions, of material resources and cultural evolution.[12] They see the value of self-expression as a necessary condition for the transition from formal to operational democracy. Enthusiasts for rational choice, action-oriented schools of strategic thinking,[13,14] and evolving notions of health governance[15,16,17] all have something to add in understanding the management of change.

How do these intricate theoretical concepts of health systems relate to the actual perceptions, and behaviour, of health policy practitioners and other social actors? The communication codes used by different health governance stakeholders do not appear to be robust enough to prevent heavy losses in translation. There is limited recognition of the need for some sense of 'meaningfulness' in order to motivate health governance players. It is also important to learn how to strike a balance where it matters; we need to be able to analyse governance critically so as to contribute to its improvement, but if we overdo the criticism we risk serious damage to its legitimacy, such that the criticism becomes counterproductive.

European health leaders become 'reformers' as they feel the need to respond to strong demands for change from public opinion. At the same time they are aware of the formidable nature of the difficulties entailed. And often they sense the naivety of government norm-setting, planning and command-and-control positivism, in dealing with the complex social systems of fragmented postmodern environments.

It was very late morning when the Minister held the press conference. Policy makers, managers, health professionals and international experts had convened over the last two days to discuss the health reform. The Berlin wall had fallen not more than two years ago. Everyone in the country was contemplating unprecedented and formidable change. The press conference was just ending when a very young journalist, seated in a far corner of the conference room, asked for the floor. His bearing was most unimpressive and he spoke unemotionally, almost timidly. 'The reform?' he asked. 'When does it start?' The Minister was hesitant for two seconds and then replied with passion, 'It has already started, aren't we working on it right now?' The Minister smiled, openly content with his answer. The audience was relieved. But the journalist came again. 'And when does it finish?' he asked. The Minister became serious and his body language expressed concern, 'You see, this is all very difficult and very complex,' he said. 'It will take a long time.' After that, and in the next few hours, things appeared to have run out of steam somewhat.

New architectures of influence

Health is a sensitive and complex domain – for individuals, the community and the political system. There are clear local and global trends, for example in increasing body mass and obesity. These call for considerable behavioural changes – from breastfeeding to an active physical and intellectual life and intelligent eating. They require more public health-friendly food markets. These problems present a clearly defined challenge to health governance. However other issues are not so clearly defined and predictable.

International and national health authorities regard preparedness for irregularly occurring health threats as of major current concern. Such contingencies highlight the need for stronger prospective thinking, and for sensitive political decisions. How much of our limited resources are we inclined to invest in preparedness for possible pandemics (the avian influenza threat), bioterrorism (the smallpox threat) or natural catastrophes (the Hurricane Katrina disaster)? Food safety and radiation threats pose similar questions. Climate change, the scarcity of water resources in some parts of the planet, the fate of tropical rainforests, all are interrelated phenomena, different from the above only because of their less acutely dramatic incidence and sudden consequences. What price are we willing to pay for what level of security? How to involve broad local thinking and action in response to such global phenomena?

European populations continue to age. At the same time the criteria for defining excessive blood pressure, blood glucose and cholesterol levels have become tighter. This means that large numbers of European citizens will be encouraged to take a daily regimen of medicines over very many years. It is claimed that from the age of 55 years, a daily intake of medicines designed to reduce blood pressure, blood lipids and blood clotting can substantially increase life expectancy.[18] It's been anticipated that such a regimen of medicines could be amalgamated into a single 'polypill'. More imaginative thinkers suggest it could well be incorporated into one's breakfast cereals or elsewhere in the daily menu.

Although not as systematically and generally as suggested above, most elderly persons in developed countries are on continuous multiple medicine regimens. Chemically supported longevity already occurs quite widely. Should these medicines continue to be seen as individual purchases at the pharmacy, or should this near universal therapeutic need rather be consider as a subject for mass public purchasing, with completely different cost and distributional implications? What sort of governance can answer such questions effectively?

The ageing of the population also implies other choices – for instance, choosing how to die. In a greying Europe, the opportunity of dying in a dignified way is an important issue. After so many battles, some won and some lost, the desire to fare well at the conclusion of life is understandable. It is not an unreasonable wish to leave behind the memory of having died a dignified death. Preparing for death, even assisting death, is a complex, controversial, value-ridden undertaking. What kind of health governance can take up this challenge?

Timely and affordable access to quality healthcare will continue to be a major concern for everyone. A growing number of diverse modalities of public–private partnerships can currently be found in many European countries. What kind of governance is necessary to ensure that these partnerships serve the public interest?

Less conspicuous conditions, such as allergies affecting the eyes, the respiratory tract and skin, those related to eating, sleeping and sexual disorders, pain and depression, also have their public health dimension. The new biology holds out the prospect of reparatory capabilities for malfunctioning organs. How to ensure easy and equitable access to such future high quality life support services?

Doctors are consistently shown to be among the most respected professions. They exercise a dominant influence in health systems. A large number of other professions are playing an increasingly important role, particularly in relation to health technologies, health promotion and long-term care. How can health governance ensure that the professional and the public health interests converge?

Social systems are influenced by a number of mechanisms.[10,19] These include command and control hierarchies in the public sector, competitive markets, cooperative networks and transactional interfaces. Hierarchies, with their command and control modes of line management, prevail in the public accountability of health systems. This is true for both traditional public administrations and for more pluralistic ones. Their involution into inefficient bureaucracies is the cause of 'state failure' in pursuing public policy objectives. So-called 'new public management' initiatives may increase efficiency, particularly at the micro level. Sometimes, however, there is the risk that if the ties are excessively loose, and organisations granted too large a degree of autonomy without the appropriate tightening of health regulations and the rigours of good governance, both public accountability and transparency will be undermined.

Markets in health may also increase efficiency when competition improves value for money in terms of health gain or quality of care. But health systems markets are often based on 'favourable' market segmentation and product differentiation. This allows economic agents to capture profitable market segments, while abandoning others to the protections of the public system. These are classic market failures that may be exacerbated by some of the specific attributes of the health system. For example, although the doctor–patient relationship is agreed to be of critical importance, in most cases there is still a gross asymmetry of information; the achievement of high levels of population immunity through vaccination programmes is based on a sense of social solidarity and community benefit, alien to market thinking.

There are very important transactional interfaces in health systems, between purchasers and providers, managers and the professionals, services and the community. These interfaces, dense bilateral exchanges across physical, organisational or cultural frontiers, have been strengthened as traditional hierarchies evolve toward more interactive modes of exchange, and take various new forms.

Knowledge–action networks are currently of critical importance in minimising research fragmentation, in optimising resource use and in bridging the gap between the production and utilisation of knowledge. Health innovation networks create and disseminate successful technological solutions. Community networks for health protection and promotion are part of broader social support networks that connect key health players in community action. Professionals have to strike an ethical balance between the quality of their services and their immediate self-interests. Social actors in health systems organise themselves around all these mechanisms, and become an integral part of these architectures of influence.

The rise of the network society is providing very powerful cultural stimuli and operational tools for networks and transactional interfaces. These are already becoming much more visible and evolving into new architectures of influence.[20,21,22]

It seems reasonable to assume that the development of a stronger role for cooperative networks in society will bring about a different kind of architecture of influence, better able to promote transparent win-win solutions in health governance. As cooperative networks expand their transactional interfaces, they become more open to public scrutiny and involvement. Public administration or regulatory hierarchies are then more likely to play a significant role in further expanding and stabilising them. Innovation – bottom-up, taking advantage of information and communication technologies, decentralised, empowering – tends to be creatively unsettling.[23,24,25] Markets may then serve better the interest of buyers, as individuals become better informed and protected from interest group capture. Professional special interests may then become more likely to engage in win-win strategies.

In health systems there is already a trend for influence and control to move from the organisation's core to its periphery. Transactional interfaces increase in relevance, and network flows become mandatory. The quality of the interface between different professional identities became as important as the very core of these identities.

A number of concomitant social and cultural changes may facilitate this transition to a different kind of architecture of influence. The ethics of appropriate negotiation and joint decision making are now receiving the sort of attention hitherto reserved for the ethics of individual health protection and autonomy. There is a move from a service to a people-centredness, and from health service information systems to citizen-centred information systems. There is a new motto: 'My time, my place, my way.'

With a move away from policy making based on bureaucratic authority to policies based on public values, 'softer' relationships are created: 'soft management' and 'soft contracting' are now becoming more widely recognised.

There remains, however, a strong but as yet unmet need to continue to address the classical socioeconomic inequalities, the extreme social exclusions in the Fourth World, and, in our so-called developed societies, the less evident inequalities in accessing quality of life support services.

Stewardship, governance and government

Two sets of notions may help explain the close relationship between current developments in health governance and the emergent features of our network society.

Firstly, the culture of the network society and its emerging new patterns of influence may be expected to have a positive effect on the traditional confrontational and negative discourse of party politics. Because of its architecture of shared information and cooperative knowledge, the network society is able to reveal new opportunities for win-win solutions. Broad-based social contracts, and their elaborate checks and balances, are part of the social machinery that sustains civilised life. In the theatre of political processes and parliamentary calendars, some political agendas lose and others win. In some ways the logic of win-win network governance can be seen as a complement to win-lose choices between competing hierarchies of values.

Secondly there is the interplay between governance and the role of government. Often in the past the word 'governance' was used largely to signify only the process of governing. However, particularly during the 1990s, a different, broader concept of governance emerged in political science. Governance is now formally defined as the set of processes by which public and private institutions interact in shaping decisions of common interest. Governance is about patterns of rule, how and why decisions are taken, and what happens then.[12,13] It goes beyond the formal rituals of government programmes, beyond the insignificant details of the machinery of government. It takes into account the role of government, but it also recognises the important influence of an array of social actors – economic agents, professional groups, non-governmental community organisations. It deals with the complexities of both top-down and bottom-up processes. It refers to anticipation and uncertainty, hierarchies and cooperative networks, innovation and markets. And its long view extends beyond narrow local or national boundaries.

Health governance can be then defined as the processes whereby collective rules about attaining health gains, more effective health services, and fairer financial contributions, are defined, drafted, negotiated, legitimised, adopted and evaluated.

In matters of health policy it is apparent that dominant social and economic actors can visibly overpower traditional forms of government and post-industrial political machineries; that modern rationality is progressively less able to explain individual health-related behaviour and community preferences; that many important health issues that are experienced both locally and nationally can only be effectively addressed at supra-national and global levels; and that intangible far-away decisions can visibly affect our local patterns of life.

Health governance brings together two complementary realities: the orderly framing of generous societal objectives and commitments in formulating health policies; and the muddling through of chaotic political processes, entailing a mix of public and private interests in setting priorities and considerable pressures from professionals and dissatisfied users, all of them impacting on resource allocation and use.

Of particular importance in network societies, governance must address the tension between cooperation and accountability. The notion of governance places public policies in a broad perspective – the interaction of government, markets and civil societies. To this, it adds a dynamic and realistic 'implementation dimension' – to muddle through and read stakeholders' agendas and values, so as to build viable platforms for change.

Good governance is essential and normative.[26,27] It reflects high-order values such as inclusion, transparency, accountability and contestability. Deep down, in its most meaningful essence, it is about a continuous search for win-win solutions, and their underlying values. It encompasses adherence to sound principles. It redefines the role of government, and points to the essential role of good stewardship.[28] Good stewardship implies that government needs to assert its responsibility and legitimacy to protect and promote population health in a way that is recognised and trusted by its citizenry.

The question of how the role of government and the effective implementation of stewardship might operate in emerging network societies deserves some tentative answers. Defining three main tasks for exercising stewardship – vision, influence and intelligence – has the advantage of simplicity and clarity.

Vision, influence and intelligence

Providing a vision, and a sense of direction, are indispensable elements of health stewardship.

The need to make sophisticated organisational arrangements for strategic analysis and direction, including the study of stakeholders' agendas and the management of policy networks,[29,30,31] is not easily recognised by political systems. The emergence of new architectures of influence, in rich and complex network exchanges, clearly calls for deep strategic thinking. It also becomes clear that in order to grasp the network nature of governance, it is necessary to understand the importance of surveying the prevailing values of communities.

There are some outstanding examples. One such is that of the Swedish Parliamentary Priorities Committee, in 1994. It concluded that societal values in relation to establishing healthcare priorities, could provide an ethical platform composed of three basic principles – human dignity, need and solidarity, and cost-effectiveness, in that order of importance.[32]

More recently, the Canadian health policy report *Building on Values*,[33] was similarly based on an extensive study of Canadian values about health. The public's appreciation of this sort of approach was reflected in an article in a popular weekly magazine that saw the report as controversial, but as having a 'distinct Canadian flavour'.

We live both in a 'risk society' and in an 'access society'. In the 'risk society'[34] the production and distribution of wealth and risk is an issue, since it seems necessary to prevent further the privatisation of wealth, and to transfer the responsibility and cost of risk to society as a whole. In the 'access society',[35] inequalities in accessing healthcare, health promotion, supportive services and health-related information are bound to be important concerns.

Vision requires anticipatory attitudes and thinking. Anticipatory thinking is indispensable for making hard choices with some confidence about their possible future impact. The English Wanless Report, 'Securing Our Future Health: Taking a Longer Term View',[36] is a good example of this. In a situation where government felt prepared, gradually but substantially, to increase NHS financing over a six-year timeframe, such a prospective view was indispensable.[37]

Stewardship is also about influence. Governance comes about with a rebalancing of traditional mechanisms of influence. Government effectiveness depends to a large extent on the capacity to fashion the right tools for action, considering at each instant both the nature of internal processes and the condition of external environments.

As organisational and managerial solutions for health promotion and health service provision become more diversified within and across European countries – involving different alliances, partnerships, foundations and agencies – the need for competent and accountable multilevel regulatory arrangements to ensure the coherence and cohesion of health systems becomes ever more obvious.

Intelligent health service purchasing, a form of influence through financing, requires a good grasp of how dense transactional interfaces operate between influential health actors. Vertical organisations affect everyday living in ways that favour specific purposes – deeply pursuing the understanding of a specific challenge, or providing some kind of specialised service. However, they often also intersect everyday living, and delay the common flows and processes that run across the frontiers of vertical organisation. People need to move expeditiously and smoothly from primary healthcare centres to hospitals, and from here to long-term healthcare facilities, and back to community settings. It has been demonstrated that appropriate use of health information can enhance the quality of such horizontal processes across health system's vertical organisational settings.[38,39]

Advanced network societies are well equipped to promote local health strategies. While international and national health strategies can be stimulating and inspirational, only genuinely local health strategies can succeed in making a visible difference.

Finally, stewardship requires health intelligence. A clear, permanently updated, picture of what is in fact happening out there is essential. This however needs to be complemented by knowledge/action networks that provide continuous learning to the full complement of social actors involved in health governance.

A parliamentary commission of an advanced western democracy concluded recently that what was needed was a permanent independent body charged with reporting annually to the public on the state of the nation's healthcare system and on the health status of country's population.[40]

Here, health governance observatories may play an important role. But they have to learn to tread a very fine line. They must stay close enough to policy makers to have a positive attitude towards the difficulties of managing change and easy access to relevant information, but, at the same time, they must distance themselves enough to preserve their independence and so ensure public credibility.

'The universe is made of stories not atoms'

Health systems are often viewed through the specific lenses of particular disciplines – biomedical, political, social and managerial. These partial insights tend to obscure the fact that they are uniquely complex, sensitive, value-driven and content-specific social systems, deeply embedded in their social and cultural environments. Improving health governance requires looking at health systems in a way that avoids fragmented 'additive' thinking – a sort of superficial collage of different scientific disciplines – as well as highly structured theoretical constructs unrelated to empirical experience.

Health systems are complex. They deal with tangible issues of common concern that are influenced by a large number of intricate factors. Health governance needs to find ways to stimulate path-finding in this complexity, combining well grounded explanations with high level communication skills and technologies.

Old habits, for example, selectively extracting the cognitive elements from reality and omitting the sensory and emotional content of common experience, as if it were the dispensable debris or impurities confounding rational clarity, is unlikely to yield effective action.

These major intellectual challenges are not always easily recognised as such by political decision makers, health professionals, health service managers and economic interest groups. And their significance is lost in the public arena, where, increasingly, well staged sophisticated political and media 'theatre' takes place.

Refined network societies are expected to combine the ability to value intangible assets – such as knowledge and intellectual capital – while at the same time displaying the capacity to respond to 'tangible' aspirations, and to produce innovative solutions that work. The notion of 'tangibility' indicates the need to address the cognitive, sensory and emotional elements of our aspirations. The need for people to have health information is widely recognised. But the importance of the emotions, the role of the senses in making individual and collective decisions, is only now being more widely appreciated. For some, happiness and wellbeing is, at least occasionally, a profound and sustained immersion in an ocean of senses.

Good stories are the ones that combine masterfully these elements of tangibility, interconnecting otherwise trivial experiences so as to reveal new meanings.

Plato's *Republic*, Thomas More's *Utopia*, Orwell's *1984* Oceania nightmare, remind us that visions about a different future, whether desirable or frightening, can remain powerful for many generations.

Various organisations as well as individual experts have been writing about the future of health. The year 2015 has been a particularly attractive destination for such prospective exercises. Some have a national focus; others remind us of global health governance.

At one extreme there is Finland – the European and world leader in competitiveness and technological innovation – implementing its Health 2015 programme. It places special emphasis on health promotion, and identifies some key challenges for Finnish health in – 'disease prevention, mental health problems, the disparities in health and welfare among different population groups'.[41] Here there is confidence that the 2015 health targets can be achieved.

At the other extreme there are more than one billion people – one-sixth of the world's population – living in extreme poverty. They lack almost everything – safe water, proper nutrition, basic healthcare and social services, hope. In such populations, 11 million children die each year from preventable diseases. The 2015 health targets of the Millennium Project do not seem to be on track. They still look quite elusive.

Scenarios about the future of health can became attractive prospective storytelling exercises and play an important role in improving health governance tangibility. The Welsh NHS Confederation[42] offers a view on how the Welsh health system might look in 2015: 'After a series of difficult but important changes to the patterns of services inherited from the mid 20th century, Wales succeeded in transforming its health system to meet the challenges of the 21st century . . . State funded health and social services are provided by a wide partnership between the NHS, local government, private providers and voluntary organizations, based on each doing what they do best.'

In one of their case studies we can read: 'One morning in early March 2015, Bronwen logged onto her home computer to find an email message from the hospital: confirmation that her eye operation will take place next month. She has chosen the date and time of the operation with the GP using a touch screen in the practice. She was amazed at the care which she had received since then as a priority patient. Not only the nursing and medical care and help from the dietitian and podiatrist, but a whole package of information and various money-off deals from Diabetes Self-Care, including the visit each month to the local group for diabetic patients.'

In this story-like vision of the future, innovation in health, communication technology and diabetes patient networks combine in promoting a more citizen-centred health system.

A very different 2015 view can be found elsewhere:[43] 'American leaders . . . unleashed the creative power of the competitively driven marketplace. These changes resulted in dramatic improvements to the US health system – lower costs, higher quality, greater efficiency and better access to care.' And this case study scenario goes on: '. . . Rodney Rogers . . . has several chronic illnesses . . . [and] . . . selects his primary medical team from a variety of providers by comparing on line their credentials, performance ranking, and pricing . . . He owns his privacy protected electronic medical record. He also chose to have a tiny, radio-frequency computer chip implanted in his abdomen that monitors his blood chemistry and blood pressure . . . He takes a single pill a day [combining medication for lowering blood glucose and cholesterol, blood clotting time] . . . [A]n evolving myocardial infarction [was diagnosed] . . . The cardiologist in the nanocath lab injects nanorobots intravenously . . . the tiny machine locates a 90% lesion . . . and repairs it . . . The insurer pays . . . [These payments] are slightly higher to this hospital . . . because of its recognized high quality . . . Rodney's deductibles and co-insurance is automatically withdrawn from his savings account. Because Rodney has met all his self-managed goals this year, he gets 10% discount on hospital deductibles.' Rodney, a homo economicus paradigm, is a sophisticated medical consumer.

The best stories, those that can best elicit interest in understanding, improving and becoming part of health governance, are about common people with their aspirations and fears, admirable and yet frequently at a loss, sometimes rational, often really not.

The Health Centre's school team was very disappointed that morning. They had invested their energies and hopes in a partnership with this apparently very cooperative schoolteacher, recently arrived at one of the neighbourhood's schools. They had just realised that he had failed completely to fulfil his commitments. They were angry and felt particularly deceived. Only the fact of having scheduled a discussion on this matter with the Health Centre's mental health team has prevented them from engaging in a sincere, hard, clarifying face-to-face conversation with that school teacher.

It was a mild, sunny, luminous Lisbon morning. The account of the school's health team was attentively listened to by the mental health expert. He was a highly respected and particularly wise figure. He had spent most of his life bringing together children, their parents, teachers, doctors, nurses, social workers and community leaders in understanding and respecting the intimate world of children – their own imaginary secret world. After listening, he spoke in his typically quiet voice. He said that we all have a face (what we are) and a mask (what we appear to be), and that there is always a certain distance between the two. But what matters here is the fact that almost always we would really like to be what we appear to be – we would like to be like our masks. Taking somebody's mask off forfeits all possibility of influencing him positively – because it is in that particular 'space' – the space between one's face and one's mask – that change takes place.[44]

The multiple, diverse, dense and constructive conversations that shape health governance in a network society deal with some of our more obvious worries.

They are also about things we are fond of listening to or imagining. They add value to what we do, and, often enough, they can make our common experiences more meaningful.

References

1 Jorgenson D (2005) *Information Technology and the G7 economies.* Paper presented in: A Sociedade em Rede e a Economia do Conhecimento: Portugal numa perspective global (The network society and the knowledge economy: Portugal in a global perspective). Presidência da República Portuguesa, Lisbon. 5–6 March 2005.

2 Granovetter M (1983) The strength of weak ties: a network theory revisited. *Sociological Theory.* 1: 1201–33.

3 Castells M (2005) *Questões em torno da sociedade em rede e da economia do conhecimento: o que sabemos e os desafios para as políticas (Questions about network society and the knowledge economy: what we know and challenges for policies)* A Sociedade em Rede e a Economia do Conhecimento: Portugal numa perspective global (The network society and the knowledge economy: Portugal in a global perspective). Presidência da República Portuguesa, Lisbon. 5–6 March 2005. Available from: http://presidenciarepublica.pt/network/home.html (accessed 9 September 2005).

4 World Health Organization (1978) Declaration of Alma-Ata: International Conference on Primary Health Care. Alma-Ata, 6–12 September 1978. Avalable from: www.who.int/hpr/NPH/docs/declaration_almaata.pdf (accessed 3 August 2005).

5 World Health Organization (2005) *The Health For All Policy Framework for the WHO European Region: 2005 update.* Regional Office for Europe, Copenhagen. Available from: www.euro.who.int (accessed 10 August 2005).

6 World Health Organization (1986) *Ottawa Charter for Health Promotion.* Regional Office for Europe, Copenhagen. Available from: www.euro.who.int/AboutWHO/Policy/20010827_2 (accessed 3 August 2005).

7 Alford R (1975) *Health Care Politics: ideology and interest group barriers to reform.* University of Chicago Press, Chicago.

8 Mossialos E and Oliver A (2005) European health systems reforms: looking backward to see forward? *J Health Polit Policy Law.* 30(1–2): 1–28.

9 Scott T, Mannion R, Davies H and Marshall M (2003) Implementing culture change in health care: theory and practice. *Int J Qual Health Care.* 15(2): 111–18.

10 Rico A and Costa-Font J (2005) Power rather than path dependency? The dynamics of institutional change under health care federalism. *Journal of Health Politics, Policy and Law.* 30(1–2): 231–52.

11 Tuohy C (1999) Dynamics of a changing health sphere: the United States, Britain and Canada. *Health Aff.* 18(3).

12 Welzel C, Inglehart R and Klingenman HD (2002) *Human Development as a Theory of Social Change: a cross-cultural perspective.* Available from: www.wvs.isr.umich.edu (accessed 15 September 2005).

13 Volberda H and Elfring T (eds) (2001) *Rethinking Strategy.* Sage Publications, London.

14 Mintzberg H and Lampel J (2000) Reflexão sobre o processo estratégico (Reflection about the strategic process). *Revista Portuguesa de Gestão* (Portuguese Magazine of Management). 15: (2).

15 Gete B (2005) Servicios publicos y gobernanza (Public services and governance). *Sistema, democracia y sector publico.* 184–5.

16 Dogson R, Lee K and Drager N (2002) Global Health Governance: a conceptual review. In: WHO (ed) *Key Issues on Global Health Governance Project.* WHO, Geneva (Discussion Paper 1).

17 Kickbusch I (2002) Perspectives on health governance in the 21st century. In: M Marinker (ed) *Health Targets in Europe: polity, progress and promise.* BMJ Books, London.

18 Wald N and Law M (2003) A strategy to reduce cardiovascular disease by more than 80%. *BMJ.* **326**: 1419–24.

19 Williamson O (1975) *Markets and Hierarchies: analysis and antitrust implications.* The Free Press, New York.

20 Jones C *et al.* (1997) A general theory of network governance: exchange conditions and social mechanisms. *Acad Manage J.* **22**(4): 911–45.

21 Mertens F *et al.* (2005) Network approach for analyzing and promoting equity in participatory ecohealth research. *EcoHealth.* **2**: 113–26.

22 Shau H *et al.* (2005) The Healthcare Network Economy: the role of internet information transfer and implications for pricing. *Industrial Marketing Management.* **34**: 147–56.

23 Foster-Fishman PG, Goodkind JR and Salem DA (2002) The adoption of innovation in collective action organizations. *American Journal of Community Psychology.* (October) **30**(5): 681–710.

24 Stubbs M and Lemon M (2001) Learning to network and networking to learn: facilitating the process of adaptative management in a local response to the UK's national air quality strategy. *Environmental Management.* **27**(8): 321–34.

25 Birchall D and Tovstiga G (2005) *Capabilities for Strategic Advantage: leading through technological innovation.* Palgrave Macmillan, Hampshire.

26 Capacity Building International, Germany (2003) *Good Governance and Health.* Available from: www.inwent.org (accessed 2 April 2003).

27 Cannac Y and Godet M (2001) La «bonne gouvernance»: l'expérience des enterprises, son utilité pour la sphère publique. *Futuribles.* **265**.

28 World Health Organization (2000) *World Health Report 2000. Health systems: improving performance.* WHO, Geneva.

29 Klijn E and Koppenjan J (2000) Public management and policy networks: foundations of a network approach to governance. *Public Management.* **2**(2): 135–58.

30 Ham C (1999) *Health Policy in Britain.* Palgrave, Hampshire.

31 Maturo A (2004) Network governance as a response to risk society. Dilemmas: a proposal from the sociology of health. *Topoi.* **23**: 195–202.

32 Swedish Ministry of Health and Social Affairs (1995) *Priorities in Health Care: ethics, economy, implementation. Final report from the Swedish Parliamentary Priorities Commission.* Swedish Ministry of Health and Social Affairs, Stockholm.

33 Commission on the Future of Health Care in Canada (2002) *Building on Values: the future of health care in Canada. Final Report.* Canadian Ministry of Health, Saskatoon.

34 Beck U (2001) La sociedad del riesgo: hacia una nova economia *(The risk society: towards a new economy).* Editorial Presença, Lisbon.

35 Rifkin J (2001) *A era do acesso: a revolução da nova economia (The age of access: the revolution of the new economy).* Editorial Presença, Lisbon.

36 Wanless D (2002) *Securing Our Future Health: taking a long-term view: Final report.* HM Treasury, London. Available from: www.hm-treasury.gov.uk (accessed 16 September 2005).

37 Wanless D (2004) *Securing Good Health for the Whole Population: Final Report.* HM Treasury, London. Available from: www.hm-treasury.gov.uk (accessed 5 August 2005).

38 Feachem R *et al.* (2002) Getting more for their dollar: a comparison of the NHS with California's Kaiser Permanente. *BMJ.* **324**: 135–43.

39 Ham C *et al.* (2003) Hospital bed utilisation in the NHS, Kaiser Permanente, and the US Medicare programme: analysis of routine data. *BMJ.* **327**: 1257.

40 Canadian Standing Senate Committee on Social Affairs, Science and Technology (2002) *Securing Good Health for the Whole Population: the health of Canadians: the federal role: final report.* Canadian Standing Senate Committee on Social Affairs, Science and Technology, Montreal.

41 Ministry of Social Affairs and Health, Finland (2001) *Government Resolution on the Health 2015 Public Health Programme.* Ministry of Social Affairs and Health, Helsinki.

42 Welsh NHS Confederation (2005) A Picture of Health: how the NHS in Wales could look in 2015. Available from www.welshconfed.org/Health2015/pictureofhealth 2015.html (accessed 15 August 2005).

43 Frist W (2005) Shattuck lecture: health care in the 21st century. *N Engl J Med.* **352**(3): 267-72.

44 Sakellarides C (2005) *De Alma a Harry: Crónica da Democratização da Saúde (From Alma to Harry: chronicle of health democratisation).* Almedina, Lisbon.

Chapter 8

Evidence

Derek Yach

Why is there a Global Fund for AIDS, malaria and tuberculosis[1] and not one for primary healthcare, or for motor vehicle injuries and death, or for tobacco control, or for depression? Was it evidence that led to the decision to create that multi-billion dollar institution? If so what evidence? And what evidence is needed to create additional institutions or generate extra funds to address other health problems?

The backdrop, against which the importance of evidence[2] for decision making has emerged, has changed over the last few years. We now have new ways of quantifying ill health, there are systematic approaches now accepted as means of assessing the effectiveness of interventions,[3] and policy makers make regular exhortations for policies to be 'science' or 'evidence' based.

New metrics have been created to capture the importance of quantifying non-fatal causes of ill health, and combining them with mortality data into a common measure – the disability adjusted life year (DALY).[4] The hope was that this would highlight the importance of conditions that cause considerable suffering and disability, but not many deaths. DALYs were to be a better way of making resource allocation decisions in respect of disease, and later in respect of risk factor-specific programmes.

The Cochrane Collaboration[5] has highlighted the importance of using methodologically sound and transparent approaches to assess the effectiveness of interventions and policies. These have tended to focus on pharmaceutical interventions. The hope has been that ineffective and unproven clinical practices and broader health policies would be displaced by those shown from meta-analyses to 'really' work.

We live in an era of heightened demands for effectiveness, efficiency and cost-effectiveness, where publicly funded interventions ought to demonstrate to the paying public that they are getting value for money. Performance matters. Rapid change matters. And transparent accounting matters. Evidence of this is that the Global Fund has recently withdrawn funds from some countries because of concerns about whether the funds reached the people for whom they were meant.[6]

Such progress in developing evidence based policies should be welcomed and actively embraced by those working in public health. However, this has not happened universally. Several concerns are being raised about the way evidence is collected, packaged, marketed and used. Additional concerns have been raised about the limits of using a randomised clinical trial (RCT) model for assessing whether all policy interventions work;[7] I will come to these later.

DALYs have helped change the way some decision makers prioritise. Mental health conditions were the major beneficiary of their use. DALYs pushed mental health almost to the top of the burden of the disease league globally and within most regions of the world. This certainly helped encourage Dr Gro Harlem Brundtland, Director General of WHO (1998–2003), to give unprecedented attention to mental health during her tenure. A special World Health Report, World Health Day and Ministerial discussion at the annual World Health Assembly were devoted to mental health.[8] Some donors shifted from their previous neglect of mental health and provided the support WHO needed to develop country-based legislative and other tools to address the stigma caused by mental health, and to integrate mental health into general health systems. But this was not sustained and did not lead to a significant increase in resources for mental health in most countries. As the political spotlight passed to another health problem, and WHO changed leadership, mental health returned to its relative invisibility as a global health priority. Yet the evidence still remains clear about the size of the problem![9]

DALYs for risk factors, first produced in the 2002 World Health Report,[10] showed that hypertension, tobacco and cholesterol were the top contributors to the global burden of disease and in countries at all levels of development. Since risk factors precede deaths or declared disease by years, it was hoped that action to address these preventable risk factors would receive high priority by WHO, and that the new evidence would lead to an increase in resources to execute programmes to address chronic disease risk factors. For a few short years this seemed possible. Tobacco received extremely high levels of political support, especially during the development of the Framework Convention on Tobacco Control.[11] No specific new support was mobilised for hypertension, and modest support allowed analytic work to complete a Global Strategy on Diet and Physical Activity.[12] Funding for follow-up work has been meagre. Beyond WHO, the broader response of funders to the evidence on the impact of risk factors, and the potential of effective prevention in preventing major epidemics, has been silence.

Why? Many decision makers take the position that risks like obesity, tobacco and physical inactivity are freely courted by informed adults, and that they should simply act more responsibly. Others argue that chronic diseases kill old people, and that therefore their prevention would be too costly and would yield few real health gains. Yet others believe (erroneously) that chronic diseases caused by these risks mainly affect affluent countries. Evidence produced to contradict these views is dismissed as self-serving. Furthermore, the reduction of tobacco use, and changes required to make healthy diets easy choices, brought WHO and the health community into conflict with many powerful corporate players. It was simply inconvenient to act upon the evidence on risk, and its potential impact on health.

Contrast this with the way in which the world has mobilised to support HIV/AIDS treatment and, to a lesser extent, prevention. Deaths from HIV/AIDS are substantially less than those from tobacco – and account for less than a third of the deaths caused by cardiovascular diseases. The age distribution of deaths from AIDS is similar to that due to injuries and violence – they both kill young adults before they reach their most productive years. Crucially, however, the epidemiological and economic evidence on the impact of HIV/AIDS[13] has been supplemented by the following arguments, where the evidence we have is contrary or at best equivocal.

- AIDS is linked to poverty and an attack on AIDS will raise populations out of poverty. This argument is advanced by Jeff Sachs[14] in the WHO Commission on Macroeconomics and Health. It is part of a general argument that holds that it is more effective to invest in health as a way of stimulating economic growth, than it is to wait for the fruits of economic development to benefit health. The evidence base for this is complex. For over 50 years, only one side of what is a complex two-way relationship between health and economic growth has been proposed. This evidence has now been well packaged and used for high level, and often laudable, advocacy reasons, like the creation of the Global Fund.
- AIDS undermines national security which in turn breeds terrorism. This rather bizarre argument has been proposed without a shred of evidence by the USA's CIA,[15] a recent high-level panel of the United Nations,[16] and many academics. Such blatant populism would normally be dismissed as such in an era when security concerns were not so pervasive.
- AIDS weakens the human resource base of developing countries, and that undermines development planning. This is a valid argument based on increasing evidence.[17] But it is also applicable to any major health problem and is not specific to AIDS. For a few selected countries, mainly in southern Africa, the argument does provide additional compelling reasons for investing in HIV and AIDS control. But once a line of reasoning has been found to be valid in one setting, it is difficult to dismiss it being used way beyond that setting.

I began by asking why there is a Global Fund for AIDS. Epidemiological evidence on the impact of the condition was important in order to raise the flag. The number of persons affected is big – and the preventive potential is big. But this is made more visible and dramatic not because there are larger numbers of AIDS sufferers than those suffering from many other health problems. The drama is created by clever advocacy and communications. AIDS activists maximised the impact of their campaigns by providing the total number of cases and deaths since the start of the epidemic, rather than by employing the more usual annual death rates. This tactic has proven to be effective in grabbing headlines, but is not one used by advocates for many other health problems, where the numbers would in fact be much larger! A prime example would be the sum total of motor vehicle deaths since the invention of the car. And potentially all these deaths would have been preventable.

From an advocacy perspective, the organisational approach to AIDS has been exemplary. AIDS rapidly displaced diarrhoea and acute respiratory infections as the major recipients of donor aid, despite the fact that these conditions are still a bigger killer of children than is AIDS. The voice for childhood conditions has weakened as the voices and faces of people with AIDS have come to dominate the public health discourse. Advocates for the AIDS agenda have brought forward real people and stories; they have reached the hearts of decision makers, not just their minds, and they have done this by forging strong relationships with the media and the entertainment industry.

Part of the success of this advocacy, which has resulted in the Fund and many other sources of funding, must be related to the fact that HIV/AIDS first became visible among gay populations in developed countries. The mobilisation of these communities, first for themselves, and later for the larger world community, was led by passionate, effective leaders who had easy access to the corridors of power, to the media and to the entertainment industry. It is doubtful that there would be Fund today if AIDS had remained a mainly African, or developing country, problem. Witness the fact that evidence suggests 850 million people in the world are hungry and undernourished. Cohort studies show that this leads to massive stunting, and, in many millions, serious cognitive impairment. This evidence should surely motivate governments to act. But it does not! The redress of hunger has few advocates in the developed countries. The solution to the complex problem of hunger cannot be packaged as simply as the solution to the problem of AIDS. There is no single industry to blame.

What can be learned from this examination of HIV/AIDS, and what does evidence have to do with values? Evidence is necessary but certainly not sufficient for action to follow. Those involved in collecting evidence are very different people from those concerned with advocacy and action. They differ in their approaches, motives and professional values. Researchers, the epidemiological, demographic, pharmaceutical and clinical scientists, do their work often isolated from the political realities of the day. Their implicit values may differ from those who advocate for change, or have the power to effect change. They are more often driven by curiosity, and a desire to advance science, than by a desire to be active participants in changing the world.

Advocates profess their values openly. These are often expressed in relation to such underlying values as equity or human rights. For them, evidence is only useful if it can be a means to the attainment of a larger value or goal. When the evidence goes against that goal it is often dismissed. Evidence is therefore selectively chosen for packaging in support of the political arguments. As for policy makers, they are most often torn between evidence and advocacy. They have to work within a system where incremental change is the norm, and where new, even compelling, evidence cannot be rapidly turned into action.

Too often those who generate evidence have limited ability to engage in how it should be used. They are most often absent when complex trade-offs are made in the hurly-burly of the policy process. This results in massive missed opportunities for their important work to influence the development of more rational policies. It leads to the situation where DALYs are rarely considered when governments decide where to invest; and it leads to a situation where the only evidence on interventions that is taken seriously is that from pharmaceutical trials.

The consequence is that the huge and growing body of evidence is still very poorly employed in the framing of policy. If it were to be fully taken into account, some believe, as I certainly do, that we would have a Fund for primary healthcare and not one for specific diseases; that mental health, chronic diseases and their risks and injuries would receive a fairer share of government and donor attention and funding; that hunger reduction would be the central reason for health NGO activism and action; and that we would have better means of reducing inequities in health in all countries.

References

1 Global Fund for AIDS, malaria and tuberculosis. Available at www.theglobalfund.org/en/ (accessed September 2005).
2 I use 'evidence' here to refer to the outcomes of epidemiological, economic and related research and surveillance activities.

3 Mandelblatt JS, Fryback DG, Weinstein MC, Russell LB and Gold MR (1997) Assessing the effectiveness of health interventions for cost-effectiveness analysis. Panel on Cost-Effectiveness in Health and Medicine. *Journal of General Internal Medicine.* **12**(9): 551–8.

4 Murray CJ and Lopez AD (1996) Evidence-based health policy – lessons from the Global Burden of Disease Study. *Science.* **274**(5288): 740–3.

5 The Cochrane Collaboration is an international not-for-profit organisation preparing, maintaining and promoting the accessibility of systematic reviews of the effects of healthcare. More info on www.cochrane.org/index0.htm.

6 Termination of Grants to Myanmar, Global Fund for AIDS, Malaria and TB. Available at www.theglobalfund.org/en/media_center/press/pr_050819_factsheet.pdf (accessed September 2005).

7 McQueen DV (2001) Strengthening the evidence base for health promotion. *Health Promotion International.* **16**(3): 261–8.

8 World Health Organization (2001) *World Health Report: mental health.* WHO, Geneva.

9 World Health Organization (2004) *Promoting Mental Health: concepts, emerging evidence, practice.* WHO, Geneva.

10 World Health Organization (2002) *The World Health Report 2002: reducing risks, promoting healthy life.* WHO, Geneva.

11 World Health Organization (2004) *WHO Framework Convention on Tobacco.* WHO, Geneva.

12 World Health Organization (2004) *Global Strategy on Diet, Physical Activity and Health.* WHO, Geneva.

13 Piot P, Bartos M, Ghys PD, Walker N and Schwartlander B (2001) The global impact of HIV/AIDS. *Nature.* **410**(6831): 968–73.

14 Commission on Macroeconomics and Health (2001) *Macroeconomics and Health: investing in health for economic development.* WHO, Geneva.

15 Gordon DF (2000) *The Global Infectious Disease Threat and its Implications for the United States.* CIA Report. Available at www.odci.gov/cia/reports/nie/report/nie99-17d.html

16 (2000) *UN Security Council Resolution 1308: on the responsibility of the Security Council in the maintenance of international peace and security: HIV/AIDS and international peacekeeping operations.* S/RES/1308.

17 United Nations Development Programme(2005) *International Cooperation at a Crossroads: aid, trade and security in an unequal world.* Human Development Report 1005. New York, NY: Hoechstetter Printing Co. www.hdr.undp.org/reports/global/2005/

Chapter 9

Efficiency

David J Hunter

> [T]he ideas of economists . . . both when they are right and when they
> are wrong, are more powerful than is commonly believed. Indeed the
> world is ruled by little else. Practical men, who believe themselves to
> be exempt from any intellectual influences, are usually the slaves of
> some defunct economist.[1]

Key concepts

The three 'Es' of economy, efficiency and effectiveness have tended to preoccupy
governments of all persuasions as they struggle to reform and modernise their
health systems. Indeed, it seems they have been adopted as the defining *raison
d'être* of government intervention in areas like healthcare. At one level, it may be
seen as testimony to the pervasive influence of economics in general, and health
economics in particular, on those devising health policy, and on successive
governments of all persuasions that have endlessly reorganised their healthcare
systems.

The dominance of the economic paradigm runs through political discourse on
health and healthcare, and an adulation of efficiency seems to arise from a view
that is rarely challenged, namely, that 'there is no alternative' but to move
towards greater economic rationality if we want to have a viable healthcare
system. This extends to repeated calls from a number of economists to be explicit
about the hard choices involved in rationing healthcare even though these are
often political, complex, contextual, and may require clinical judgement.[2]

For many economists, productivity is the best measure of economic efficiency
even if this means ignoring the fact that productivity alone does not make what
Gray terms 'a humanly acceptable economy'.[3] Because health resources are
scarce, we are told, it would be morally wrong to waste them. An inefficient
use of resources in one area leads inevitably to other areas being deprived of
services they need. There is therefore a moral imperative to find the most efficient
organisation of services.[4] Hence the persuasive power of introducing economic
rationality to health services and their management. Who could possibly be
against it since to do so might imply condoning inefficient practices?

Efficiency is something of a weasel word – there are many ways of defining it,
none of them value-free. Moreover, there may be other essential requirements
on organisations concerned with healthcare in addition to efficiency, especially
when measured in terms of productivity.[5] For instance, the stewardship role of
government has been defined more broadly by WHO as 'the careful and respons-

ible management of the wellbeing of the population'.[6] It recognises that achieving and sustaining the health and wellbeing of the population is a key task for government at all levels, and for a range of agencies at each level. All their activities should be directed towards this ultimate goal which, WHO argues, is 'the very essence of good government'. Stewardship comprises six domains – generation of intelligence, formulating strategic policy direction, ensuring tools for implementation, coalition-building, ensuring a fit between policy objectives and organisational structure and culture, ensuring accountability.[7] While efficiency in the use of resources may be a component of effective stewardship, it is not singled out for special mention and is far from being the defining reason for government action.

This chapter reviews the concept of efficiency and its application in the management of healthcare. As noted, the term is slippery and is sometimes used to embrace both means (i.e. efficiency) and ends (i.e. effectiveness). More commonly it is taken to mean something separate from effectiveness. Cochrane, in his classic monograph, distinguishes between the two terms.[8] He employs 'effectiveness' to measure the effect of a particular medical action on altering the natural history of a disease for the better (i.e. the intervention is evidence based) while the term 'efficiency' is employed to cover the optimum use of personnel and materials in achieving the effective results of treatment. Whereas the first meaning entails both means and ends, the second meaning is concerned only with means.

The two concepts which relate to these issues are allocative efficiency and managerial efficiency respectively. Allocative efficiency assumes the functioning of perfect competition in a free market in which consumer, rather than producer, sovereignty prevails. It implies a 'want-regarding' view of interests, namely, that the consumer knows best. But in healthcare, where information asymmetry operates to confound consumer sovereignty, and where needs rather than wants are the currency of resource allocation, the role of professionals becomes vital as a proxy for consumer sovereignty. The professional acts on behalf of, or in co-production with, the user.

The most important technique which endeavours to respond to allocative efficiency is cost-benefit analysis (CBA). This entails the enumeration and evaluation of all the relevant costs and benefits. The value of CBA in improving allocative efficiency lies in giving a local optimisation within the limits of the studied areas, e.g. the best mix of kidney transplantation, and home and hospital dialysis.

The concept of allocative efficiency may be applied to healthcare at two distinct levels. The first addresses the question of whether the resources devoted to healthcare within a society would produce greater benefits if allocated to some other sector of the economy, and vice versa. This is a huge undertaking and in practice does not happen for a variety of technical and political reasons. The second level concerns the allocation of new resources within the healthcare system, with a view to improving allocative efficiency. But, even here, the concept of managerial efficiency is dominant.

Managerial efficiency is a less radical concept than allocative efficiency. It is not concerned with whether some organisational activity is worth undertaking at all, but with the least costly means of provision.[9] In healthcare systems, it is the notion of managerial efficiency which largely prevails since healthcare organisations are not examples of perfect competition and securing allocative efficiency is riven with value judgements and technical difficulties that preclude its adoption other than in theoretical terms.

The interpretation adopted here is restricted to the notion of managerial efficiency since in most healthcare systems attention is concentrated on means rather than ends. For example, the British National Health Service (NHS) is currently experiencing unprecedented investment after many years of alleged underfunding although no attempt is being made to measure its impact on health outcomes. Indeed, were such an attempt to be made (an example of the first level of allocative efficiency described above) it might be argued that the additional funds would be more effectively spent on closing the wealth gap between social groups (i.e. on social justice rather than specifically on healthcare) or on improved housing for people living in damp premises in poor repair, social conditions that contribute to their poor health and, in turn, to the growing demand for healthcare services. Instead of adopting such a 'whole systems' perspective, the focus of reformers is on the efficiency with which the funds are being allocated to meet centrally determined targets that are centred on inputs and processes rather than on outcomes. So, the focus is on reducing waiting lists, improving access to hospital beds and achieving balanced budgets, although these are means to an end and not ends in themselves.

But even trying to take a broad all-encompassing view of efficiency encounters pitfalls and 'deep conceptual problems'.[10] The task of measuring the value of the many diverse benefits of different healthcare interventions and activities, and then feeding these into a cost-benefit calculation, is an impossible one. For a start, it is not possible to know with precision how specific healthcare interventions affect the lives of diverse patients; attributing causation remains a problem. Moreover, often incommensurable values are being dealt with. How, for example, can one choose between more staff for the special care baby unit and additional care assistants for elderly mentally infirm people? Although having nothing in common, both may be equally deserving. If benefits are hard to identify and measure then so are costs, especially if these are not all financial.

The narrow view of efficiency described above, which is decoupled from effectiveness, manifests itself in a British context through a particular approach to performance management and one that is essentially mechanistic and top-down in conception and application. Elements of such a system may be found in other countries, but the British NHS is almost unique in the degree to which central control of its activities is possible. Visitors from our neighbours elsewhere in Europe marvel (or baulk) at the way successive national governments can impose their will on such a complex undertaking, and in effect seek to micro-manage it from the centre.

In the specific context of the search for efficiency, it is argued that the prevailing narrow conception of the term has been informed by what has been described as the economic colonisation, or imperialism, that underpins much health policy.[11] Of course, many economists would distance themselves from the focus, evident in health systems, on a narrow conception of cost containment and efficiency, arguing that it amounts to a travesty of their discipline, which is concerned as much with benefits (i.e. effectiveness) as with costs, i.e. with allocative efficiency. Nonetheless, since many of the special advisers who now constitute a crucial feature of British policy making are economists, or have had economics training, and since many of the outpourings of policy 'think tanks' are derived from the work of economists, it cannot be denied that the influence of economics thinking on policy, however partisan, is considerable.

As an example of such thinking, this chapter reviews the 'new public management' doctrine that, since the 1990s, has held sway, pervading successive healthcare reorganisations, and considers its limitations. The notion of 'complex adaptive systems' is introduced to show that an alternative conception of the management challenge in health systems is both possible and urgently needed to counter much of the simplistic thinking arising from a focus on the twin gods of efficiency and productivity that are driven by a concern for cost control, and the desire to remain competitive in a global economy. This neo-liberal ideology seems to be in the ascendant in all developed countries and yet largely goes unchallenged. Critics of the new orthodoxy assert that these are political constructs, not predetermined, not inevitable, not iron laws of economics, and that there are alternative conceptions of modernity.

Having briefly considered these larger global concerns, the chapter concludes that too narrow and reductionist a conception of efficiency is potentially dysfunctional in complex systems like health, where there is a need for high levels of flexibility and adaptability to particular circumstances that are both highly contextual and often hard to foresee. Indeed, the notion of professionalism is derived to a degree from such a recognition, such that groups of skilled practitioners, e.g. doctors and nurses, are accorded a degree of trust and autonomy to exercise judgement over how resources are used in the pursuit of health gain for their patients and populations.

Efficiency in health systems

In what sense should health systems be efficient? In the current British NHS, for example, what has been termed 'myopic cost-cutting' has led to an attempt to maximise patient throughput, with the result that there is inadequate spare bed capacity at times of high seasonal demand.[12] More recently, it has been argued that the rise in rates of hospital-acquired infections, notably MRSA, has been exacerbated, if not actually caused, by the intense pressure on hospital beds and the high turnover of patients. Elsewhere, the move to contracting out services like hospital cleaning, in order to reduce costs and improve efficiency, is also claimed to have resulted in dirty wards, a further factor in increasing infection rates.

Efficiency has been likened to 'a state of grace: something to which all aspire, but which few achieve and then only fleetingly'.[13] But though efficiency may be universally regarded as a good thing, there is no general agreement about its nature.

In considering efficiency it is important to take into account any loss of benefit that results from cutting cost. No sensible discussion of efficiency is possible if only costs are considered. The benefits associated with alternative policies need to be made explicit before their efficiency can be assessed although, as was pointed out in the last section, this is notoriously difficult to do. Cost control is important, but it cannot be an end in itself, decoupled from any consideration of benefits. In this regard even a term like 'value for money' is value-laden if used to reduce costs without regard for the unintended changes in the provision and distribution of benefits. Benefits need to be evaluated independently of costs before rational decisions can be taken about what benefits a healthcare system can afford to provide. To this end, the evaluation of benefits should receive at least as much attention as the assessment of costs.

In practice, the issue of benefits and costs are often muddled up in ways that are neither explicit nor clear. For example, the tendency of governments to worry about lengths of waiting lists and access to care may give rise to unintended consequences which could prove deleterious to high quality care. Moreover, often waiting lists serve a clinical purpose in terms of assessing priorities for treatment. This becomes distorted when government sets a rigid target that those delivering care are required to meet within a specified timescale. Such issues go to the heart of successive health system reform initiatives in many countries, and suggest that a particular model of performance management has been applied, concerned with a rather narrow conception of efficiency that does not allow for its impact on benefits and their distribution.

The search for ways of defining, measuring and improving the performance of health services has been a consistent and persistent theme of successive re-organisations in many countries in recent decades. In the British NHS, which has gone further than most European countries in reforming its healthcare system, the cult of 'managerialism' that came to the fore at the time of the first major reform in 1974 has remained a key theme of every restructuring since. Governments have progressively sought to tighten their grip on cost control, and on the uses to which resources have been put. Such an approach has been described as management 'by spreadsheets and tick-boxes' full of 'target-setting and pro-duction-line values'.[14] An unintended consequence of such an approach to management has been evidence of cheating, manipulating the data and 'gaming', i.e. employing a variety of stratagems to ensure that performance improves and targets are met, thereby delivering – on paper at any rate – the performance improvements sought by government. The unintended con-sequences and transaction costs arising from implementing a particular type of performance regime are rarely quantified. For example, under the payment by results system being introduced in England, hospitals will get paid according to the number and type of patients they treat. Game-playing is almost guaranteed in order to maximise income. This will take many forms. A common ploy is to discharge patients early where there is a high risk of readmission that will result in additional income. Also, early discharge will reduce average length of stay which will make the hospital appear efficient and enable it to meet activity targets.

Managing for efficiency

Economists and others have long argued that healthcare services tend to be inefficient. Among the reasons advanced are: that they are inherently biased in favour of producers (i.e. doctors); that they suffer from endless political inter-ference that is both counterproductive and inefficient; that they lack incentives to use resources efficiently, thereby pursuing ends that have an organisational, professional or political logic that many economists would regard as 'irrational'. The history of reform in many healthcare systems in recent decades has been predicated on an analysis of their weaknesses and failings that is largely derived from economics. Similarly, the proposals advanced to remedy such deficiencies in order to render healthcare services more efficient in terms of cost control, and maximising benefits, have their origins in economic theories. Indeed, the evidence for this is especially apparent in the doctrinal basis of the form of hard-line managerialism that has come to be known as 'new public management' (NPM). NPM thinking is dominated by the language of economics and by economic concepts such as markets, competition, incentives, devolved budgeting, the celebration of enterprise, and so on. The economic catchphrases of 'efficiency', 'choice', 'value for money' and 'rationalisation' are well to the fore in NPM.

The arrival of NPM in the 1990s, described as 'one of the most striking international trends in public administration',[15] has had a major impact on the management and delivery of healthcare. It continues to be influential. NPM arouses powerful emotions among both its supporters and detractors. The former believe that it has succeeded in replacing the old administrative mindset that permeated most governmental bureaucracies, with a 'modern' management ethos. Its critics, however, consider that NPM, borrowing practices from the business sector and private companies, has done great violence to the notion of a distinctive public service ethic and culture.[16] They would not dismiss the importance of efficiency but would seek to have it pursued in the context of an agreed set of values appropriate for a public service like healthcare. What they take issue with is the use of efficiency as a proxy for what amounts to market-style solutions. These overlook competing frameworks, such as the notion of professionalism, whereby the decisions about resource use rely on a mix of evidence, judgement and tacit knowledge. These are of the very essence of good professional practice, and underpinned the original conception of clinical governance.[17]

There are seven doctrinal components that go to make up NPM thinking.[18] These are:

- 'hands-on professional management' in the public sector (i.e. a commitment to action);
- explicit standards and measures of performance (i.e. efficiency requires a 'hard look' at objectives);
- greater emphasis on output controls (i.e. a stress on results rather than processes);
- shift to disaggregation of units in the public sector (i.e. separating commissioning from provision, achieving efficiency gains by contracting);
- shift to greater competition in public sector (i.e. competition is the key to lower costs and improved quality);
- stress on private sector styles of management practice (i.e. their application to public sector will improve efficiency and performance);
- stress on greater discipline and parsimony in resource use (i.e. need to 'do more with less').

NPM is derived from various influences. Notable among them is the business-type managerialism in the public sector in the tradition of the international scientific management movement.[19,20,21] It can primarily be understood as an expression of values that emphasise cutting costs, and doing more for less as a result of improved management and structural redesign.

The critics of NPM profoundly reject this sort of analysis.

They consider that public services like healthcare cannot be run like commercial undertakings. Their objectives are complex and multiple, whereas many private companies have simpler objectives, and are primarily motivated by profit and stakeholder value. Moreover, in health systems a relatively high degree of 'slack' is necessary in order to provide spare capacity for learning, or deployment in a crisis. This is in contrast to the NPM tenets for a lean and tight organisation that eliminates waste and slack. Finally, instead of narrow compartmentalising or segmenting activities in separate silos, health services require a 'whole systems' perspective. For example, in healthcare many of the challenges in the twenty-first century focus on chronic disease or long-term conditions, and public health issues.[22] These require a systems-wide approach to management where collaboration, rather than competition, is uppermost, and where there is effective management of pathways across the primary, secondary and social care interfaces.

Limits to new public management

Whatever its achievements, and these are not easy to quantify or separate from the rhetorical claims emanating from government policy makers, arguably NPM and its focus on efficiency and economic reason has contributed to the emergence of a raft of problems with regard to the effective delivery of healthcare services. These include: the opening up of a cultural rift between managers and clinicians, as power is perceived to have shifted from the latter to the former with managers being regarded as little more than the agents of government; growing fragmentation between the component parts of the health system as organisations are unbundled and disaggregated into semi-autonomous units (e.g. foundation hospitals in the British NHS); a focus on individual choice and consumerism as making for more efficient provision, rather than on collective decisions that are informed by, and benefit, whole communities and groups of citizens. As Broadbent and Loughlin[23] put it, the application of Taylor's scientific management tenets to professional craft processes could result in the loss of skills necessary to enhance social welfare. This arises in particular from what they term the 'accounting logic' that runs through NPM, combining elements of 'task control, characteristic of classical management, alongside a market approach'. The effect has been to reduce the independence and scope for judgement of the professional.

It is also questionable whether in fact NPM has succeeded in tackling the very inefficiencies which it was introduced to confront. Seddon for one believes that the current focus on efficiency measures and activity targets misses the point and is contributing to the problem and creating disorder.[24] If services are poorly designed, then the current system of performance management to raise efficiency levels and volume of patients seen does nothing to tackle that. Indeed, it achieves precisely the opposite. It fuels calls for more resources (human and/or financial) that may well not be needed if the redesign of services to improve patient care and population health were to be made the goal. So-called 'waste-busting' initiatives will not help in a system that is managed and measured with targets, since the targets are themselves a major cause of waste, consuming people's time in artificial activity, and deflecting attention from what they ought to be doing. As Seddon points out, waste and inefficiency can only be removed 'when managers learn to manage the overall flow of work, rather than the functions within it'. This means ignoring targets and efficiency measures which are functional and activity-related (e.g. numbers of operations cancelled, or appointments met within specified times – the very things now being targeted).

Assuming that the diagnosis of the problem in healthcare (that NPM is designed to address) is accepted, even in part, there remain crucial questions about the nature of the prescription being adopted in many countries and its appropriateness. As already mentioned, few would doubt the importance of efficiency as a component of health policy. What is at issue is the precise definition of efficiency that should prevail. The danger stems from the dominance of a particular approach to economics theory, in what should be an essentially political discourse, an approach that dismisses dissent from its tenets as representing irrational vested interests.

In particular, we need to know if an accounting logic is detrimental to good professional work, or whether the claimed gains outweigh the benefits of professional independent judgement even if the importance of, and necessity for, such judgement has become discredited and unfashionable. No such public debate appears likely, and the discussion proceeds using technocratic language to cloak what are, at root, value judgements and political constructs with major implications for the distribution of power and for the outputs and outcomes arising from investment in healthcare.

Taken to its extreme, we are left with a notion of the purely economic rational man who, in Sen's words, 'must be a bit of a fool . . . a social moron. Economic theory has been much preoccupied with this rational fool decked in the glory of his one all-purpose preference ordering.'[25] In reality, there are many types of rationality, and choices are made within complex contexts where conflicting objectives are unavoidable, and trade-offs need to be made. Healthcare systems are riven with such features, and decision making in such contexts is invariably messy and imperfect. In Simon's words, decision makers seek to 'satisfice' rather than 'optimise'.[26]

Critics of NPM maintain that it has opted to put a 'spotlight' on problems rather than to act as a 'lighthouse beam'; that it oversimplifies both the complexity of the problem, and the solutions required to address it.[27] Complex social problems that cross organisational boundaries require a lighthouse beam to illuminate the terrain; in contrast, spotlights focus on particular facets of a problem and fail to see the interconnections. For example, producing more doctors and nurses to do more of the same thing will not bring about the redesign of services that require that they should work differently. Indeed, it might reinforce and entrench the forces against change. And it might be that, were doctors and nurses to work differently, their numbers might not need to rise by much, if at all.

The difficulty arises when only one aspect of the problem is dealt with in isolation from the whole. NPM thinking suffers from a tendency to concentrate on the parts rather than the whole thereby resembling Newton's 'clockwork universe' in which big problems are broken down into smaller ones, analysed, and solved by rational deduction.[28] Chapman makes the same point when he argues that, 'the current model of public policy making, based on the reduction of complex problems into separate, rationally manageable components, is no longer appropriate to the challenges faced by governments.'[29]

Possibly the most serious charge levelled against NPM, and its narrow focus on managerial and organisational efficiency, is its inability to comprehend 'wicked issues', that is, issues that are multi-faceted and have no clear boundaries. They are 'the deeply intractable issues which are imperfectly understood and to which solutions are not clear'.[30] Generally under NPM, according to Stewart, there is a tendency to simplify management tasks in the belief that clear targets, and separation of roles, can clarify responsibility and release management initiative. Simplification has been achieved by the separation of policy from implementation, by the development of contracts, by quasi-contracts or targets governing relationships, and their enforcement by performance management. In short, NPM remains rooted in an industrial, mechanistic, top-down model of organisation and management that owes a great deal to the management philosophy of FW Taylor and his theory of scientific management.[31]

From NPM to complexity

An alternative to the pursuit of efficiency through NPM-type approaches is to view health systems as examples of complex adaptive systems.[32,33,34] A complex adaptive system has been defined as a collection of individual agents with freedom to act in ways that are not totally predictable, and whose actions are interconnected, so that the actions of one agent change the context for others.[35]

The pursuit of efficiency, along the lines described earlier, is at odds with such a view of policy and practice. It can be seen as lending legitimacy to inefficiency as a necessary by-product of delivering appropriate healthcare in a context of uncertainty, a context in which it is impossible to be precise about needs, and how these can best be met. This constitutes a paradox – to be efficient in the sense of also being effective actually requires acknowledging, and intentionally building in, a degree of inefficiency.

The assumption that there are universal ways of managing needs to be challenged. This is especially true in respect of complex public policy sectors like health, dealing with messes or 'wicked issues'. Applying ideas derived from complex adaptive systems to health cases in Canada, Glouberman[36] sought to draw out lessons for policy makers. A number of important themes emerged, including the following.

- Complex systems are adaptive – a side effect of complexity and of managing messes is that such systems will self-organise to evolve and regain stability.
- Making decisions under conditions of uncertainty is unavoidable since there are real limits to the amount of certainty that is possible; decisions need to be made with best available, or good enough, rather than perfect, data.
- Reverting to rational planning remains a constant temptation to those raised or trained in, or drawn to, such a culture. It often leads to decisions to streamline systems in the belief that they become more efficient. even though by doing so the risk of unintended consequences or even of failure can be increased.
- Effective management does not hinge on a single individual (i.e. the notion of the 'heroic' leader) or group – it is a collective enterprise. In the words of Warren Bennis: 'None of us is as smart as all of us. The Lone Ranger is dead.'[37]

Under a systems approach, policy would proceed in a very different manner from that adopted by a classic scientific management approach. In particular, interventions would introduce learning processes rather than specifying outcomes or targets. The key to establishing learning systems is an increased tolerance of failure, continuous feedback on effectiveness, and a willingness to foster diversity and innovation.[38] The emphasis would be on improving general system effectiveness, which cannot be accomplished by using simple quantitative measures of performance. There would be a premium placed on being non-prescriptive. So, for example, resources would be allocated, but without specifying, for a reasonably long period of time, how they must be used, so as to allow innovation to occur. Finally, practitioners would be directly engaged in generating service-level innovation.

The marketisation of health policy in a global context

In his epic work, *The Shield of Achilles*, Philip Bobbitt[39] writes of the emergence of the market state. The characteristics of the market state are its dependence on the international capital markets and on the modern multinational business network to create stability in the world economy. This is in preference to management by national or trans-national political bodies. The overriding goal is the maintenance of material wellbeing and the prevention of social instability. In a market state, the marketplace becomes the economic arena in which we are all consumers, not producers. Different cultures will adapt the market state in distinct ways, ranging from a US-style focus on individual rights and personal liberty to a Scandinavian-style emphasis on citizenship and collective responsibility, involving what Bobbitt terms 'a state-inflected market'.

Critics of the more extreme versions of the market state suggest that there are alternatives, that there is nothing inevitable about the neo-liberal view of the world, even though at present it seems to be the only view of efficiency and progress on offer, or which holds mass appeal.

David Marquand suggests we are caught in a clash between two different conceptions of modernity. One is the managerial, economic, determinist and top-down conception, implicit in the Washington Consensus, cherished by global businesses, increasingly espoused by public sector managers who ought to know better, and propagated by most of the media and all mainstream political parties and, for that matter, the European Commission. The other is a humanistic, decentralist, 'green', and pluralistic conception which commands increasing support in civil society, particularly among the young, but is almost squeezed out of formal politics.[40]

In his critique of the growth fetish, Hamilton seeks to articulate an alternative scenario – the 'post-growth society'.[41] He argues that we need to look beyond the pursuit of growth, however efficient, as an end in itself, and focus attention and public policies on those things that contribute to wellbeing. Sectors like health and healthcare would no longer be sacrificed on the altar of growth and managerial efficiency.

Conclusion

On the face of it, the global considerations described in the preceding section may seem to have little to do with the pursuit of efficiency in health policy, especially at a micro level. But this would be to misunderstand the close interconnections between globalisation, the emerging neo-liberal consensus (sometimes referred to as the Anglo-Saxon model), and the doctrines underpinning new public management that draw heavily on mechanistic business models owing much to concepts like Taylor's theory of scientific management, which rely on particular notions of how work should be conducted to maximise efficiency. In contrast, notions of complexity and pluralism offer an alternative way of looking at health policy, and seek to encourage rather than stifle improvement and innovation.

If we are to move away from the narrow conception of efficiency that seems to dominate much health policy making, and to preoccupy policy makers and managers wedded to NPM thinking, then it is essential that these wider connections are appreciated. Moreover, the pursuit of efficiency through performance targets and top-down micro-management is self-defeating in the long run, since it induces systemic distortions, dysfunctional behaviour, and elaborate forms of 'gaming' and 'cheating' that are anything but efficient when they divert managers' energies and talents from the task in hand.[42,43] As Seddon puts it: 'People who work in our public services want to focus on their purpose . . . They need help with measures and means, not cajoling to focus on arbitrary activities through hierarchical dictat.'

If we are to break free from the shackles of efficiency and an economistic view of modernity, then we need to look to a new paradigm that regards health systems as complex entities that require a 'whole systems' perspective in the pursuit of the goal of improved population health. Complex adaptive systems are not unconcerned about efficiency – they just go about achieving it in a different way that places responsibility, and the locus of control for achieving it, where it needs to be, that is, with those who do the work, and who themselves will need to change. In the case of healthcare, this means clinicians, nurses and others, who need to establish measures that, in their view, help them understand and improve performance. But not performance viewed in isolation from purposes or outcomes. These are the measures by which efficient healthcare and policies must be truly judged.

References

1 Keynes M (1973) *Collected Writings of John Maynard Keynes, vol. VII: The General Theory of Employment, Interest and Money.* Macmillan/St Martin's Press, London.
2 Hunter DJ (1997) *Desperately Seeking Solutions: rationing health care.* Longman, London.
3 Gray J (2003) *Al Qaeda and What it Means to be Modern.* Faber and Faber, London.
4 Williams A (1992) Cost-effective analysis: is it ethical? *Journal of Medical Ethics.* 18: 7–11.
5 Loughlin M (2002) *Ethics, Management and Mythology.* Radcliffe Medical Press, Oxford.
6 World Health Organization (2000) *The World Health Report 2000 – health systems: improving performance.* WHO, Geneva.
7 Travis P, Egger D, Davies P and Mechbal A (2002) *Towards Better Stewardship: concepts and critical issues. Evidence and Information for Policy.* WHO/EIP/DP 02.48. WHO, Geneva.
8 Cochrane AL (1972) *Effectiveness and Efficiency: random reflections on health services.* Nuffield Provincial Hospitals Trust, London.
9 Brooks R (1985) Effiency in health care. In: AF Long and S Harrison (eds) *Health Services Performance: effectiveness and efficiency.* Croom Helm, London
10 Loughlin M (2002) *Ethics, Management and Mythology.* Radcliffe Medical Press, Oxford.
11 Ashmore M, Mulkay M and Pinch T (1989) *Health & Efficiency: a sociology of health economics.* Open University Press, Milton Keynes.
12 The Commission on the NHS (2000) *New Life for Health.* Vintage, London. World Health Organization (2000) *The World Health Report 2000 – health systems: improving performance.* WHO, Geneva.

13 Brooks R (1985) Effiency in health care. In: AF Long and S Harrison (eds) *Health Services Performance: effectiveness and efficiency*. Croom Helm, London

14 Seddon J (2003) *Freedom from Command & Control: a better way to make the work work*. Vanguard Education, Buckingham.

15 Hood C (1991) A public management for all seasons? *Public Administration.* **69**: 3–19.

16 Ferlie E, Pettigrew A, Ashburner L and Fitzgerald L (1996) *The New Public Management in Action*. Oxford University Press, Oxford.

17 Scally G and Donaldson L (1998) Clinical governance and the drive for quality improvement in the new NHS in England. *BMJ.* **317**: 61–5.

18 Hood C (1991) A public management for all seasons? *Public Administration.* **69**: 3–19.

19 Peters TJ and Waterman RH (1982) *In Search of Excellence: lessons from America's best-run companies*. Harper & Row, New York.

20 Pollitt CJ (1990) *Managerialism and the Public Services: the Anglo-American experience*. Blackwell, Oxford.

21 McLaughlin K, Osborne SP and Ferlie E (eds) *New Public Management: current trends and future prospects*. Routledge, London.

22 Strong K, Mathers C, Leeder S and Beaglehole R (2005) Preventing chronic diseases: how many lives can we save? *Lancet.* **366**: 1578–82.

23 Broadbent J and Loughlin R (2002) Public service professionals and the New Public Management: control of the professions in the public services. In: K McLaughlin, SP Osborne and E Ferlie (eds) *New Public Management: current trends and future prospects*. Routledge, London.

24 Seddon J (2003) *Freedom from Command & Control: a better way to make the work work*. Vanguard Education, Buckingham.

25 Sen AK (1979) Rational fools. In: F Hahn and M Hollis M (eds) *Philosophy and Economic Theory*. Oxford University Press, Oxford.

26 Simon HA (1957) *Administrative Behaviour*. Free Press, New York.

27 Society of Local Authority Chief Executives (SOLACE) (1995) *Lighthouses not Spotlights*. SOLACE, Birmingham.

28 Plsek PE and Greenhalgh T (2001) The challenge of complexity in health care. *BMJ.* **323**: 625–8.

29 Chapman J (2004) *System Failure: why governments must learn to think differently* (4e). Demos, London.

30 Stewart J (1998) Advance or retreat: from the traditions of public administration to the new public management and beyond. *Public Policy and Administration.* **13**: 12–27.

31 Taylor FW (1913) *The Principles of Scientific Management*. Harper and Brothers, New York.

32 Chapman J (2002) *System Failure: why governments must learn to think differently*. Demos, London.

33 Seddon J (2003) *Freedom from Command & Control: a better way to make the work work*. Vanguard Education, Buckingham.

34 Hunter DJ (2003) England. In: M Marinker (ed) *Health Targets in Europe: polity, progress and promise*. BMJ Books, London; Hunter DJ (2003) *Public Health Policy*. Polity, Cambridge.

35 Plsek PE and Greenhalgh T (2001) The challenge of complexity in health care. *BMJ.* **323**: 625–8.

36 Glouberman S (2000) *Towards a New Perspective on Health and Health Policy: a synthesis document of the health network*. Canadian Policy Research Networks, Ottawa.

37 Bennis W (1998) *On Becoming a Leader*. Arrow, London.

38 Chapman J (2002) *System Failure: why governments must learn to think differently*. Demos, London.

39 Bobbitt P (2003) *The Shield of Achilles: war, peace and the course of history*. Penguin Books, London.

40 Marquand D (2005) Monarchy, state and dystopia. *The Political Quarterly.* **76**: 333–6.

41 Hamilton C (2004) *Growth Fetish*. Pluto Press, London.

42 Hunter DJ (2003) *Public Health Policy*. Polity, Cambridge.

43 Seddon J (2003) *Freedom from Command & Control: a better way to make the work work*. Vanguard Education, Buckingham.

Chapter 10

Synergy

Morton Warner

Introduction

'How can we achieve better organisational integration in the search for health gain for individuals and their communities?' The one-word title of this chapter suggests the answer to this question. But despite its brevity it is a complex and not a simple answer. To introduce the complexity involved consider the following familiar story which echoes Einstein's observation 'that we should make things as simple as possible, but not simpler'. It is worth retelling in full because it helps our understanding of a number of the essential facets of synergy.

The scene is a farmyard, looked after for 50 years by a farmer who is about to retire. He has always treated his animals well. This particular morning sees a small gathering – a chicken, a cow and a pig. They lament the farmer's retirement, but are determined to give him a real send off. 'Let's make him a good breakfast,' says the chicken; and the others readily agree that eggs and bacon with a glass of fresh milk would be just perfect. A day later they meet again: the chicken and the cow notice the pig is not so enthusiastic. He explains his problem about the breakfast: 'It's alright for you two,' he says, 'you only have to *participate*, but I have to be *committed*!'

The intention of the animals was to work synergistically – in a cooperative way, where the effects would be produced by actions coming together through a common sense of purpose. Synergy refers to an expression that can be traced back to Aristotle in the Metaphysics,[1] 'the whole is greater that the sum of the parts', or $2 + 2 = 5$.

But is it as straightforward as this? Can synergy be assumed always to result in additional positive effects? The literature on this suggests that synergies can be positive (functional synergy), negative (dysfunctional) or neutral in their impact. The farmyard scene illustrates all of these possibilities. The idea of providing a good breakfast created initial positive synergy. The sudden realisation by the pig of the need to be *involved* was dysfunctional. And the self-interest of the chicken and the cow was served by participation not commitment, at best a neutral role. Note also that 'breakfast' has no connotation of higher moral value. In this instance $1 + 1 + 1 = 0$, or at best 2!

In contrast with the natural world of, for example, particle physics or molecular biology where the underlying 'laws' are derived through relentless reductionism, the social world of the farmyard displays profound and aggregative complexity by way of interactions, interrelations and time specificity.

'Systems theory' using cybernetics and feedback models, and now 'complexity theory' drawing on chaos models and hypotheses of 'self-organisation' have been favoured as disciplines better able than reductionist approaches to provide an understanding of social institutional arrangements. Corning[2] says that 'there seems to be a growing appreciation of the inextricable relationship between (and within) wholes and parts which necessitates multi-levelled, multi-disciplinary, "interactional" analyses', and he proposes a typology of synergies.

Adopting a translational approach

Corning's work, undertaken at the Institute for the Study of Complex Systems in Palo Alto, is a very important representation of recent attempts to bridge the theoretical chasm between holism and reductionism. The pursuit of 'health', as the aspiration of a civilised and technological society, involves multiple layers and requires us to bridge this chasm. The spectrum of activity in health stretches from the reductionist value-free natural world of molecular biology, to the holistic most often value-laden delivery of services.

Essentially, the approach used by Corning is to set out a 'conceptual re-visioning' of the phenomenal world – a paradigm shift – which directs our attention to an underlying causal principle that is concerned with structural and functional relationships of various kinds and with the concrete consequences or effects they produce'.[3] Two broad concepts to understand the development of the natural world are described: natural selection and hierarchies. Synergy, in the different guises shortly to be described, flows through these.

Whilst the focus of this chapter is on synergy *per se*, natural selection and hierarchies have considerable relevance, acting as often hidden or quietly 'under-stood' fundamentals that surround and influence synergistic activities. Translation of behaviour observed in the natural world is not without its hazards. By translation I mean the attempt to draw an analogy from things going on in one domain (here, the natural world) to explain things going on in another (the phenomenal world), and so in health systems. However, the habit of rigorous thinking that characterises natural sciences can help us to think more clearly about such social constructs as organisational complexity, and to propose approaches to achieving organisational integration.

Natural selection

In nature, selection refers to factors responsible for the differential survival and reproduction of genes, species and populations. The theory does not allow us to make predictions about the overall course of evolution or the future of any given species. For analogous reasons, and also because of the complexity of the interactive forces, it can be as hard to predict the effects of health policy on organisations concerned with health, as on health itself. Politicians everywhere constantly surprise with their reorganisation of services, with a penchant for destruction and renewal of institutions in equal measure. However, in the many parts of the world where managed healthcare markets dominate, actual extinction of a 'species' is a rare occurrence.

Hierarchies

There are a number of ways of thinking about hierarchies, and each offers much to our understanding of how synergies can be functional, dysfunctional or functionally neutral.

In natural history a taxonomic hierarchy categorises species (genera, families, orders, etc). By analogy, 'orders' could be equated with the 120 or so occupational groups that typically work in the health field in western countries. Every one has certain characteristics and evolutionary relationships. Physiologists associate the term 'hierarchy' with a nested set of functioning part-wholes, or silos. Something similar can be seen in health services too – formed for example by the professional colleges or chambers, each with its system of special interest sections. Political scientists think of hierarchies in somewhat the same way, referring to structured relationships of power, rule and authority at different levels of control.

Many biologists go one stage further and link genealogy with ecological hierarchies. This can be applied to health systems as well. Within European countries, health, social care and the voluntary sector (NGOs, civil society) all have a different genealogy, developmental history and contexts within which they function. In addition, there are major secondary differences such as election or political appointment to their boards. In order to describe the taxonomic hierarchy of these systems, it is necessary to relate all these disparate elements, and I attempt to do so later.

This general discussion illustrates the difficulties that might be expected when organisations of different origins are required to cooperate in an integrated way, as is often the case in the healthcare world. Anticipating the exact nature of organisational resistance is difficult, but it must be attempted if synergies are to be functional.

Synergy types and their translation to the world of healthcare

Synergy, a fundamental and all-pervasive aspect of the natural world, describes a coming together of different elements to produce unique powerful effects. As with the primitive drives of insects, or chemical attraction in the case of molecules, no sense of motivation is involved! But the descriptive terminology used by various scientific disciplines to describe synergy is only one stage away from this – *ordering* (quantum physics), *cooperation and coordination* (biophysics and developmental biology), *functional integration* (biochemistry), *mutualism and cooperation* (ecology and behavioural biology), *cooperation* (anthropology). All can be thought of as having their genesis in the social world, and being translated to the natural world. This is an important consideration underpinning the reasonableness of reversing the application.

Next, I will list a number of synergy types occurring in the natural world, and provide analogies with contemporary health systems where they have, by commission, produced some particular effects, often with unexpected consequences.

Linear or additive phenomena

The simple cause–effect is that larger size may provide collective advantage. This is easier said than done, however, and the expected results of such synergies in health systems often fail to materialise. The expressions 'takeover' and 'merger' are often confused; and especially in public sector reorganisations 'new partnership' is the preferred term, indicating, sometimes falsely, a consensus by all parties.

Set alongside natural selection, the application of linear synergy suggests a prey can be consumed or destroyed. Often in the public sector, however, the 'prey' remains unstated, not clearly identified or elusive. Clarity is not necessarily helpful! The effects are, however, more visible in the private sector where balance sheet and bottom lines mark success, for example in the increased profitability that can result from newly merged health insurance funds. But performance management in many state-run healthcare systems often fails to be able to attribute success in a timely way, and certainly in terms of what is really important – reducing morbidity and mortality, increasing and achieving greater efficiencies.

Frequency or density-dependent phenomena

This is a variety of the first synergy type, but the effect here lies in the size of the organisation *and* the density (i.e. the multi-layered complexity) of its activities to make a difference. As in the natural world, in health systems there can be both functional and dysfunctional synergies at play. The perceptions of the public count for a lot in determining whether the synergistic effects are well thought of or not.

Euregios[4] are involved in formal cross-state border cooperation in the provision of health services for two or more regions. They often increase the density of services, or provide a greater range of specialisation, for each of their resident populations.

Clinical networks so popular with politicians, and an example of virtual organisations, have been brought into play as a means of promoting higher quality of care (as governments claim), but also to manage manpower and skills shortages (a consumer claim). By and large, they have not received much public attention. Many professionals go along with the concept, but are not wholly persuaded either on quality grounds, or on the grounds that they overcame the scarcity of resources. As a synergy, clinical networks are viewed quite neutrally.

In the UK, the National Institute for Health and Clinical Excellence[5] is an example of an innovation perceived as being associated with dysfunctional synergy. Set up by the government in 2000 as evidence based medicine came of age, it has emerged as the focal point for bringing together the fruits of research into the effectiveness and efficiency of healthcare interventions; and it is the senior advisory body on the introduction of new treatments and medicines into the NHS. Even though its aims to be science-based are laudable, and its transactions increasingly transparent, it has not been able to shake off the perception of being the rationing arm of government, rather than an attempt to incorporate the best findings from research into clinical practice.

Emergent phenomena

Generally, in terms of the natural world, 'emergence' is restricted to describing how synergies result in the appearance of new physical 'wholes'. This is also very familiar to the world of healthcare, and often occurs through a process referred to as 'substitution'.

Substitution has been defined as 'the continual regrouping of resources across and within care settings, to exploit the best and least costly solutions in the face of changing needs and demands'.[6] Health sector staff, skills, equipment, information and facilities can be reengineered to achieve better clinical, financial or patient-related outcomes. New and successful physical 'wholes' in recent times have included dedicated day surgery suites, medical assessment units, robotic pharmacy dispensaries, and the movement and adaptation of services, relocating them from secondary to primary care. Such synergy is often made possible or dictated by access to new technologies. The effects of the synergies involved here are mainly regarded as positive, although workforce substitution is sometimes initially challenged, not least by those directly affected.

Division (or combinations) of labour

Although part of substitution, division of labour is an important synergy in its own right. For example, the benefits of creating specialised units for patients with rarely occurring disease, so that they can be cared for by relevant, highly specialised health professionals, are well recognised. Indeed, compartmentalisation and specialisation of functions, an important example of synergy in the natural world, is a wide-ranging and frequently occurring feature of healthcare systems.

But this reductionist approach can also be dysfunctional to 'whole person' integrative medicine, especially where general practice has not been well developed or is only of poor quality. It is perhaps with the broader-based care in the community that the effects of division of labour can be most difficult to manage, and major coordinative effort is needed to control transaction costs. A recent alternative strategy has been to multitask health and social care professionals, to reduce the gaps that often exist between service organisations and to improve efficiency.

Mutual enhancement

In the area of biochemistry, 'cooperativity theory'[7] focuses on a range of synergies of this nature. Production and correction occur simultaneously, resulting in stable chemicals fit for the body's use.

Within hospitals, too, integrated functioning of clinical governance, risk management and audit board-level committees can be mutually enhancing and result in corrections being applied in a timely way where there are breakdowns. Achieving a balance between unthinking heavyhandedness and the light touch implied in cooperativity can be difficult, and the synergy very easily becomes dysfunctional.

For a number of European countries, at the inter-organisational level, there is the complexity of the 'commissioning' (as opposed to the more limited 'purchasing') process, where population need and care provision are carefully matched, often to meet socially predefined objectives. Health commissioning agencies rarely have sufficient expertise to undertake the process well without calling on the specialist knowledge-base resident in provider organisations to guide them. And the providers quite reasonably will do this to ensure contracts are put into place where price best matches need and demand.

Perhaps, ideally, in both cases the integrative actions should be seen as having a neutral synergistic effect for the immediate parties, although the benefits to patients and the public should be positive. However, lack of trust often results in dysfunction and failure to achieve benefit.

'Bio-economic' efficiencies

In the animal kingdom, instinctively coming together to reduce individual energy expenditure is common in cold climates. This could well serve as a metaphor for the providers of healthcare in many countries. Indeed this can be an alternative *unforced* mechanism in order to bring some hoped-for collective advantage. It is in contrast with, for example, legislative requirements to reorganise by merger or takeover – a linear synergy.

Bio-economic efficiencies, involving cost and/or risk sharing, information sharing or joint environmental exposure (for example, a joint venture in a new market or world location), can all be seen as elements in takeovers. But they can also be at the top of an agenda for provider organisations seeking, under government or commissioner pressure, to be more efficient.

In the case of provision of clinical services, the cooperative relationships between organisations working in the same overall health field is one of the most difficult to handle; and failure to provide integrated care is very often the result. Imagine the interface between two organisations. With goodwill both organisations attempt to blur their boundaries and cooperate, but often they fail to close the gap. In other circumstances they may compete and overlap. Rarely do they intertwine completely to coordinate functions and attain a high level of efficiency. Bio-economic synergies are very difficult to achieve without merger or takeover, but they can be instigated at an inter-organisational level as will be seen later. For now, clinical pathway developments are about as close as it gets in attempting to achieve integrated care, but, even so, major questions of efficiency remain unanswered in their respect.

Information sharing, as a particular aspect of bio-economic activity, can be highly synergistic. Occurring wittingly or otherwise, a few rather diverse examples may serve to illustrate this.

Health professionals draw down on information sources (journals, Medline, Google, etc.) and disseminate knowledge 'horizontally' through personal relationships with colleagues and patients, and 'vertically' through management, clinical governance, regulatory and professional lines. The synergy 'scatter' is sometimes positive, bringing improved standards of care, for example reducing the use of grommets for glue ear, and sometimes negative, for example creating public alarm by misleading claims from poor science (the MMR vaccination scare).

Of growing importance is the notion of the co-production of health.[8] This was somewhat anticipated by the medical historian Henry Sigerist in 1942 when he presaged the WHO slogan of total physical and social wellbeing and added 'and individuals will want to take responsibility for their own health'.[9] But how are they to do this? Engagement with health professionals as partners to achieve higher levels of health literacy is one way. The use of the Internet by patient support groups is another. And there is a growing appreciation of the fact that patients themselves are experts. Diabetes sufferers were amongst the first to be thought of in this way. Many new partnerships based on an explicit co-production of health gain are beginning to emerge. These are regarded as a positive by many, but not all, health professionals.

Next, an example of dysfunctional synergy. In the UK, failures of information sharing across health and social service agencies was viewed as so serious and difficult an issue that, in the case of child protection cases, information exchange was made mandatory by law several years ago. Now a requirement for 'unified assessment' – a common agency record for patients and clients – is posing major challenges to long-held practices of confidentiality, particularly those of medical practitioners. This is a difficult issue, but unified assessment is key to information sharing and to enabling integrated care to be developed inter-organisationally.

In reaching this point where the translation of synergy types is complete, an important difference needs to be identified which sets the phenomenal human world apart from its reductionist neighbour. In the natural world synergy is value-neutral (although we can become confused by the use of some technical terms particular to the field of biology, like 'mutualism' and 'altruism'). In the human world synergistic activity positively buzzes with values: they underpin our thoughts and heavily influence the actions of individuals and organisations alike. The value of values cannot be understated in the analysis of complexity.

The health hierarchy: why integration is difficult

It is time now to bring a number of the elements of the discussion together, and this is done through Figure 10.1. Earlier I suggested that it would be possible to develop a taxonomic hierarchy – a classification of 'species'. The complexity of the phenomenal world requires a certain flexing of the term species, but its use seems broadly reasonable. Politicians, for example, are only a homogenous group in name; they are differentiated in terms of party affiliation, social sympathies and so on. And to imagine a concept such as 'effectiveness' as a species may be a little far-fetched, until we think about the evidence based medicine coterie who haunt every academic and scientific meeting nowadays!

The figure, in its vertical column, is grouped in terms of the 'aspirational' and the 'observable'. The aspirational aspects cannot be quantified, tending to be but gleams in the political, academic and philosophical eye. In terms of the observable, there are the perspectives of a variety of stakeholders, together with the instruments they use to support and enforce them.[10] At the heart of this part of the taxonomy are organisations, a matter which will become self-evidently important in the final part of the chapter; but their form is optional, though mostly they are hierarchical.

Turning then to the horizontal plane. Here it is the synergistic *choices* exercised by the various stakeholders that will determine organisational form, together with the types of instrumentation to be used to support it. The synergistic *effects* come from an involvement of all stakeholders. However, some are more powerful than others, and often it is difficult to anticipate accurately the outcomes.

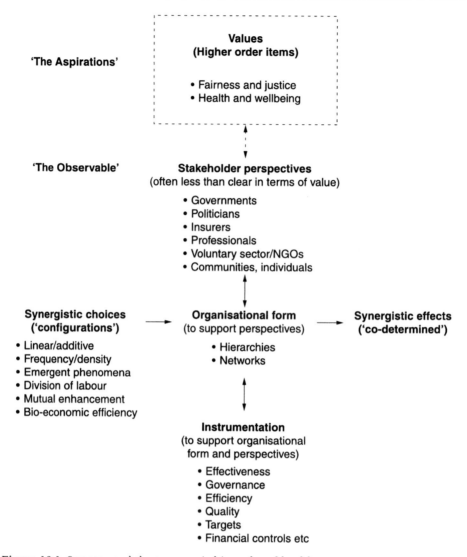

Figure 10.1 Synergy and the taxonomic hierarchy of health systems.

Stakeholder perspectives

These are at the heart of difficulties in achieving integrated organisational activity. Particularly true for civil service settings, 'territorial defence' is a central tenet of day-to-day life, and most public employees will recognise the 'natural' or 'primitive' forces at work as organisations defend themselves.

In contrast, 'territorial attack' is often the entrepreneurial choice of private sector groups, where 'forced' integration is not without its enthusiasts and its losers. Intention to increase synergistically the concentration of activities is not limited to either the public or private sector, but their bottom lines are different – money on the one hand and political capital on the other.

The stakeholder list in Figure 10.1 implies a hierarchy of its own, with differential levels of power accruing across the list; and this often varies between stakeholders and at different points in time. Currently in many parts of Europe politicians are deeply distrusted by their constituents, who then scrutinise the thinking of professional associations and actively seek their advice. The result? Governments seek to reduce the power of these professional groups by increasing regulation on the one hand, and emphasising consumer choice on the other. This perhaps serves to illustrate a major point. The constantly shifting levels of power of different stakeholder groups bring great strain to the organisational tectonics, with often unforeseeable results. There are, some would say, positive aspects to living life on the organisational boundary between these colliding tectonic plates. Paul Tillich writes: 'The border line is the truly propitious place for acquiring knowledge'[11] and 'Boundaries are as windows and doors, not prison walls.'[12]

Through all this, timing and time specificity are important considerations. Stakeholder groups may well behave differently in the face of a particular threat or promise at different points in time during negotiations. And in achieving consensus about mutual benefit – an integration of views – timing is everything. It is, however, very difficult to manage this timing within any one organisation, let alone across several.

Instruments

In one way the list of instruments set out in Figure 10.1 would not be considered controversial in almost any country across Europe, or beyond. The difference between countries is more a matter of the degree of emphasis, and the interpretation given to any one of them, as well as to how sanctions related to their non-application are applied.

As an example, all developed countries have access to the results of scientific investigations into the effectiveness of clinical interventions. Where governments are the funders of services, generating and sharing this knowledge assists them to allocate resources. But for NGOs, concerned with a particular group of disease sufferers such as those with multiple sclerosis, a decision such as one not to prescribe beta-interferon[13] made the conflict of perspectives dramatically clear. Technical, political, professional and common sense rationalities do not sit easily together; and the total synergistic effect may be neutral at best or even negative in the eyes of some.

Target setting is another contentious issue, the full extent of which is dealt with elsewhere.[14] But Van Herten and Gunning-Schepers[15] have drawn attention to the need to create an optimal balance, setting technocratic and participative approaches against each other on one axis, and policy makers and professionals on the other.

It is not so much the 'what' of instrumentation that is of concern, as the 'how' of implementation. In the policy debate, because of the dominance of such issues as the volume of the supply side and how it is to be organised, there is little or no attempt to address the higher order issues concerning values, and so little common ground within which the vested interests of stakeholders can, even temporarily, be put to one side.

Aspirations and values

These have been included only with broken line connections to the stakeholder perspectives. Why is this? Well, the history of placing the achievement of health gain as an object of health investment and integrated action is quite recent. WHO Europe did this first in the late 1980s,[16] and reviewed their approaches in the 1990s.[17] Many countries in Europe followed the lead in strategy documents, but there was little action on the ground.

In more recent times, with increasing acceptance of the role of health in furthering peace and harmony has come a realisation of the value of 'values' in promoting fairness, and this has not gone unnoticed amongst national and international stakeholders (think of the position of AIDS medication in Southern Africa).[18,19,20] And at local level the appeal for joint working in health and social care requires some higher order idea to come into play if it is to be successful. Health and social gain may be useful starting points, but they are insufficient. Altruism, justice and fairness must also be present; and an acceptance that mutualism is the vehicle.

Organisational form

The private sector, in its quest for profit making, has been quite adept in employing formal network (horizontal) approaches alongside hierarchical vertical arrangements. The public sector, by contrast, is very hierarchical, finding it difficult to network across organisational boundaries in a formal way. Only recently have there been positive moves forward on this; but the health sector generally does not have clarity about its aspirations or the way forward to achieve an optimum return on public investment. The understandable tendency is to focus on shorter waiting times for surgery, rather than engage in a longer-term venture to achieve a reduction in health inequalities.

Network arrangements are superior to hierarchical approaches when the issues to be tackled are complex and require integrated cross-agency action for their solution. And it is the various types of synergy acting *in concert* which form the bedrock of network activity. In a short case study, the final part of the chapter explores how the challenges of problem complexity and agency fragmentation were managed synergistically to improve the quality of life of one important group in the community.

The management of synergies to achieve inter-organisational integration

Dahlgren and Whitehead in their classic work for WHO[21] set out all the aspects of life that determine good health, from the broadest of global conditions to individual DNA. They involve the state of economic development, cross-sectoral organisational capacity, community and social networks, and genes. This clarifies the 'what' of good health. But the 'how' to achieve it has been elusive.

The challenges to integration, and by extension to inter-sectoral working, were for many years thought of in terms of overcoming or removing the range of barriers set out in Figure 10.2.[22]

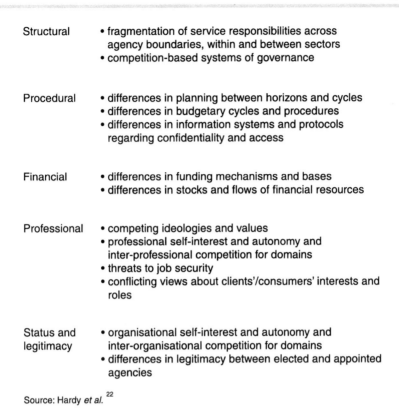

Structural	• fragmentation of service responsibilities across agency boundaries, within and between sectors • competition-based systems of governance
Procedural	• differences in planning between horizons and cycles • differences in budgetary cycles and procedures • differences in information systems and protocols regarding confidentiality and access
Financial	• differences in funding mechanisms and bases • differences in stocks and flows of financial resources
Professional	• competing ideologies and values • professional self-interest and autonomy and inter-professional competition for domains • threats to job security • conflicting views about clients'/consumers' interests and roles
Status and legitimacy	• organisational self-interest and autonomy and inter-organisational competition for domains • differences in legitimacy between elected and appointed agencies

Source: Hardy *et al.* [22]

Figure 10.2 Barriers to integration.

Two principal approaches have been tried: formal mergers, for example of health and social care programmes; and co-location of services. The first has very frequently failed due to the persistence of previous professional barriers, and the second because of communication and coordination problems.

In more recent times attention has turned to 'boundaries' and 'boundary spanning', with useful development and empirical research undertaken by Aldrich.[23,24,25] Barriers and boundaries are legitimate and useful: they guard organisational rights and define possibilities, and must be respected. However, barriers are also described as impenetrable, exhibiting great resistance to change. Boundaries, by contrast, can be elastic or permeable, offering the possibility of adjustment, diffusion and exchange.

Three major questions require an answer. What kind of activity is appropriate for the boundary territory? How is it to be orchestrated? What sort of mechanisms are to be put in place to link the boundary territory with the parent organisations?

Project CHAIN (Community Health Alliances through Integrated Networks)

Operating in the UK in the South Wales Valleys from 2001 to 2004, CHAIN was an action research project dedicated to improving the quality of life of older people.[26] CHAIN had two main objectives: addressing the population determinants of health of older people; and improving the delivery of care services. Two innovations formed the centrepiece of the project. First, with respect to boundaries, the visual metaphor of a 'white space' was developed to represent an opportunity territory for creative service redesign. Second, the role of 'Virtual Organisation Coordinator' (VOC) was created to 'manage' activity in the white space.[27]

The white space

An organisational chart is depicted visually as a number of boxes, normally interconnected. The central area between the boxes indicates an absence of organisational activity, and this was titled as the neutral 'white space'. There are precedents for this idea: in network theory, Burt[28] has pioneered the concept of 'structural holes', which both impose constraints and offer opportunities.

In this new territory, untrammelled by organisational preconditions and assumptions, creative network activity took place which resulted in the redesign of service. The network activities were sustained through governance arrangements which involved social mechanisms such as trust, commitment and the threat of exclusion from the network.[29] Even though governance suggests a means of regulating activity in the white space, for practical purposes we are forced back to the problem of 'who' or 'what' is to be responsible for coordination.

The Virtual Organisation Coordinator

A VOC was charged with managing white space activities, where necessary in a hierarchical way. What did this entail? Because they have no statutory diktats, span-of-control or immediate institutional authority, coordinators of partnerships, alliances and networks require a new toolbox to make things happen. The role was created to deliver CHAIN's aims by developing new styles of management.

Over time, the VOC engaged in the following three core activities:

- **attracting:** a key function of developing a virtual organisation through its supporting networks;
- **guiding:** keeping uncertainty within reasonable limits, involving constant movement between stakeholders, recognising the complex interrelatedness of the barriers;
- **brokering:** which was lightly applied in the early stages, but became stronger later as coordination became necessary to agree protocols and reallocate funds.

In all this it was necessary to explore the total range of synergistic options. Figure 10.3[30] sets out the coordinative role in more detail, and as it emerged over about 18 months.

A number of networks functioned in the white space. They focused on concerns that, were they tackled in an integrated way, would improve the quality of life for older people in the locality. These were: income sufficiency; increased mobility through good local transport; reducing the fear of crime; the development of a unified health and social care record; reducing the incidence of falls; reducing many problems associated with medication, such as polypharmacy, and the wide range of social factors – loneliness, depression and the like – that contribute to older people requiring medication in the first place.

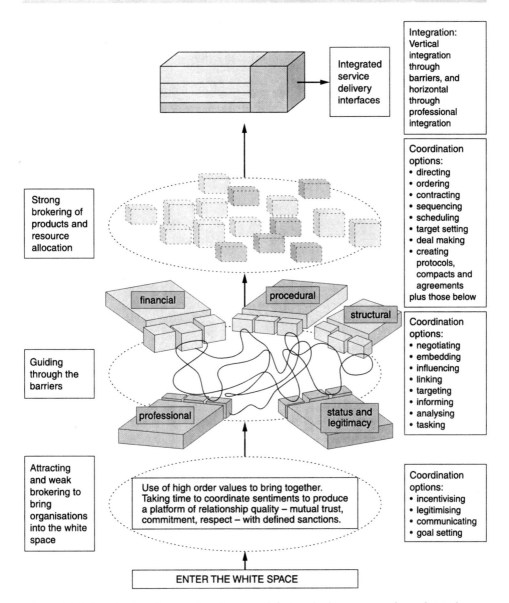

Figure 10.3 Developing the coordination possibilities of white space – from dependency to integration.[30]

It should be observed that the umbrella expression 'quality of life' represented a strong, morally persuasive higher order value. And, as such, it acted as a motivating force for both individuals and organisations to become involved.

Coordinating the medication network

Figure 10.4 takes the barriers to integration set out earlier and identifies some specific issues that arose throughout the year-long life of the Medication Network.

Individual and Inter-organisational Platform			
Coordinating sentiments to produce relationship quality – mutual trust, commitment, respect, with defined sanctions for breaching arrangements.			
Time sequence of barrier presentation	Barriers to integration (actual and potential)	Virtual organisation coordinator response	Synergy types employed by the VOC, (a)–(f)
1	**Structural** – fragmentation of service responsibilities across agency boundaries, within and between sectors	Recognising all medication interests and identifying a network core.	(b) Failure of population coverage and access (e) Representations of agencies required improvement (f) Need to risk share solutions in face of emerging policy initiative from government
2	**Status and legitimacy** – organisational self-interest and autonomy and inter-organisational competition for domains	Need for protracted negotiations with organisation with a core commissioning interest in medication since it was concerned with loss of control.	As in 1, plus (d) Negative inappropriate division of labour, with need for enhancement across agencies
3	**Professional** – threats to job security	Bringing network core lead to a recognition that the present arrangements were a threat – and not just to job security.	(e) Failure to act would result in further questions about lead agency professionals, a negative synergy
4	**Professional** – professional self-interest and autonomy and inter-professional competition for domains	This has similarities to barrier number 2. Through extensive communicating with colleagues the VOC progressively identified dependent, interdependent and independent activities. This formed the basis for non-conflictual interactions.	As in 2, but also (e) Identifying discrete activities for individual professionals in networks to undertake
5	**Status and legitimacy** – differences in legitimacy between elected and appointed agencies	VOC invoked a greater form of legitimacy – CHAIN was given legitimacy by the initial partnership arrangement and, most critically, the support and stated needs of older people themselves. This was a mandate for goal setting.	(a) CHAIN itself (an emergent phenomena) has an added ingredient which was given and gave legitimacy to the networks
6	**Professional** – conflicting views about clients'/ consumers' interests and roles	As interactions became increasingly embedded within a culture of trust, the VOC was able to harmonise these differences.	(e) Trust became the organisational glue and gave comfort, all organisations would be winners
7	**Procedural** – differences in information systems and protocols regarding confidentiality and access	Many issues here, often with a legal basis. Extensive fact finding and statement of legal responsibilities lead to clear demarcation between the possible and impossible.	(f) Some efficiencies possible, but barriers were also legitimate because of legal and fiduciary responsibilities
8	**Structural** – competition-based systems of governance	This was of limited significance, except for the community pharmacists operating in their own market. The VOC lobbied for the principle of equity in the provision of funding for their inputs.	(a) (f) Participating agencies responded because of a government requirement to produce joint plans for their area in areas seen by their constituents as a priority
9	**Procedural** – differences in planning horizons and cycles	This translated more in terms of getting medication problems recognised by decision makers and established as a priority.	(f) Taking a neutral view on the need to align agencies' financial cycles and procedures
10	**Procedural** – differences in budgetary and operational plan cycles or definitions	Differences in procedures partly between local government (LG) and healthcare providers were significant. The VOC had to guard against any service re-design that would require LG policy changes since this would take considerable time.	(b) (e) (f) Through more creative use of pooled budgets
11	**Financial** – differences in funding bases and mechanisms	Not a barrier. In fact the different bases provided alternative potential sources of funding for service re-design.	(b) (e) (f) Through more creative use of pooled budgets
12	**Financial** – differences in stocks and flows of financial resources	Also not a barrier. Accessing money designed for joint health and social care projects (flexibilities) provides one way to re-direct financial resources.	The value/moral imperative of health and social gain and synergy in its own right

Synergy types:
(a) Linear/additive (b) Frequency or density dependent (c) Emergent phenomena (d) Division of labour
(e) Mutual enhancement (f) Bio-economic efficiencies

Figure 10.4 Medication Network – synergistic choices for integrated service design. Adapted from Warner and Gould (2004).[31]

The platform which the VOC built amongst the Medication Network members was important, highlighted by the reticence of one key individual to participate in the first instance. This person maintained that the area of competence of their organisation was being improperly challenged, as was their own professional integrity. This was in the face of wide-scale concerns about medication amongst many of the (more than 120) people interviewed across all agencies that had dealings with older people in the locality.

The parent organisation of the individual concerned was still immature in terms of its development and functioning. It is of interest to speculate whether attachment theory[32] might play a part in the ease, or otherwise, with which individuals feel they can move into the white space. Immature or malfunctioning organisations are unlikely to develop the secure environment – the good parenting – that their employees need if they are to feel comfortable in exploring the boundary territory and beyond. Of course, it is equally true that the failure of any individual to attach may result from their own personal experience in detaching, and subsequent non-integrational behaviour.[33]

From a contentious beginning, the Medication Network (made up of a hospital and a community pharmacist, general practitioner, local authority representative, commissioning organisation pharmaceutical adviser, and voluntary sector member) was ultimately able to reach agreement on joint action on a number of complex issues which had long been unresolved. These included: ways of reducing hospital admissions caused by polypharmacy; agreement on district nurse prescribing; cross-agency responsibilities for homecare training for patients and their relatives in medicines use and administration; and improvement of access for older people needing to have prescriptions filled. Integrated service redesign took place on a wide front, and there were winners all around.

To conclude

Let me end with another story. A senior public servant goes on holiday to the east coast of England. One day he sits on the cliff top, gazes across the North Sea and falls asleep. He dreams that the Almighty tells him he can have anything he wants. So he asks for a bridge to be built to the Netherlands. 'I was thinking of something a little less ambitious' says the Almighty. The public servant thinks for a while and realises this is a really great opportunity for a big idea. 'Could you bring about the successful integration of health and social care services?' he asks. The Almighty is quick to answer: 'How many lanes do you want on the bridge?'

Organisational integration is a complex matter; but then, complexity *per se* is a pervasive feature of both the natural and the phenomenal worlds. At all organisational levels, in agencies where individuals often have very different perspectives, and organisations have differing working cultures, the use of synergies can play a key part in reordering our approaches to solving human problems.

Acknowledgements

The author would like to recognise the work and insight of his Co-researcher in Project CHAIN, Nicholas Gould of the Welsh Institute for Health and Social Care at the University of Glamorgan, and Angela Jones, who pioneered the role of

Virtual Organisation Coordinator. Marina Roberts engineered the drafts with her usual skill and good humour.[34]

References

1 Aristotle (1998) (Lawson-Tancred H, translator) *The Metaphysics*. Penguin, London.
2 Corning P (1998) The synergism hypothesis – on the concept of synergy and its role in the evolution of complex systems. *Journal of Social and Evolutionary Systems*. 21(2). www.complexsystems.org/publications/synhypo.html.
3 Corning P (1998) The synergism hypothesis – on the concept of synergy and its role in the evolution of complex systems. *Journal of Social and Evolutionary Systems*. 21(3). www.complexsystems.org/publications/synhypo.html.
4 An expression used by the European Union to describe where a region from within a country joins with one or more from other countries to deliver some form of integrated service (not just health services, but perhaps transportation). Euregios often make sense of the historical accidents which befell communities as the result of conflicts and subsequent boundary adjustments.
5 www.nice.org.uk.
6 Warner M (1997) Implementing health care reforms through substitution: implications for the primary care sector. In: Saltman RB and Figueras J. *European Health Care Reforms: analysis of current strategies*. WHO Regional Publications, European Series, No. 72. WHO Regional Office for Europe, Copenhagen.
7 Salthe SN (1985) *Evolving Hierarchical Systems*. Columbia University Press, New York.
8 Hart J (1999) Could an alternative economy and culture originate from health care? In: B Schmacke (ed) *Gesundheit und Demokratie: von der Utopie der Soziale Medizin*. Hans-Ulrich Deppe zum 60 geburtstag. VAS, Frankfurt.
9 Sigerist H (1942) *Bulletin of the History of Medicine*. AAHM, Philadelphia.
10 For a discussion on stakeholder perspectives, *see* Warner MM (2002) A European view. In: M Marinker (ed) *Health Targets in Europe: polity, progress and promise*. BMJ Books, London.
11 Tillich P (1926) *Religiöse Verwirklichung*. Furche Verlag, Berlin.
12 Tillich P (1936) *The Interpretation of History*. Part one trans. by NA Rasetski; parts two, three and four trans. by Elsa L Talmey. New York and London..
13 *See*: www.nice.org.uk: Final appraisal determination – beta-interferon and glatiramer for Multiple Sclerosis, 30 October 2001, which was made final formally on 14 November 2004, when Ministers intervened. (Multiple Sclerosis – beta-interferon and glatiramer acetate (No.32).)
14 Marinker M (2002) *Health Targets in Europe: polity, progress and promise*. BMJ Books, London.
15 Van Herten LM and Gunning-Schepers LJ (2000) Targets as a tool in health policy: guidelines for application. *Health Policy*. 53: 13–23.
16 WHO (1985) *Targets for Health For All*. European Health for All Series No. 1. WHO Regional Office for Europe, Copenhagen.
17 WHO (1991) *Health For All Targets: the health policy for Europe*. WHO Regional Office for Europe, Copenhagen.
18 Najman D (2003) The future of Europe in the light of geopolitical and economical developments. In: K Barnard (ed) *The Future of Health: health of the future*. Fourth European Consultation on Future Trends. The Nuffield Trust on behalf of WHO Europe, London.
19 World Bank (1993) *World Development Report 1993 – Investing in health*. World Bank, Washington DC.
20 Kickbusch I (2004) *The Need for Common Values, Principles and Objectives for Health Policy in a Changing Europe*. Paper presented at the European Health Forum Gastein 2004.

21 Dahlgren G and Whitehead M (1992) *Policies and Strategies to Promote Equity in Health.* WHO Regional Office for Europe, Copenhagen.

22 Hardy B, Mur-Veemanu I, Steenbergen M and Wistow G (1999) Inter-agency services in England and the Netherlands. A comparative study of integrated care development and delivery. *Health Policy.* **48**: 87–105.

23 Aldrich H and Reiss A Jr (1971) Police officers as boundary personnel. In: H Hahn (ed) *Police in Urban Society*: 193–208. Sage, Beverly Hills, CA.

24 Aldrich H and Herker D (1977) Boundary spanning roles and organisation structure. *Academy of Management Review.* **77**(2): 217–30.

25 Aldrich H and Whetten DA (1981) Organization-sets, action sets and networks: making the most of simplicity. In: PC Nystrom and WH Starbuck (eds) *Handbook of Organizational Design. Volume 1: adapting organizations to their environments.* Oxford University Press, New York.

26 Warner M and Gould N (2003) Integrated care networks and quality of life: linking theory and practice. *International Journal of Integrated Care.* **3**. www.ijic.org.

27 Warner M and Gould N (2004) *Virtual Co-ordination: re-framing systems' management.* International Journal of Integrated Care Conference, February 2004, Birmingham, UK.

28 Burt R (1992) *Structural Holes: the social structure of competition.* Harvard University Press, Cambridge, MA.

29 Jones C, Hesterly WS and Borgatti SP (1997) A general theory of network governance: exchange conditions and social mechanisms. *Academy of Management Review* **22**(4): 911–45.

30 Warner M and Gould N (2003) Integrated care networks and quality of life linking theory and practice. *International Journal of Integrated Care.* **3**. www.ijic.org.

31 Warner M and Gould N (2004) *Virtual Co-ordination: re-framing systems' management.* IJIC Integrated Care Conference, Birmingham. WIHSC, Pontypridd.

32 Bowlby J (1953) *Child Care and the Growth of Love.* Pelican Books, London. This is the popular version of Bowlby J (1951) *Maternal Care and Mental Health.* World Health Organization, Geneva.

33 Keller T (2003) Parental images as a guide to leadership sensemaking: an attachment perspective on implicit leadership theories. *The Leadership Quarterly.* **14**: 141–60.

34 Warner M and Gould N (2003) Integrated care networks and quality of life linking theory and practice. *International Journal of Integrated Care.* **3**. www.ijic.org.

Chapter 11

Sustainability

Mihály Kökény

The idea of sustainability emerged in the 1980s in the borderland between ecology and social policy. It has become a very widely used concept today, finding its way into social sciences and even everyday parlance. In 1983 the General Assembly of the United Nations Organization, responding to the environmental crisis threatening the Earth, invited Mrs Gro Harlem Brundtland, then Prime Minister of Norway, to develop a comprehensive programme for change. The Commission she headed made its report in 1987. This seminal document formulated the principles and requirements for sustainable development as follows: 'Development that meets the needs of the present generation without compromising the ability of future generations to meet their own needs.'[1] Five years later at the Earth Summit in Rio de Janeiro[2] 178 countries adopted the declaration which came to be known as Agenda 21. This became the blueprint for UN member states on how to achieve sustainable development.

The Rio Earth Summit, as well as the World Summit on Sustainable Development convened in Johannesburg ten years later, extended the concept of sustainable development to include not only environmental concerns but also quality of life issues, fairness between generations, and social justice. In the decade between the Rio and Johannesburg declarations other world conferences addressed further social issues affecting health: population (Cairo), habitat (Istanbul), social development (Copenhagen), and so on. Important environmental health treaties were signed (for example, the Kyoto Protocol[3]), though their persistent implementation is far from smooth. However, Agenda 21 contains more than 200 references to health, and clearly indicates that sustainable development depends on the role that health will come to play in public thinking, for example as a major consideration in general policy making, or, more specifically, in securing the conditions and infrastructure for the most efficient means of restoring and promoting health.

The term 'sustainable health' first appeared in the literature in the early 1990s.[4] But even before this, since the First International Conference on Health Promotion in Ottawa in 1986 an increasing number of WHO documents have attempted to define the concept and scope of a sustainable health policy.

Accordingly, health policy is considered sustainable if it:

- aims at eliminating socioeconomic factors that have a negative impact on health, and at neutralising other factors detrimental to health;
- is capable of implementing policies in support of health outside the health sector;
- provides responsible and balanced information, enabling people to opt for health;
- offers participation to NGOs and local communities.[5,6]

The above considerations formulate the criteria for a socially acceptable health system, and the conditions for the political sustainability of health policy. However, many political and social developments that have taken place in the last third of the twentieth century have shattered the social models that emerged in Europe following the Second World War. In most European states, irrespective of the method of financing, whether based on the Bismarck or Beveridge or the state-socialist models, access to quasi-free healthcare, with very wide availability, became a generally acquired right. Fundamental values such as justice and equity underpinned these expectations. However, with the advent of technological developments and demographic trends, they became increasingly difficult to satisfy.

In recent years there has been a critical analysis of the relationship between globalisation and health policy. As a result the Charter adopted at the 6th Global Conference on Health Promotion in Bangkok[7] warns that increasing inequalities within and between countries, new patterns of consumption and communi-cation, and the commercialisation and privatisation of health services may all have an adverse effect on health.

One major difficulty is that important issues are often decided at forums such as world trade conferences and security policy institutions, where health promotion experts have hardly any influence and where health policy itself is not even considered. For this reason the participants at the Bangkok Conference urged the promotion of dialogue and cooperation among nation states, civil society and the private sector.

Sustainability as a value and requirement has been increasingly emphasised in many European Union policies. These approach public health issues from the angle of consumer protection, from the perspective of clients, the potential patients with health impairment. The Commission also acknowledges the emer-gence of a 'knowledge-based society' which is capable of radically transforming our living conditions. As a consequence of this, the roles of those constituents hitherto seen as the basis for economic growth – labour, natural resources and financial capital – are on the wane. In their place, the main driving engine of future economic growth is now seen to be the knowledge necessary for innovation, and the educational and training qualifications of the citizenry. This insight is the linchpin of the European Union's Lisbon Strategy.[8]

Consequently there is increasing recognition of the importance of the indi-vidual as 'human capital' in all of the institutionalised creatures of man – the economy, politics and the state. It is also becomes clear that this human capital is at its most efficient, that people can best adapt to changing conditions, that they are best capable of lifelong learning, and can perform at their best, if they are healthy, if health hazards can be minimised. It is in this sense that health is considered to be a driver of economic competitiveness and growth.

The concept of sustainable development has been expanded to specify the requirements necessary for the long-term growth of organisations or socio-economic systems.[9] Such growth is generally based on the following three conditions:

- the organisation or system should not use up its own resources;
- the end- or by-products of the organisation should not have adverse effects (the organisation should not be self-destructive);

- the operational goals of the system should be recognised socially and politically. Society should be prepared to make sacrifices that are needed for the sake of sustainability.

Of course, to meet this last condition, citizens and communities would need to be in possession of appropriate knowledge and information to be able to judge the quality of the system's operation, or at least to be able to have realistic expectations as to its performance.

How are the above criteria in the health sector? In other words, what are the boundary conditions for the sustainable development of health systems?

Supply of resources

The most general, non-systemic, problem is the supply of funds. A basic feature of modern health systems is scarcity. The supply of funds essentially lags behind the opportunities provided by scientific and technological development, and also behind objectively assessed health needs, worldwide. Consequently, the allocation of resources has presented an escalating problem in the health sector. There are many international examples of this mismatch between needs and resources, and it seems that increasing needs cannot be met solely by stepping up funding. To achieve a sustainable health system, this must go hand in hand with limitations on the expenditures side of the equation.

The main political tools for controlling expenditures are:

- defining the package of services that fall within the scope of public finance;
- regulating use, for example by establishing rules for the referral of patients to specialists, creating waiting lists;
- regulating the application of technologies by insisting on 'evidence based' decisions;
- limiting the goods that are to be paid for by public funds;
- improving both technical and allocation efficiency;
- improving the cost-sensitivity of all three actors (the funders, the providers and the users).

Each health system uses these tools in differing combinations, and to differing degrees.

Sustainable development in the health sector is also threatened by problems with the supply of human resources. This is a growing concern. For example, in Hungary until recently there was a problem of oversupply of physicians. Today there is an evident shortage in certain areas and this trend seems to be rising. The serious, and global, nature of the problem is illustrated by the fact that one of the reasons for the shortage in Hungary has been the migration of its own physicians to other EU member states.

There are many reasons for this shortage of human resources in healthcare. The first is the increase in demand for services, explained partly by a real increase in the need for services. The second is that technological advances in healthcare do not lessen the manpower burden, but actually increase the demand for specialist staff. The third and consequent reason is that, in contrast to the provision of funds, human resources cannot be quickly supplied by means of a political decision. Training of adequately qualified and experienced doctors takes six to ten years. The fourth is the problem of keeping people in a health career, motivating them and securing the appropriate material and moral recognition by society.

There is a related problem: the absence of a social consensus about what should be the tasks and capabilities of the health system. Without such consensus, healthcare staff are directly exposed to the public's frustrations with the gap between demand and capabilities. Also there are doubts about the return to society from the considerable costs of lengthy specialist training. How is this return to be measured? How can we optimise the distribution between the various specialists and general practitioners?

Sustainability and health technology

The sustainability of enterprises is threatened by the trend to self-destruction as a consequence of over-production and over-consumption. This appears not to apply to health systems because health, the finished product, is neither harmful nor self-destructive. Nonetheless the development of public health systems can generate such a huge increase in perceived needs and demands that the ability of governments to supply the resources required to create sustainability is jeopardised. For this reason governments must impose certain restraints on the introduction of new technologies. The introduction of new health technologies and services cannot be undertaken without limitation. To do so would be to compromise the ability of governments to supply resources, to threaten political acceptance and support, and to render the system unsustainable.

Another, often less appreciated, problem with new technologies is that their short- and long-term consequences may be expressly detrimental both to the individual and to the community. Examples are the growing resistance to antibiotics because of overuse, and the teratogenic effect of diagnostic and therapeutic applications of radiating energies.

Social and political acceptance

Social and political acceptance of a health system is a fundamental criterion of sustainability. To gain such acceptance the health sector must take account of the profound changes that have occurred in society, and become a modern branch of the service sector, adapted to respond to the needs and expectations of the population. This process is already in progress, such that the previously passive and vulnerable patient emerges as an informed and value-conscious consumer whose safety and quality of care is guaranteed by the mechanisms of consumer protection.

In such a consumerist model, however, the requirements made of the health system have to be realistic and people made aware of the (public financial) consequences of their demands. In other words, the public's high expectations can only be met by government policies when these are linked to greater public, and individual, responsibility and self-sacrifice.

All this necessitates a transformation in public thinking. The impossible (and unfulfilled) myth of a full-fledged free and high quality health service must be abandoned once and for all. Western European market economies seem to be haunted still by the spirit of state socialism. Rapidly increasing needs and expectations are barely, if ever, accompanied by a willingness to pay, almost irrespective of whether payments for health services are made directly by the patient or indirectly through taxation.[10,11]

The state cannot be healthy for anyone. Health and healthcare should not be seen as the sole responsibility of the state. These are responsibilities that must also be shouldered by the individual so that demands remain realistic and the sharing of burdens efficient, with all stakeholders accountable.

Why is sustainability a value in health policy?

In the wake of ever faster advances in medicine and technology, we are left with the old problem of reconciling the technically possible with the economically possible. This is exacerbated everywhere by the inevitable increase in needs resulting from the ageing of societies, and consequently the growing numbers of people with chronic diseases and disabilities requiring long-term care.

The pattern of morbidity has also changed. The familiar infectious diseases have been joined by new and dangerous epidemics. New threats appear (AIDS, SARS, avian influenza), capable of spreading worldwide, and at a pace so far unprecedented, because of the globalisation of trade and transport. There are changes also in the challenges posed by chronic non-infectious diseases.[12] In Sweden, low back pain alone causes more economic damage annually than industrial action. Smoking kills five million people a year. In addition to the depredations of malnutrition, developing countries are faced with the consequence of mass obesity. The number of diabetic patients is expected to double by 2030. Worsening environmental pollution, galloping deterioration of biodiversity, climate change, increasing incidence of diseases related to environmental pollution (allergies, skin cancer, chronic pulmonary diseases, etc.) are all threats be taken into account.

We have also to face the unprecedented scale of mental illness. One in five teenagers in Europe has some kind of mental problem. Among the ageing population diseases leading to dementia are expected to increase. Unemployment, work-related stress, alcoholism, abuse of illicit drugs, different forms of violence and accidents also constitute health hazards. Further, local wars and ethnic and religious fanaticism constitute major threats to health. All these changes in the structure of health impairment reflect the social, political and economic processes that are taking place all over the world.

It is beyond question that the task of finding solutions to these emerging health problems is far beyond the competence and capabilities of the health system alone. This is a task and duty for the state and society as a whole, indeed it is also an overarching international task. The Ottawa Charter pointed out that 'the prerequisites and prospects for health cannot be ensured by the health sector alone'. The promotion of health calls for a multi-sectoral health policy. Health is a depiction of the age; the health status of a society is an imprint of a given period. The challenge is to ensure the sustainability of our endeavours.

Expectations, demands and needs

It is important to keep in mind the differences between the parts played by public expectations and individual demands on the one hand, and the professional estimation of need on the other. By 'demand' here I refer to the unregulated use of services, to the widest choice of which services to use, and to free access to goods and services not proven to have a positive influence on health outcome. Examples would include the wish for an attractive room in a private hospital; having a test or intervention carried out at the facility of the patient's choice; fast access to interventions not classified as urgent from the medical point of view; access to procedures or medicines where there is no proven relationship between the costs and expected benefit – for example the use of PET-CT for screening. The overall reinforcement of consumerism in our societies and culture makes certain that, whatever the professional and political estimations of need, public demands can confidently be expected to grow.

Citizens ought to be happy to have their legitimate needs met. Differences between individual demands and professionally assessed needs are bound to lead to dissatisfaction, even in situations where the technical quality and benefits of services is uncontested. But often the problem of dissatisfaction is rooted in the failure of politicians to make citizens realise that, given the inevitable limits of funding, no health system is able to meet all demands.

This problem of disparity between public and individual wants, and governmental beliefs about 'legitimate needs' is exacerbated by the competition induced by globalisation, and by a period of global recession being keenly experienced by many European states. Inevitably this will put strains on the availability of public funds which are further exacerbated by the changing age pyramid, the increasing disparity between society's dependants requiring increasingly expensive services, and the falling number of tax and social security contribution payers.

In the late twentieth and early twenty-first centuries the traditional values of health systems underwent rapid change. It became more and more evident that, given the limits of public funding, the previously indivisible three key desiderata – comprehensive services, equal access to them, and good quality – compete with one another. Any one of these could only be maximised at the expense of another. The result was a general crisis in health systems. And this is why the question of sustainability and, in the interest of sustainability, efficiency and cost control, have been put on the agenda in almost every country.

Throughout Europe, health reforms propose the imposition of governmental controls on the consumption of health services and goods. This involves considerable political risk. Differences in the direction of particular reforms depend on the person undertaking the task of limiting the availability of services and goods, the tools to be used for achieving this, and on the nature of the groups targeted for these limitations – both providers and patients.

One typical solution to the demand/need conundrum that has been gaining ground is cost sharing. Increasingly patients are expected to contribute from their own resources to the cost of services and goods provided by social security services. Germany and Slovakia have chosen this course. However, this solution is a double-edged sword. While co-payment certainly curbs the use of services, it does so selectively on the grounds of income. Since poverty and sickness generally go hand in hand, the most vulnerable may therefore be blocked from the accessing the services they need. Even so, systems of co-payment are worth considering, provided always that they can be coupled with targeted compensation mechanisms and incentives to promote additional personal health insurance or personal savings.

A second solution proposed to deal with the demand/need/public funds problem has been to improve the efficiency of health systems by encouraging competition between different insurance companies. This approach, however, has not justified the high hopes reposed in it. The benefits have not materialised, for a number of reasons. The complex, multi-actor systems generate unexpectedly high operating costs, and there is the moral hazard of risk-based selection of patients and communities, so that social solidarity and the sense of a 'national risk community' is weakened. Today the multiple insurance company model survives in Europe (for example, in the Netherlands, Germany and the Czech Republic), but largely as a historical tradition characterised by a dwindling number of actors, convergence of companies, and concentration in smaller numbers of larger outfits.

A third approach consists of systems based on providers' cost-sensitivity, where efficiency is improved through both the supply and demand sides. Its main tool is the provision of incentives to providers. The model emerged in the United States – Health Maintenance Organisations (HMOs and other managed care programmes), and in later in England – General Practice Fund Holding. A similar approach seems to be developing in Spain, Austria and Hungary.[13,14]

The essence of this model is that health providers create organisations in geographic areas, either on a voluntary basis or by force of statutory provisions, and aim to be cost-effective by rationalising patient pathways. In return they are free to use any savings made for further service development and to provide staff incentives.

The responsibility of policy makers

It is a perennial problem in democracies that when a new government comes into power, the reforms of the previous administration are swept away or actually reversed. This can produce turmoil both for the health system and for the public. Therefore, in attempting reform, the difficult aim must be to gain the support of public opinion of as many as possible of the professional actors, and, as was the case in Germany in 2003, by building a political consensus beyond the governing majority.

Whatever the social system, people still largely seem to foster the deep-rooted belief that the state has virtually unlimited responsibility to provide health services, and that users have virtually unlimited rights and choices. Also, in many European countries citizens appear to have a vested interest in getting out of their obligation to contribute to common financing, and so to fulfilling their common responsibilities.

When we need to use health services, everybody expects to receive the most and best. The rules of our systems are often 'soft' and permit an ill-defined level of demand. A distribution mechanism which is not based on social responsibility creates its own inequities. Patients may be offered health services of indifferent quality not only because of an uneven distribution of capacities, but because the more socially powerful the patients, the more easily they will find their way, sometimes through semi-legal channels, to 'privileged handling' and the best services available. It is the responsibility of the policy makers to change all this, however delicate the issues, however unpopular it may be to argue in favour of reforms, and however hard it is to persist even when difficult action will only bear fruit in the long term.

Policy makers are unwilling to take steps in an unstable force field full of uncertainties. It is a great deal to ask for courageous policies when the appropriate actions involve political risk. Consequently Members of Parliament in the party of government can court popularity, and secure their re-election, by inaugurating hi-tech diagnostic laboratories, which are political rather than health priorities. And those in opposition parties can score points by soapbox rhetoric, obstructing the difficult and unpopular reforms which they know full well are much needed. Civil society and its advocates must become stronger, they must seek political pacts that can bring about substantive reform in health policy.

Health goods are not private goods, they are not just goods in the market-place. People's health is not a private affair. A strong and competitive society should consist of individuals who are able and willing to maintain their health, and are willing to use the services provided by the health system in a reasonable fashion. In this sense, health is a public domain, though not solely a public responsibility.

Modern health policy relies on the principle of responsible partnership. There is no social or national responsibility detached from individual responsibility. People who are not willing to undertake responsibility for themselves, their families and institutions, cannot constitute a responsible society. If we reject the idea of individual responsibility in the matter of health, we perpetuate a state socialism mentality. I believe it was Ralf Dahrendorf who said that change in the political system could be carried out in six months, and in the economy in six years, but that the public mentality will not change for sixty.

Sustainable development relies on two preconditions. Firstly, the adaptability of the health system to rapidly changing needs and expectations, emerging technologies and increasing patient mobility. Secondly, the transformation of the public's attitude to a publicly provided service.

References

1 World Commission on Environment and Development (1987) *Our Common Future.* Oxford University Press, Oxford.
2 United Nations (1993) *Earth Summit – Agenda 21.* UN Department of Public Information, New York.
3 (1997) *Kyoto Protocol to the United Nations Framework Convention On Climate Change.* Available from: http://unfccc.int/resource/docs/convkp/kpeng.html.
4 King M (1990) Health is a sustainable state. *Lancet.* **336**: 664–7.
5 (1986) *The Ottawa Charter for Health Promotion.* Available from: www.who.int/health promotion/conferences/previous/ottawa/en/index.html.
6 (1998) *HEALTH21: the health for all policy framework for the WHO European Region.* WHO Regional Office for Europe, Copenhagen. (European Health for All Series, No. 6.) Available from: www.who.dk/document/health21/wa540ga199heeng.pdf.
7 (2005) *The Bangkok Charter for Health Promotion in a Globalized World.* Available from: www.who.int/entity/healthpromotion/conferences/6gchp/bangkok_charter/en.
8 Byrne D (2004) *Enabling Good Health for All. A reflection process for a new EU Health Strategy.* 15 July 2004. Available from: http://europa.eu.int/comm/health/ph_overview/Documents/byrne_reflection_en.pdf.

 9 Kincses G (2005) Sustainable development and health care. *Egészségügyi Gazdasági Szemle.* **43**(5): 5–8.

10 Anton S. *et al.* (2005) Exploring possibilities for consumer choice in German health care system. *Eurohealth.* **11**(1): 14–18.

11 Schut FT, Gress S and Wasem J (2003) Consumer price sensitivity and social health insurer choice in Germany and the Netherlands. *International Journal of Health Care Finance and Economics.* **3**: 117–38.

12 Kickbusch I (2004) The Leawell lecture – The end of public health as we know it: constructing global health in the 21st century. *Promotion & Education.* **XI**(4): 206–11.

13 Fairfield G *et al.* (1997) Managed care: origins, principles and evolution. *BMJ.* **314**: 1823.

14 Lagoe R, Aspling DL and Westert GP (2005) Current and future developments in managed care in the United States and implications for Europe. *Health Research Policy and Systems.* **3**: 4.

Chapter 12

Interdependence

Graham Lister

'With globalisation, a single microbial sea washes all of humankind. There are no health sanctuaries.' So said Dr Gro Harlem Brundtland[1] in her 2000 Reith Lecture. International travel enables not only microbes to cross borders but also scarce health workers. The aeroplanes that carry them exemplify the threat posed by global warming and pollution. While in the first class cabin the executives of global corporations may be seen as vectors of health and disease, bringing employment, increased prosperity and health but also working conditions, products and lifestyles with profound impacts on non-communicable disease. The poor farmer looking up at their vapour trails, unable to afford medicines for her family because she cannot compete in highly subsidised agricultural markets, reminds us of the impact of trade policy on the determinants of health.

This chapter examines different perspectives that shape our understanding of the value of the interdependence of global health – as a threat to national interests and security, as a basic human right, as a global public good and as a product of globalisation. In each case the implications for international policy and action are explored by means of a specific country case study. The case studies examine how the value of interdependence in global health can be reconciled with other elements of aid, trade and foreign policy as well as other values for health.

Global health as a threat to national interests and security

International efforts to address global health in the nineteenth century, dating from the first international sanitary conference of 1851, attempted to address the threat to the health and trade of rich countries[2] posed by the spread of epidemics of cholera and yellow fever. It seems that the scope for action on such issues was limited by a fear that they could become impediments to trade, a view that was later reflected in debate at the World Trade Organization (see below).

The concept of global health being centred on the threat of infectious disease also found a later echo in the 1997 report of the American Institute of Medicine on global health, subtitled 'Protecting our People, Enhancing our Economy and Advancing our International Interests'.[3] This report influenced thinking in both Clinton and Bush Administrations. It led to the elaboration of global health issues in US foreign policy and a redefinition of national security issues to include global health threats.

At international level, HIV/AIDS has become a core issue for the UN Security Council and an issue of 'hemispheric security' for the Americas.[4] In Africa, three heads of state have commented that HIV/AIDS threatens to make their countries ungovernable. David Feachem has noted that failure to halt the spread of the pandemic in the Indian subcontinent could have massive implications for the stability of the region.[5] David Fidler describes how the positioning of global health as a threat to national interests and security has raised it to 'high policy' status in US international relations.[6]

The frank recognition of the importance of global health to national interests and security was clearly a factor in increasing US government commitment to international aid. It resulted in an increase in expenditure on official development assistance (ODA) from 0.11% to 0.16% of gross national product (GNP) between 2001 and 2005 with the highest rate of increase in health-related aid. US ODA rose to $19 billion in 2004, of which some 35% was directed to low-income countries; the amount allocated to health is believed to have risen from less than 5% to over 8%.[7] It was also a factor in the increase in private US philanthropic aid, which is estimated at some $14 billion in 2002, excluding personal remittances and scholarships.[8]

Emphasis on the threat posed by infectious diseases has resulted in increased investment in disease-specific programmes, such as HIV/AIDS prevention and treatment; tuberculosis treatment, including measures to counter the spread of multi-drug-resistant strains; the eradication of polio; and measures to monitor and control influenza (including avian flu) and new and re-emergent diseases such as SARS. All of these are diseases posing a direct threat to health in OECD countries. When the Global Fund was established, its remit was extended to include not only HIV/AIDS and TB but also malaria, perhaps to ensure that the interests of donor countries were not seen to predominate over the needs of the recipients.

Disease-based vertical programmes are claimed to be more effective in counter-ing specific threats, because they make it possible to develop and apply systematic approaches and resources through partnership between government, voluntary and private sector. The disadvantage of such programmes is that they can impose high coordination costs on recipient health ministries and may divert doctors and other resources from basic health services.

US policies towards global health also reflect national self-interests and security in other ways. The Millennium Development Account is a mechanism to link general budgetary support aid to the performance of recipient countries in respect of measures of 'ruling justly', 'investing in people' and 'economic freedom'. The President's Emergency Plan for AIDS Relief (PEPFAR) reflects US values in its focus on faith-based organisations and the ABC approach (abstinence, be faithful, use a condom). PEPFAR has also insisted on the use of US patented anti-retroviral medicines rather than cheaper generic versions. US health aid is constrained by the so called 'gag rule' that prohibits funding of any organisation that performs abortions or advocates for the liberalisation of abortion laws in other countries.

There has also been an increasing focus on the importance of aid, particularly health aid, in projecting what has been described, in reference to US foreign policy, as 'soft power' – the ability to influence people's thinking and perception to want the things you want.[9] Thus US aid is now made more apparent to recipients and more prominent in international meetings. For example, while the US provides far less health aid than the EU and its member states, it appears to dominate and lead action against HIV/AIDS and other aspects of international health aid, both by the positioning of President Bush, and by the role played by American philanthropists Bill and Melinda Gates.

Health as a human right

The UN Charter declaration of human rights of 1948 refers to the right to a standard of living adequate for health and wellbeing, and a universal right to life. However, the preamble to the World Health Organization constitution, prepared at the same time, states that: 'The enjoyment of the highest attainable standard of health is one of the fundamental rights of every human being.' The interpretation of this value depends on the perspective of the commentator. Many refer to health as a human right, reflecting the principle of solidarity which is the basis for healthcare systems in most countries. Where access to healthcare is not universal within the national system, as in the US, this may be less obvious.

The acceptance of health as a human right implies a value of solidarity not only between members of national communities but as an element of global citizenship that people should be able to demand from their governments and from the international community. As Kofi Annan has stated, 'It is my aspiration that health will finally be seen not as a blessing to be wished for but as a human right to be fought for.'

In practice, commitment to this value seems limited; even within the European Region of WHO, life expectancy varies by more than 15 years and annual expenditure on health ranges from $3500 per capita in Switzerland, to less than $50 per head in Tajikistan.[10] Global comparisons are even more stark, with life expectancy varying from 80 years in Sweden to 45 years in Uganda. G7 countries spend an average of $2400 per capita on health, whereas low-income countries spend $18 per capita on average.[11]

The Millennium Development Goals can be seen as a statement of compromise on the value of health and other human rights. They set goals with respect to poverty, education and health which were designed to reduce but not eliminate some of the worst deficits in human rights. These targets were intended to be affordable within the resources committed to aid. It was signed by 189 countries of the United Nations and included the following clause: 'We urge developed countries that have not done so to make concrete efforts towards the target of 0.7% of gross national product (GNP) as official development assistance (ODA) to developing countries . . .'

The target for ODA was set in 1970 following the Pearson Commission Report, with the intention of achieving total flows of assistance to developing countries of 1% of GNP, of which ODA would contribute 0.7%. This compares with expenditure on ODA in 2004 of 0.36% of GDP for the EU and 0.16% for the US. Over the 35 years in which this target has been adopted, expenditure on aid rose in real terms over the first 15 years, then reduced for the next 15 and is now once more increasing in real terms, to some extent reflecting increases in expenditure in health. The proportion of aid devoted to health has risen rapidly, from less than 5% in 2000[12] to 9% of total aid of $78.6 billion in 2004.[13]

The Commission on Macroeconomics and Health (CMH) of 2001 identified a 'set of essential interventions' for basic health at a cost of $34 per capita, to be funded from a combination of aid and local funding, enabled by debt reduction programmes.[14] This compares with the WHO 2002 estimate of per capita health spend of $18 per capita (44 per cent being out-of-pocket expenses) in low-income countries. The specific target for health aid indicated by the CMH was to achieve annual flows of $27 billion by 2007, rising to $38 billion by 2015. This compares with the current total ODA for health of around $6 billion.

Jeffrey Sachs has pointed out that in comparison with military expenditure the sums required to address global health issues are minor, while the benefits are immense.[15] Nevertheless it is now clear that both the essential interventions identified by the CMH and the 'affordable' MDG targets are likely to be grossly underfunded. At the 'Making Globalisation Work for All' conference in February 2004, the UK Chancellor Gordon Brown said, 'With the prevailing air of apathy many of the [MDG] goals are unlikely to be met within the next 100 years, let alone by the planned date of 2015.' Goals that are least likely to be met are those relating to health in Africa, to reduce child mortality by two-thirds, reduce maternal mortality by three-quarters, and to halt the spread of HIV/AIDS, malaria and tuberculosis.[16]

Since the 2002 International Development Act, virtually all UK ODA must be provided for the purpose of either furthering sustainable development or promoting the welfare of people in a way that is likely to contribute to the reduction of poverty. ODA includes bilateral and multilateral aid and debt relief. Health is seen as a key to improving life chances and hence achieving poverty reduction as a human rights issue. Total UK ODA in 2004 is estimated at $7.8 billion, of which 43% is multilateral aid and 55% is bilateral. Health aid has increased as a percentage of total UK bilateral ODA from 11.4% in 1996/7 to 16.5% in 2003/4. At the same time, most aspects of poverty reduction also lead to health improvements through better education, safe water, improved nutrition and employment opportunities. The main operational policies for UK ODA have been to provide general budgetary support and debt relief to the poorest countries. Currently 80% of UK bilateral aid goes to low-income countries.

Health as a global public good

The concept of global public goods as those which affect all countries and regions, which may have intergenerational impacts, which all may share and from which none can be excluded, was first mooted by Inge Kaul[17] in 1999, though its origins in the discussion of public goods can be traced back to the 1950s. Specific health measures which may be regarded as global public goods, applying a narrow definition of the term, include: shared health research knowledge, surveillance for diseases, measures to prevent, control and eliminate global diseases, and measures to reduce or counter global pollution and climate change.

Ilona Kickbusch applies a broader interpretation of health as a global public good, seeing common commitment to health as defining values of global citizenship and global governance.[18] Strengthened global governance for health is seen as key to global health security and international justice for health. It requires new forms of international funding and greater capacity at WHO and elsewhere to identify health threats, including the health impacts of actions by governments or international corporations, and to intervene to protect global health goods and rights. This in turn requires that health should be a key social responsibility of governments and business, backed by international charter. These measures would underpin the health rights of global citizens in a globalising world.

International financing of global goods is a crucial first step towards this vision. The options for international financing include the issuance of special drawing rights by the International Monetary Fund, carbon taxes and the so called Tobin Tax proposal for taxation of the international movement of finance.[19] As yet, there has been no international commitment to the adoption of any of these measures.

Perhaps the country which best exemplifies the values of global health as a global public good is the Netherlands. In 2004, Netherlands ODA amounted to $4.2 billion, which was 0.8% of GNP. They have a longstanding commitment to sustainable development and poverty alleviation and were the first country to meet the 20/20 Commitment agreed at the World Summit for Social Development, held in Copenhagen in March 1995, which agreed to match developing country spending of 20% of government budget on social services with a matching 20% of aid. Some 55% of ODA is directed to low-income countries and 73% is bilateral, 27% multilateral. They are a supporter of UN bodies in providing un-earmarked funding for their operations. Human rights are also strongly embedded in Dutch development assistance with clear rules that prohibit funding for countries which breach human rights.

In recent years, Dutch bilateral ODA has been targeted at and monitored against the achievement of the MDGs. ODA is coordinated by the Netherlands Ministry of Foreign Affairs, under one budget head known as the Homogeneous Budget for International Cooperation.

The aid implementation agency 'Netherlands Development Assistance' works in cooperation with other ministries, institutes and partnerships. For example, the HIV/AIDS programme is jointly managed by the Ministry of Heath, Welfare and Sport (VWS) and the Dutch AIDS Fund. VWS has its own International Affairs Directorate within which is a department responsible for global health issues.

Alongside these commitments the Netherlands has played a major role in programmes of research and support on global health issues, through its research and training institutes, and particularly in respect of tuberculosis control and treatment. A conference on global health issues held by the VWS in December 2003 recognised that there are many reasons for supporting action on global health. While not detracting from the focus on the MDGs, there are also good reasons to work on public health measures with Eastern European countries, since these are seen as the health defences – 'the health polders' – for the Netherlands and Europe.

It is also recognised as politically important to build social and cultural links with countries that have substantial voting rights in the new EU. Moreover it is recognised that these countries produce an excess of clinical staff, who could be valuable to the Netherlands, which suffers from medical staff shortages. Recruitment of nurses to the Netherlands from poorer countries has led to public criticism of the damage this does to health in the countries from which staff are taken.[20] For these reasons the Netherlands has led more EU and bilateral assistance programmes with EU accession states than any other country.

Global health impacts of globalisation

The conceptual framework for the analysis of the impacts of globalisation on global health was put forward by Kelley Lee in 1998.[21] This examines the processes that are intensifying human interaction, reducing the barriers of time, space and ideas which have separated people and nations in a number of spheres of action including economic, environmental, social and cultural, knowledge and technology, and political and institutional, each of which has a profound impact on health.

These interdependencies were identified and explored in the Nuffield Trust programme 'Global Health: a local issue'.[22] Even within a single field of action the impact of globalisation was found to be complex. Thus, while economic globalisation can bring employment, greater prosperity and health, it may also result in the weakening of workplace health and environmental controls as countries compete in a 'race to the bottom' to attract investment.[23] It largely results in the creation of employment for women, who, without further support, may suffer a double burden as wage earners and the main resource for family health and care.[24]

The price of entry to global markets, demanded by the General Agreement on Trade and Services (GATS) and the World Trade Organization (WTO), was particularly high for the health sector. Liberalisation of trade has opened healthcare markets to the privatisation of profitable sectors, resulting in an undermining of state health systems by the drain on resources and personnel both to the private sector and to other countries.[25] Some countries lost 90% of locally trained doctors to international migration;[26] almost 5000 doctors were recruited to the UK in 2000/1 from non-EU countries. The Trade Related International Property Rights Agreement (TRIPs) required the observation of international patents, which threatened to make some drugs unaffordable.[27] When economic problems hit, the price of assistance from the International Monetary Fund (IMF) also fell heavily on health services through imposed limitations on public spending.[28]

Internationalisation of local markets has exposed developing countries to a wide range of lifestyle, smoking, alcohol and diet-related non-communicable diseases, including diabetes, heart disease, and lung and bowel cancer.[29] Furthermore, the conflicting demands of different cultural influences may have been a factor in the rapid growth of mental illness.

Many middle-income countries have felt that the economic benefits of globalisation have outweighed the health costs, and globalisation remains a highly valued principle for many such countries.[30] However, the poorest countries have experienced costs, in terms of increased environmental damage and extreme weather conditions, rapid increases in non-communicable disease, and migration of health workers, but have had little or no economic benefit. The exclusion of agriculture from trade liberalisation meant that they were unable to compete in international markets and their farmers could be impoverished by the importation of subsidised produce from rich countries. It is estimated that agricultural subsidies amount to some $300 billion per year and restrict world economic growth by about $500 billion,[31] creating economic losses to developing country producers of approximately one-third of this level – twice the level of aid to developing countries.

A more exhaustive analysis of models of the consequences of globalisation for global health is provided by Ronald Labonte and Renee Torgeson.[32]

UK policies for development recognised the complex interdependence of globalisation and the determinants of global poverty and health in the White Paper launched in 2000, 'Making Globalisation Work for the Poor'.[33] This committed the UK government to action on issues such as: reducing agricultural subsidies; increasing access to essential medicines; improving information to consumers about environmental and working conditions; supporting the development of global civil society; and ensuring that poverty reduction programmes were environmentally sustainable.

Since 2000 the UK government has taken a wide range of policy initiatives and leadership actions which reflect this broad-based approach. These include a leading role in the Doha trade round negotiations and G8 summits, to broker agreement on revision to TRIPs to improve access to essential medicine,[34] to address the unfairness of agricultural subsidies,[35] to achieve international agreement to increase debt relief and aid,[36] and to develop comprehensive proposals to address the problems of development in Africa.[37] The aim of increasing aid to achieve the UN target of 0.7% of GNP by 2013 was announced in 2004.

A broad-based evaluation of the contribution of OECD countries to development is provided by the 2004 Commitment to Development Index prepared by the Center for Global Development.[38] This index scores seven factors: aid, trade, investment, migration, environment, security and technology. A score derived from these factors shows that in 2005 the UK was rated tenth in relation to 21 OECD countries, due to low scores in respect of security and migration.

Specific actions on global health include an international programme on HIV/ AIDS, which was launched in 2004 as a cross-government, cross-sector initiative[39] led by the Department for International Development (DfID). Action to limit direct overseas recruitment from vulnerable countries was announced by the Department of Health (DH) in 2001; however, the effectiveness of this measure has been questioned since it applies only to direct recruitment to the NHS.[40] The DH sponsors the Health Protection Agency, which in 2004 developed a strategy to support international health (through its laboratory and advisory services). DH also put forward measures to assist NHS Trusts to form twinning relationships and exchange staff and know-how with developing countries. The Department of Health is preparing a UK strategy to support global health, the US already has such a strategy and Switzerland is producing its own national strategy for global health.

Treasury-supported actions for global health include tax relief for drug donation programmes, and tax incentives to promote research and development on diseases predominantly affecting developing countries,[41] oriented towards research on vaccines. The International Finance Facility and an Advanced Purchase Fund for medicines have both been launched in 2005 as pilot programmes. In addition, Gordon Brown as Chair of the Finance Committee of the IMF has made recommendations to increase aid funding, write off debt and mitigate the impact of IMF restrictions on public sector spending for indebted countries.

Understanding of interdependence as a value for global health

Clare Short, the former UK Secretary of State for International Development, drew parallels between the emergence of the welfare state, in response to the industrial revolution, and the need to establish global governance to respond to globalisation. The agenda for the necessary reinvention of public health to develop global governance was set out by Ilona Kickbusch in her keynote speech to the World Federation of Public Health Associations conference in 2004.[42]

This transition requires a careful re-examination of the values that guide health governance, to ensure they are fit for this new purpose. The Madrid Framework[43] explores the values in health policy, the tensions between them, and their resonance with current and future health policy.

The juxtaposition of health values and current policy makes it possible to question the tension between some of the Dimensions of the Framework. As examples, how much is the health and wellbeing of others valued in relation to self-interest or expenditure on our own health? What are the limits to equity and social justice when considering other people's health? How much democracy is there in the international institutions that govern our globalising world? These are uncomfortable questions.

This chapter has explored the dimension of interdependence, first in relation to self-interest – the realisation that global health cannot be separated from protection of 'homeland' health security. It considers where such an approach may lead by way of a case study of US global health policy. Although we may find the notion of interdependence in global health stemming from a common human right more appealing, a case study shows how limited action has been in response to this approach. Consideration of health as a shared global good is also attractive, and the case study of the Netherlands suggests that it can encompass both acceptance of the human rights of others and recognition of local health interests. Finally the interdependencies of global health in a globalising world were explored with a further UK case study. The lesson here seems to be that such a perspective requires us to rethink the boundaries of global health governance, to understand that the engagement of the whole of government and whole of society is essential to match the scale and complexity of this challenge. Even so, it is clear that many of the implications for action point us beyond national government to international institutions.

The conclusion for action is that a strategy for global health is required at European Union level, that it should give practical expression to values for health, and that it should encompass a 'whole of society' approach.

References

1 Bruntland GH (2000) *Respect for the Earth: health and population.* Reith Lecture, BBC, London.
2 Loughlin K and Berridge V (2002) *Global Health Governance: historical dimensions of global governance.* Centre on Global Change and Health LSHTM and WHO, Geneva.
3 Institute of Medicine (1997) *America's Vital Interest in Global Health: protecting our people, enhancing our economy, and advancing our international interests.* Institute of Medicine, Washington.
4 Panisset U (2002) *Health and Hemispheric Security.* PAHO, WHO, Geneva.
5 Russell S (2004) AIDS In India – Unanswered Questions – Epidemic imperils the future – Nation could face Africa-like disaster. *San Francisco Chronicle.* 8 July 2004.
6 Fidler D (2004) Germs, norms and power: global health's political revolution. *Law, Social Justice & Global Development Journal (LGD).* (On-line journal.)
7 Shah A (2005) The US and foreign aid assistance: sustainable development. *Global Issues.* 20 August 2005.

8 Adelman C (2002) Aid and comfort. *Tech Central Station*. 21 August 2002. www.tcsdaily. com/article.aspx?id=082102N

9 Nye J (2005) Soft power: the means to success in world politics. *Public Affairs*. **June**.

10 WHO (2002) *Core Health Indicators: per capita total expenditure on health in international dollars*. WHO, Geneva.

11 Labonte R, Schrecker T, Sanders D and Meeus W (2004) *Fatal Indifference: the G8, Africa, and global health*. University of Cape Town Press/IDRC, Cape Town.

12 Labonte R, Schrecker T, Sanders D and Meeus W (2004) *Fatal Indifference: the G8, Africa, and global health*. University of Cape Town Press/IDRC.

13 Fisher H (2005) Official Development Assistance increases further – but 2006 targets still a challenge. OECD Press release 11 April 2005.

14 Commission on Macroeconomics and Health (2001) *Macroeconomics and Health: investing in health for economic development*. WHO, Geneva.

15 Sachs JD (2003) *Achieving the Millennium Development Goals: health in the developing world*. Speech at the Second Global Consultation of the Commission on Macroeconomics and Health. Geneva, 29 October 2003.

16 Department for International Development (2004) *DfID Annual Report 2003*. HMSO, London.

17 Kaul I, Grunberg I and Stern MA (1999) Defining global public goods. In: I Kaul, I Grunberg and MA Stern (eds) *Global Public Goods: international cooperation in the 21st century*. Oxford University Press, New York.

18 Kickbusch I (2004) *The End of Public Health As We Know It: constructing global health in the 21st century*. Keynote speech WFPHA 10th Annual Conference Brighton.

19 Ukabiala J (2001) Can the financing gap be closed? UN panel suggests new international taxes to help fund development. *Africa Recovery*. **15**(4): 22.

20 Tjadens F (2002) Health care shortages: where globalisation, nurses and migration meet. *EuroHealth*. **8**(3): 33–6.

21 Lee K (1998) *Globalisation and Health Policy: a review of the literature and proposed research and policy agenda*. London School of Hygiene and Tropical Medicine, London.

22 Parsons L and Lister G (1999) *Global Health: a local issue*. The Nuffield Trust, London.

23 Greider W, Nader R (ed) and Atwood ME (1993) *The Case Against Free Trade: GATT, NAFTA, and the globalization of corporate power*. Earth Island Press, San Francisco.

24 Pande A (2003) *Nimble Fingers, Tired Bodies*. Nuffield Trust, London. www.ukglobal health.org/Default.aspx?textID=543&cSectionID=6

25 Woodward D (2003) *Trading Health for Profit: the implications of the GATS and trade in health services for health in developing countries*. Nuffield Trust, UK Partnership for Global Health, London. www.ukglobalhealth.org/Default.aspx?textID=512

26 Buchan J and Dovlo D (2004) *International Recruitment of Health Workers to the UK: a report for DfID*. DfID Resource Centre, London.

27 Commission on Intellectual Property Rights (2002) *Integrating Intellectual Property Rights and Development Policy*. Commission on Intellectual Property Rights, London.

28 Stiglitz J (2002) *Globalization and its Discontents*. WW Norton, New York.

29 Yach D and Puska P (2002) *Globalization, Diets and Noncommunicable Diseases*. WHO, Geneva.

30 Dollar D (2003) The poor like globalization. *YaleGlobal*. 23 June 2003.

31 HM Treasury (2004) *Trade and the Global Economy: the role of international trade in productivity, economic reform and growth*. HMSO, London.

32 Labonte R and Torgeson R (2003) *Frameworks for Analysing the Links between Globalization and Health*. WHO, Geneva.

33 DfID (2000) *Eliminating Poverty: making globalisation work for the poor*. The Stationery Office, London.

34 DfID (2002) *Access to Essential Medicines: report to the Prime Minister*. HMSO, London.

35 DfID (2004) *Working Group Report to the Prime Minister on Increasing Access to Essential Medicines in the Developing World: UK Government plans and actions*. HMSO, London.

36 HMT and DfID (2003) *International Finance Facility*. HMSO, London.

37 Commission for Africa (2005) *Report*. Office of the Prime Minister, London.

38 Center for Global Development (2005) *Ranking the Rich: the 2004 Commitment to Global Development Index*. Center for Global Development, Washington. www.cgdev.org/section/initiatives/_active/cdi

39 DfID (2004) *Taking Action: the UK's strategy for tackling HIV and AIDS in the developing world*. HMSO, London.

40 Buchan J and Dovlo D (2004) *International Recruitment of Health Workers to the UK: a report for DFID*. DFID Resource Centre, London.

41 HM Treasury (2001) *Budget Report 2001*. HMSO, London.

42 Kickbusch I (2004) *The End of Public Health As We Know It: constructing global health in the 21st century*. Keynote speech, WFPHA 10th Annual Conference, Brighton.

43 Marinker M (2004) *The Madrid Framework of Health Policy and Governance*. Paper presented at the European Health Forum Gastein.

Chapter 13

Creativity

Miquel Porta

According to the wine and food magazine *Wine Spectator*, the Catalan chef Ferran Adrià 'is changing the way the world thinks about dining'.[1] Quite a claim! 'His exquisite and provocative dishes are technical marvels, visual works of art, as rich with humour and cultural references as they are with exotic ingredients and shocking flavours. Adrià invented ethereal foams and other ''states of matter'' flavoured with fruits, vegetables, wood smoke. Liquids are hot on top, cold on the bottom. A cold powder dissolves in chicken broth and adds the earthy flavour of foie gras.' In his workshop *El Taller* ('not a restaurant, neither just a laboratory') Adrià asserts: 'We take advantage of technology, but the most important tools are our imaginations and our palates.' This is not that far from health policy making . . .

Ferran Adrià puts the effort in context. 'Nouvelle cuisine was creative. My approach is to investigate. It's not the same. This takes a team, equipment, money, time. We have one rule here. It has to be new. It may be good, but not if we've done it before.'

Let us look at Box 13.1. As in public health, so in today's cooking, it seems that very little can be invented. Yet doesn't what Adrià does seem much closer to the tasks of public health than one would at first expect?

Box 13.1 As in public health, in today's cooking very little can be invented, but . . .

Adrià is now working with a powdered form of cellulose. He's blending it with water and varying amounts of sugar, trying to make a 'creamless cream'. He bakes it, steams it, microwaves it, just to see what happens. The chemist is writing down the proportions, keeping track of the results. They like it when it has the consistency of a meringue. Ferran sticks a spoon into it, tastes. 'We're tasting for texture,' he explains. The cellulose cream is one of half a dozen experiments in progress this day. The chefs keep track of their ideas in thick notebooks. The atmosphere seems relaxed, but the chefs are relentless in their pursuit of new ideas. 'Talk is easy,' a colleague adds. 'Doing is hard. That's why we're here working like crazy people. Sometimes weeks go by and nothing comes. We think we're idiots. Then we stumble on something like the hot gelatines. And it's all worth it.'

Ferran estimates that from 5000 experiments at *El Taller*, the team might create some 500 dishes, which will then be distilled into the 25 to 50 dishes that will make up the year's core degustation menu at their restaurant, *El Bulli*.

This may all sound far too stylish or pretentious to you, but, believe me, I've eaten at *El Bulli* a few times, and these descriptions are not exaggerations. The following dishes illustrate what creativity may do to something as commonplace as food.

'Gin fizz frozen caliente' has the citrus tang and juniper snap of the traditional cocktail; but it's also a study in contrasts: a warm, sweet foam sits atop cold, tart juice. Taste buds snap to attention.

'Golden egg': a mysterious appearance, then the shock of the contrasts – crunchy/liquid, cold/warm, sweet/salty. There is technical breakthrough here, allowing the caramel to envelop the raw egg and cook it, just enough, inside the crunchy wrapper. There is humour, the play of ideas – the egg in its candy 'shell'. And there is the element of didacticism.

'Olive oil soup': it's an evocation of Andalucia, the sun-drenched, Arab-influenced south of Spain. First, the waiters bring white balloons and snip off the ends. A stream of air escapes, scented with orange blossom, perfuming the table as it does the countryside around Seville when the orange groves bloom. The soup is a kind of thickened olive oil, flavourful but not at all greasy, dotted with blood orange sections. The dish's references are as much cultural as they are culinary.

Source: Wine Spectator Online.[1]

Perhaps it does not seem a close analogy . . . if so, much of this may appear to be too frivolous or pretentious. Yet, I'm sure that there are many people more glamorous than Ferran Adrià working today in public health and public policy. I also suspect that far too many of us do not believe that creativity is important in public health.

Of course avant-garde 'research cooking' does seem rather far removed from public health policy. But the relevant question is: How do we creatively 'blend, bake or amalgamate the ingredients' in making public health work?

Quite analogous to Adrià's inventiveness in cooking, the most creative public health concept that I kept in mind while thinking about this chapter was Geoffrey Rose's 'big idea'.[2,3,4] Rose's fundamental insight was that changing the population distribution of a risk factor does more to reduce the burden of disease than targeting people at high risk.

Figure 13.1 is probably one of the most creative and most frequently reproduced graphs in the recent history of public health. The applications of this insight have been rich, and the societal implications vast.[5,6] There surely are other ideas in epidemiology and public health that are both as innovative and as relevant.

Figure 13.1 demonstrates that even though the *individual* risk of death is higher among people in the highest categories of the risk factor, in a given *population* most cases occur among people who have moderate values of the risk factor; this so-called 'prevention paradox' occurs because the prevalence of those intermediate values is much higher than that of the highest values. Therefore, the coherent strategy, from a population perspective, is to try to shift the whole distribution of the risk factor towards the left; in the example above, the challenge is to decrease

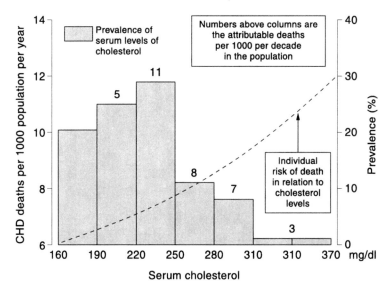

Figure 13.1 The dominance of deaths in those with average levels of a risk factor. Source: World Health Organization, Technical Report Series 678 (1982). Reproduced with permission.

serum cholesterol for the entire population. This population shift is in fact now attempted by many health programmes that target the more distal, societal causes of harmful living conditions. It may not be glamorous, but it takes a lot of creativity to make the shift real. 'Prevention paradoxes' such as the one summarised in Figure 13.1 are indeed 'managed' every day by clinicians and policy makers.

Creativity and the causes of disease

It has been proposed that Rose's approach is even more relevant in respect of certain environmental contaminants, such as some persistent toxic substances (PTS), which are 'invisible' but frequently present at low concentrations in many fatty foods.[7,8,9,10] The main reason for this proposition is that there is virtually nothing an individual can do to change his or her own levels of these environmental compounds. This is in sharp contrast with 'exposures' such as dietary cholesterol, obesity or cigarette smoking, which are amenable to control both by individuals' change of behaviour, and by societal interventions.

PTS epitomise the problem of widely prevalent environmental hazards that result from cultural and economic processes that are deeply rooted in our societies. Hence, PTS pose profound challenges to creative policy making. Figure 13.2 illustrates some of them; it shows the distribution of the concentrations in amniotic fluid of the pesticide p,p'-DDT in three different cohorts: children born in 1965, in 1985 and in 2005. The shift of the distributions of the pesticide towards lower levels is positive for the entire population: it decreases the population mean, and it decreases the number of individuals in the higher categories of exposure. Figure 13.2 might seem just 'technical', but I think it exemplifies a suitable blending of public health thinking and scientific creativity.

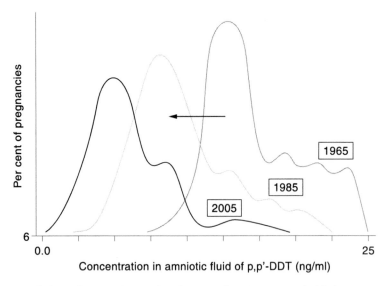

Figure 13.2 Shifting the population distribution of environmental risk factors.

The curves are estimates based on data from the literature.[11,12,13,14,15] They apply primarily to Spain, though similar scenarios are plausible for other countries. There is strong evidence of the presence of low doses of PTS during pregnancy, and throughout life, for virtually all populations around the globe – truly a 'glocal' issue.[16] However, information based on representative population samples is surprisingly scarce, and hence for most populations the actual distributions are unknown. This exemplifies the wide gaps in the information available in our so-called 'information societies'. Because the causes and consequences of 'glocal' contamination by PTS are profound, it will take a lot of creativity, and courage, and more, as we shall see below, to shift the distributions in the healthy direction.

The need to focus on distal causes of the societal burden of illness has long been obvious. Yet, some healthcare policy makers still have conflicting feelings about such need. Perhaps creativity only finds its role in changing the social and environmental causes of disease when we internalise – and externalise – the imperative to act on the basis of all three components of the triad of scientific evidence, moral values, and political will.[17]

Creativity: beyond aesthetics and subjectivism

Emotions reveal rules indispensable to social organisation. Emotions arise when socially needed values we are attached to are threatened. Morals or 'prosocial emotions' function to regulate social behaviours, more often for the long-term interest of a social group than the short-term interests of the individual.[18]

But let us not get too lyrical. As the previous examples show, in public health policy creativity does not necessarily involve what we look for in the arts – for example, aesthetics and emotions. Often what is required most is a skilful and creative management of power, usually the power of *others*. Or, to be more precise, the capacity – yes, creative – to gather socially relevant scientific evidence, to persuade the many actors and stakeholders involved, to build alliances and synergies, and to achieve agreements between often strongly opposed economic and other power interests. Agreements, for instance, such as those that made possible the huge success of reducing lead in gasoline, and so of lead concentrations in the blood of many populations around the globe.[19]

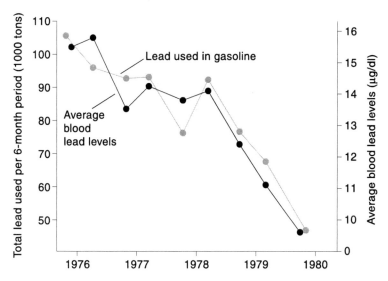

Figure 13.3 A lot of creativity, political skills and social pedagogy were necessary to progressively reduce lead used in gasoline, and so blood lead levels in the US population. Source: Stolley and Lasky.[19] Reproduced with permission.

Figure 13.3 is also one of the graphs that has most influenced the minds, and modified the actions, of policy makers within and outwith the health sector. The graph also reminds us of other graphs which, though much needed, are missing – that is, of analyses of social and environmental processes whose influence on human health is unmeasured, and hence unknown. I had thought to place another Figure in the text here, a Figure with nothing on it – this as a reminder of the gaps in our knowledge and information. But instead an allusion to the Beatles' *White Album* will suffice.[20]

Pedagogic, diplomatic and political skills can be the allies of aesthetics and art – and vice versa. Good taste and persuasiveness are evident, for instance, in many posters and pamphlets long used in many (not all) public health campaigns.[21,22] In our visually oriented era, creativity is particularly needed in order to connect with the social imagination. An ingenious use of some artistic forms, such as film/video, photography and painting, is hence important in order to change social beliefs about health and about the structural determinants of health.[23]

The pitfalls are many, of course. It suffices only to recall the widespread use (and abuse) of PowerPoint,[24] the beguiling power (and limits) of 'googling' and other uses of the Internet, or the peculiar reading habits of our younger constituencies and 'target populations'. Figure 13.4 reflects some of this.[25] With its subtle beauty, the black and white photograph contrasts classic wisdom (the Parthenon) with the modern ravages of war (the spread of a cholera epidemic by flies) and the naïveté with which we humans have too often embraced new technologies; in this case, our recent friend/pest, DDT.

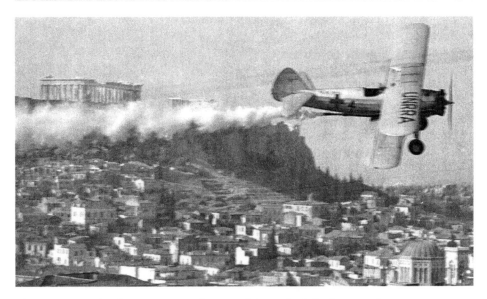

Figure 13.4 A plea for a more creative use of (meaningful) photographs.
Source: *Nature – Associated Press.*[25] © EMPICS, reproduced with permission.

The splendid graphic works of Edward R Tufte provide other examples of what is feasible in combining beauty and meaning.[26,27,28] Newspaper cartoonists are capable of this too (Figure 13.5).

Even political and public health publicity provide abundant examples of such creativity. Of particular relevance to public health, some environmental organisations have an interesting record of scientific and social pedagogy (Figure 13.6).

Admittedly, the creations of Ferran Adrià, Geoffrey Rose and Edward Tufte are not among the main preoccupations of the average public health officer or civil servant. More influential in their professional lives are the routines of daily work, the more or less hierarchical culture of their organisations and, rightly so, the adherence to standard protocols in field work, the office or the laboratory. I will come back to this later. It is time to sketch the less obvious reasons for this chapter.

Why creativity?

Does it not still sound a bit superfluous or frivolous? Perhaps, but in the following introduction to the Madrid Framework the inclusion of creativity in social policy is appropriately posited.[33] 'Health policy and governance are not securely predictable and linear exercises: many of the contextual factors may change over time – sometimes quite rapidly and unexpectedly. Tightly specified ends are not necessarily achieved by tightly specified means, and public health challenges may not be solved by current and conventional approaches. Successful implementation requires imagination, experimentation, innovation and flexibility on the part of stakeholders and institutions.' Compelling reasons . . .

We might probably also agree that 'the practice of public health is both a

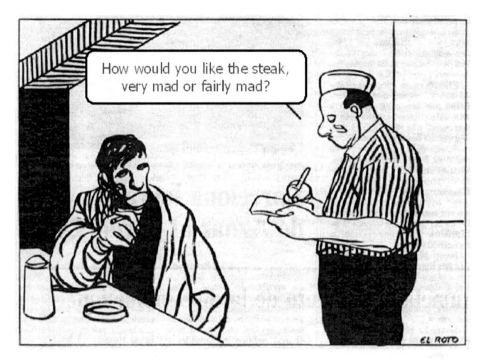

Figure 13.5 In the midst of the 'mad-cow crisis', a reminder that any individual has a limited capacity to protect himself from certain social and environmental hazards.[29,30,31] Source: Andrés Rábago, El Roto. *El País* (4 July 1997).[32] Reproduced with permission.

science and an art'.[17] Nonetheless, these pages are written as if this book was only about the science of health policies and not at all about art. Yet, while differences abound, there are also vital similarities. For instance, both in policy making and in art the inner world matters hugely; not only the inner worlds of individuals but also, and perhaps more relevantly, the inner worlds of institutions. Many private companies around the world are far ahead of most public administrations in their successful creation of positive inner environments, companies with working cultures that encourage freedom of thought, constructive criticism, imagination and innovative solutions. But, as poignantly noted by Crown and Gunning-Schepers:[34] '. . . it is difficult nowadays for public health practitioners to fulfil crucial functions as the "conscience of the organisation", the "poet in residence", or the "critic of the system".' Not just difficult, but often unthinkable.

In other words, our health organisations reproduce the metaphors by which their leaders choose to operate.[33] And oh, well, the common metaphors are not very inspiring, or conducive to creativity. Lewontin[35] (writing about genetics) says: 'It is not possible to do the work of science without using a language that is filled with metaphors.' Paraphrasing Lewontin we may say: it is not possible to promote health policies – or carry out any other socially relevant work – without using metaphors. Hence the crafting of public health policy metaphors – persuasive, powerful, touching metaphors that are also evidence based, morally coherent and culturally sustainable – is a task where creativity is a must.[30,33,36]

Metaphors, similes, images, analogies, slogans are virtually all used in public health programmes for 'consumption by the public'. Although in the process of

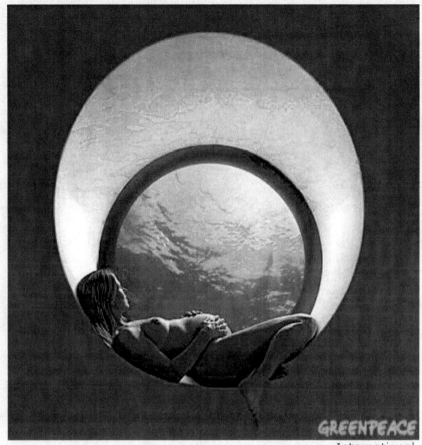

Our children inherit the toxic burden of our planet.

Figure 13.6 Even highly sensitive processes can be explained sensibly. Certain lipophilic persistent toxic substances are transmitted from mother to child during pregnancy and lactation. Source: Greenpeace. Reproduced with permission.

artistic creation some artists profess to care nothing for the outer world, most ultimately wish to interest, if not also to seduce, their audiences. The desire (in this sense) to seduce active, mature, sensitive and sensible citizens should be much stronger than is commonly the case when public health policies are being thought out, designed and offered for implementation. Many initiatives in clinical medicine, public health and ecology fail because they do not truly aim or succeed at touching, seducing, and conquering the hearts and minds of those for whom their initiatives are designed. It is hence not surprising that these rarely permeate the wider social imagination.[7,8]

Compared with the input of the mass media, the insights of public health and the other life and social sciences play a relatively minor part in the social construction of risks. How then can we influence the social agendas, the output of the mass media, government budgets or health targeting in this regard? The wish to be influential is certainly also common in public health; this is a strength. However, there rarely seem to be concomitant ideas about how exactly to listen, or to share. Perhaps because the source of the ambition to be influential is too often paternalistic. The public voice of public health too often sounds authoritarian, however well meant the message. 'We' know what's good for 'them' – which is to obey doctors' orders, to quit smoking, exercise more, eat less fat, and so on. Yet, in the process of policy formulation, if we wish to seduce our audiences, we are in fact in a much better position than most artists. Government units have so many means to enable public participation, to let the creativity of its advocates flow into the civic stream of public health policies.

This desire to entice, this wish to share, to do so creatively, is this not too subjective an ambition for policy makers? Too insubstantial? Too postmodern? Honestly, I believe the answer is 'no'. It is not insubstantial, quite the opposite, as can be seen throughout this book. The Madrid Framework itself is a metaphor.[33] And metaphors are not simple ornamental devices, flowery vases for contemplation. They are meant to persuade, to create complicities and alliances . . . for action.[36] True, tough choices must not be shunned; in the words of John Kenneth Galbraith: 'Politics is not the art of the possible. It consists in choosing between the disastrous and the unpalatable.' Well, even when things are as dramatic as that, a real, practical question remains: What does it take today to be creative in health policy? Again, I mean both at the individual and at the organisational levels.

A serene, peaceful and balanced spirit is not a prerequisite for creativity. In *The Guermantes Way* Marcel Proust wrote:[37,38] 'Everything we think of as great has come to us from neurotics. It is they and they alone who have founded religions and created great works of art.' We might add, '. . . and proposed grandiose health policies.'

Both in art and in policy making, harmony is not a prerequisite for creativity. Though it often helps, to be creative, one doesn't really need to be at peace with oneself (or with other units in the Department of Health). Feeling worried, angry, desperate or just misunderstood may work as well. (Anger, or at least irritation, may be even more prevalent among our public administrators than it is said to be among artists.) By contrast, it is hard to be creative if one feels indifferent, unsympathetic, apathetic or unmoved. Fortunately, for the most part public health professionals do feel involved, concerned, and committed. We care about equity, justice and solidarity, for instance, about the efficient use of available resources, about the values written about in this book.[33]

Nevertheless, it may be that the reader will still judge these paragraphs to be excessively naïve! And it may be true that survival in public health administration and politics sometimes depends on keeping expectations as down to earth as possible – really low.

Recently, on the bus to work, I was skimming through a paper dealing with the 'survival benefits' that premenopausal women with early breast cancer require, in order to accept the side effects of adjuvant endocrine treatments.[39] But rather than the specific results of the study, what struck me was the concept of 'cognitive dissonance reduction'. It turns out that comparisons of treatment preferences of those who have had treatment, and those who are about to commence treatment, may be biased by the phenomenon of cognitive dissonance reduction – the tendency to make current attitudes and beliefs consonant with previously taken decisions.[39] There are all sorts of dissonances that relentlessly we try to reduce – disappointments, disillusions, frustrations, embarrassments, reprimands. The message to all those creative people working in public health services, in hospitals, in many commercial companies, and in the 'invisible colleges', seems to be '*Lasciate ogne speranza voi ch'intrate!* (Abandon all hope, you who enter here!)' – Dante's infamous inscription at the entrance to Hell.[40] Abandon all hope of creativity and stick to your business, just keep a low profile, listen to political reason, don't mess up and, please, don't come up with any more ideas.

In spite of the cultural, economic and organisational constraints often found 'inherent' in public service, a certain wish to be creative is essential in health policy making. We want to produce ideas and projects that are both novel, or original and worthwhile, or appropriate, useful, attractive, meaningful . . . Can the definitions in Box 13.2 be adapted to health policy? Are we able, for instance, '. . . to construct public health systems that exhibit creative behaviour . . . '? This chapter could have started with these definitions, of course, but I think they are more evocative in the context of what has gone before.

Box 13.2 As in Raymond Carver's book of stories *What we talk about when we talk about love* . . . what do we talk about when we talk about creativity?

creativity n. The production of ideas and objects that are both novel or original and worthwhile or appropriate, that is, useful, attractive, meaningful, or correct. According to some researchers, in order to qualify as creative, a process of production must in addition be heuristic or open-ended rather than algorithmic (having a definite path to a unique solution). [*A Dictionary of Psychology*. Andrew M. Colman. Oxford University Press, 2001.]

    creativity n. Inventiveness, imagination, imaginativeness, innovation, innovativeness, originality, individuality; artistry, inspiration, vision; enterprise, initiative, resourcefulness. [*The Oxford Paperback Thesaurus*. Ed. Maurice Waite. Oxford University Press, 2001.]

    creative adj. Relating to or involving the use of imagination or original ideas in order to create something. [*The Concise Oxford English Dictionary*. Ed. Catherine Soanes and Angus Stevenson. Oxford University Press, 2004.]

    creativity A subfield of artificial intelligence that covers the computational study of the creative mind and the construction of systems that exhibit creative behaviour. Topics covered include all forms of creative reasoning (e.g. music, art, literature), computational models of creative processes, and the philosophy of computational creativity. [*A Dictionary of Computing*. Oxford University Press, 2004.]

Source: *Oxford Reference Online*, Oxford University Press.

In the context of this book we could also discuss healthy creativity, sociopolitical creativity, community-sensitive creativity, practical creativity, meaningless creativity . . . Indeed, 'Eminent creativity, everyday creativity, and health'[41] is the title of a book based on research previously published, as you may have guessed, in the *Creativity Research Journal* (http://gort.ucsd.edu/newjour/c/msg03406.html).

Creativity is in the air, in the field

Remember the song 'Love is in the air . . .'? So is creativity. Perhaps it is not as widespread as we would wish, but still, as the following two Internet searches suggest, there are many examples.

Box 13.3 Creativity . . . of course there is a lot of noise, but let us search . . .

Search 1. The database Scirus (http://www.scirus.com) is linked to Elsevier's ScienceDirect (http://www.sciencedirect.com) and includes documents from BioMed Central and MEDLINE/PubMed; it portends to be 'for scientific information only'. A search in Scirus for any of the 2 words ('creativity' or 'creative') and 'public health', limited to the period 1996–2006, yielded the astonishing figure of 931 058 items, of which 9798 were journal results (most of the rest were 'web results'). True, there are many duplications – fortunately.

Restricting search 1 to 'decision making' yielded a total of 861 553 items, of which 9025 were journal results. Similarly, restricting search 1 to 'health policy' yielded 847 252 items (8890 journal results). A search for all the following words: creativity OR creative AND (public AND health) AND 'social inequalities' found 849 317 items (15 896 journal results).

Search 2. A division of the Stanford University Libraries, HighWire Press (http://highwire.stanford.edu/) claims to 'host the largest repository of free, full-text, peer-reviewed content, with 878 journals and 979 504 free, full-text articles online'. A search similar to above but using only keywords ['(creativity OR creative) AND public AND health'] and restricted to High-Wire-hosted articles found 85 900 articles.

And the searches could meaningfully be expanded to include synonyms of creativity, or closely related words. Even if we discard documents suggesting purely rhetorical uses of 'creativity', the very large figures in Box 13.3 suggest that there are many efforts out there to be creative in health policy. Perhaps a greater challenge is implementation on larger scales, beyond small 'case studies' and 'demonstration projects'. Nonetheless, some examples follow.

The Center for Global Development in the Philippines[42] bears testimony of 'proven successes in global health', as shown in particular by the analyses of 17 effective projects. They conclude: 'In developing countries, life expectancy has risen from 40 to 65 years, and the chance that a child will survive to the age of five has doubled. In addition to directly improving people's lives, this progress contributes to economic growth. While some of the improvements in health are the result of overall social and economic gains, about half of it is due to specific efforts to address major causes of disease and disability.'

Another example of practical creativity is Oral Rehydration Therapy (ORT).[43,44] ORT involves the administration of a Oral Rehydration Solution (ORS) containing sodium chloride, potassium chloride, trisodium citrate and glucose dissolved in drinking water, as a replacement of vital body salts and fluid lost in many debilitating diarrhoeal illnesses. It was first developed by researchers in Bangladesh and India, and by 1979 it had become the cornerstone of WHO's global effort to reduce deaths associated with cholera and other diarrhoeal diseases. As William Foege[45] puts it, 'The health problems of the world often seem overwhelming, complex, expensive and intractable. It is refreshing when an answer is so simple that it approaches the unbelievable.'

There are creative strategies such as the Integrated Management of Childhood Illness (IMCI),[46,47] which is fostering a holistic approach to child health and development. The core intervention of IMCI is a set of preventive and therapeutic interventions for the integrated management of the five most important causes of childhood deaths: acute respiratory infections, diarrhoeal diseases, measles, malaria and malnutrition. The essential pillars include improvement in the case management skills of health personnel, improvement in health systems, and improvement in family and community practices. IMCI has reportedly been introduced in more than 80 countries.

There are creative methodological proposals for policy analysis like the 'simple and rapid approach' to aid formulation and implementation of 'Health for All' policies.[48] Based on the selection of a small number of tracers (such as HIV/AIDS, traffic injuries, ageing-related disabilities), it contains three dimensions – timing (early or late policy options), action level (individuals or social focus), and equity (social class, gender and ethnic groups). The methodology makes it possible to map the formulation of health strategies, compare different geographical areas and forecast policies' impact.

There are also powerful alliances between private companies and public institutions such as the 'Grand Challenges in Global Health'[49] initiative, a major effort to achieve scientific breakthroughs against diseases that kill millions of people each year in the world's poorest countries. The ultimate goal of the initiative is to create deliverable technologies – health tools that are not only effective, but also inexpensive to produce, easy to distribute, and simple to use in developing countries. In 2005 it offered 43 grants totalling over $400 million for a broad range of innovative research projects involving scientists in 33 countries. In partnership with the US National Institutes of Health, the initiative is supported by a $450 million commitment from the Bill and Melinda Gates Foundation, $27 million from the Wellcome Trust, and $4.5 million from the Canadian Institutes of Health Research. Many of the projects include scientists who had never before focused on global health. Examples of the projects include heat-stable vaccines, single-dose vaccines, mosquito control to prevent dengue, more nutritious staple crops, new HIV vaccine strategies, and diagnostics for the developing world.

The Centers for Disease Control and Prevention (CDC) Assessment Initiative[50] provides funds to states to promote the development of innovative partnerships between traditional public health agencies and other public and private partners. Novel and creative approaches and methods of assessment are being developed to monitor progress toward achieving measurable national, state, and community health objectives.

Relevant, too, for a wider perspective on creativity, are analyses of innovation intensity and the 'national innovative capacity',[51] the ability of a country to produce and commercialise a flow of innovative technology over the long term. It was found, for instance, that while a great deal of variation across countries is due to differences in the level of inputs devoted to innovation (R&D manpower and spending), an important role is played by factors associated with differences in R&D productivity (including policy choices, the share of research performed by the academic sector and funded by the private sector, the degree of technological specialisation, and each country's knowledge stock). Further, there has been convergence among OECD countries in terms of the estimated level of innovative capacity over the past quarter-century. Technological creativity is indeed contributing hugely to public health; e.g. by helping control the concentration of chemicals in air, water and food.

The potential for more creative health policies

In closing, I echo our editor, who wrote this on the process of writing. 'I have written this chapter not to say what I know but to find out what I think and feel.'[17] I would add, '. . . and to evoke paths for creativity; foremost, a state of mind and spirit.'

If one takes a broad look at health and social policies it is often difficult not to feel fairly bad. As in: 'Virchow has died, Rose has died, and I myself don't feel too well.' But we may look at this from a positive side: the gods and their dogmas are gone and we are at last free. As in: 'Just when the gods had ceased to be and the Christ had not yet come, there was a unique moment in history, between Cicero and Marcus Aurelius, when man stood alone.'[52]

True, in many ways the world is a shambles. Yet, many Berlin Walls have crumbled. Many dogmatisms (economic and political, if not yet religious ones) have lost ground, and some are only residual now.[16,17,53,54] Even the construct 'globalisation' has lost some of its sex appeal. Today public policies are less static: they fail or succeed, but they evolve; they succeed or fail, and then change again.[33] While no individual or organisation is ever free from internal and external constraints, today we possess unprecedented cultural and ideological freedom to innovate: the potential for more creative health policies may seldom have been so deep.

Acknowledgements

I am deeply grateful to Ferran Ballester, Ana García, Alfonso Hernández, Marisa Rebagliato, Fernando Benavides, Estefanía Blount, Núria Ribas, Jordi Sunyer, Tomàs López, Eli Puigdomènech, Javi Selva and José Pumarega for many creative discussions on the environmental and social issues addressed in this paper. Warm thanks are also due to Isabel Egea and Puri Barbas for technical assistance. The work of our unit (www.imim.es/URECMC/eng.htm) is partly supported by research grants from the Catalan Government (Generalitat de Catalunya – CIRIT SGR 0241, SGR 0078); 'Red temática de investigación cooperativa de centros en Cáncer' (C03/10); and 'Red temática de investigación cooperativa de centros en Epidemiología y salud pública' (C03/09), Instituto de Salud Carlos III, Ministry of Health, Madrid.

Notes and references

1 Matthews T (2004) Ferran Adrià and the cuisine of tomorrow. *Wine Spectator Online*. 15 December 2004. www.winespectator.com. Accessed 20 January 2006.

2 Hofman A and Vandenbroucke JP (1992) Geoffrey Rose's big idea. *BMJ*. 305: 1519–20.

3 Rose G (1992) *The Strategy of Preventive Medicine*. Oxford University Press, Oxford.

4 Rose G (1985) Sick individuals and sick populations. *Int J Epidemiol.* 14: 32–8. Reprinted: (2001) *Int J Epidemiol.* 30: 427–32 (with commentaries).

5 Rose G and Day S (1990) The population mean predicts the number of deviant individuals. *BMJ.* 301: 1031–4.

6 Porta M (2004) Persistent toxic substances: exposed individuals and exposed populations. *J Epidemiol Community Health.* 58: 534–5.

7 Porta M (2002) Bovine spongiform encephalopathy, persistent organic pollutants and the achievable utopias. *J Epidemiol Community Health.* 56: 806–7.

8 Porta M and Zumeta E (2002) Implementing the Stockholm Treaty on POPs [editorial]. *Occup Environ Medicine.* 59: 651–2.

9 Schafer KS and Kegley SE (2002) Persistent toxic chemicals in the food supply. *J Epidemiol Community Health.* 56: 813–17.

10 Lang T (1998) The new globalisation, food and health: is public health receiving its due emphasis? *J Epidemiol Community Health.* 52: 538–9.

11 Foster W, Chan S, Platt L and Hughes C (2000) Detection of endocrine disrupting chemicals in samples of second trimester human amniotic fluid. *J Clin Endocrinol Metab.* 85: 2954–7.

12 Lackmann GM (2005) Neonatal serum p,p′-DDE concentrations in Germany: chronological changes during the past 20 years and proposed tolerance level. *Paediatr Perinat Epidemiol.* 19: 31–5.

13 Sala M, Ribas-Fitó N, Cardo E, de Muga ME, Marco E, Mazon C et al. (2001) Levels of hexachlorobenzene and other organochlorine compounds in cord blood: exposure across placenta. *Chemosphere.* 43: 895–901.

14 Ribas-Fitó N, Grimalt JO, Marco E, Sala M, Mazon C and Sunyer J (2005) Breastfeeding and concentrations of HCB and p,p′-DDE at the age of 1 year. *Environ Res.* 98: 8–13.

15 Porta M, Kogevinas M, Zumeta E, Sunyer J and Ribas-Fitó N (2002) Concentraciones de compuestos tóxicos persistentes en la población española: el rompecabezas sin piezas y la protección de la salud pública. *Gac Sanit.* 16: 257–66.

16 Kickbusch I (1999) Global + local = glocal public health. *J Epidemiol Community Health.* 53: 451–2.

17 Marinker M (2002) Evidence and imagination. In: M Marinker *Health Targets in Europe: polity, progress and promise.* BMJ Books, London.

18 Tassy S, Gorincour G and Le Coz P (2005) Prenatal research: a very sensitive field. *Lancet.* 366: 1162.

19 Stolley PD and Lasky T (1995) *Investigating Disease Patterns: the science of epidemiology.* Scientific American Library, New York.

20 Known as the *White Album* because its cover was plain white, left blank without the traditional photographs, pictures and words to be expected on record covers, the two-record album was released by the then newly formed Apple label. Recording sessions started with the song *Revolution* in May 1968, and concluded with *Julia* in October 1968. Mixing for the album was completed in five days (source: www.beatletracks. com/btwhite.html). The Beatles were creative, worked quickly and were widely accepted. The lesson for health policy makers is clear. The *White Album* is the Beatles' best selling album, and the eighth best selling album of all time in the United States (source: http://en.wikipedia.org).

21 Weed DL (1995) Epidemiology, the humanities, and public health. *Am J Public Health.* 85: 914–18.

22 Boyle E, Rhee Y, Woynowski K and Helfand WH. *To Your Health: an exhibition of posters for contemporary public health issues.* National Library of Medicine, History of Medicine Division. Available at: www.nlm.nih.gov/exhibition/visualculture/vchome.html. Accessed 20 January 2006.

23 Eames P (2003) *Creative Solutions and Social Inclusion: culture and the community.* Steele Roberts, Wellington.

24 Tufte ER (2003) *The Cognitive Style of PowerPoint. A pamphlet*. Graphics Press, Chesire, CT.

25 Sharpe RM (1995) Another DDT connection. *Nature-Associated Press*. **375**: 538–9.

26 Tufte ER (2001) *The Visual Display of Quantitative Information* (2e). Graphics Press, Chesire, CT and at www.edwardtufte.com/tufte/.

27 Tufte ER (1990) *Envisioning Information*. Graphics Press, Chesire, CT.

28 Tufte ER (1997) *Visual Explanations: images and quantities, evidence and narrative*. Graphics Press, Chesire, CT.

29 McKee M, Lang T and Roberts JA (1996) Deregulating health: policy lessons from the BSE affair. *J R Soc Med*. **89**: 424–6.

30 Porta M and Morabia A (2004) Why aren't we more ahead? The risk of variant Creutzfeldt-Jakob Disease from eating Bovine Spongiform Encephalopathy – infected foods, eight years after: still undetermined [editorial]. *Eur J Epidemiol*. **19**: 287–9.

31 McMichael AJ (1999) Dioxins in Belgian feed and food: chickens and eggs. *J Epidemiol Community Health*. **53**: 742–3.

32 Rábago A, El Roto (2004) *El libro de los desórdenes*. Reservoir Books – Mondadori, Barcelona.

33 Marinker M (2006) Health policy and the constructive conversationalist. In: M Marinker (ed) *Constructive Conversations About Health: policy and values*. Radcliffe Publishing, Oxford.

34 Crown J and Gunning-Schepers L (1996) The challenge to public health advocacy. In: M Marinker (ed) *Sense and Sensibility in Health Care*. BMJ Books, London.

35 Lewontin RC (2000) *The Triple Helix: gene, organism, and environment*. Harvard University Press, Cambridge, MA.

36 Porta M (2003) The genome sequence is a jazz score. *Int J Epidemiol*. **32**: 29–31.

37 Proust M (1994) *Le côté de Guermantes* (*A la recherche du temps perdu*, III) [1920]. Collection Folio classique, No. 2658. Gallimard, Paris. In fact, Proust does not write of *'néurotiques'* but of *'nerveux'*: *'Tout ce que nous connaissons de grand nous vient des nerveux.'* The usual translation of *'nerveux'* as 'neurotics' in this passage takes the meaning a bit further away from us than it actually is: nervous, volatile, highly strung people are rather prevalent in daily life . . . Sometimes to the good.

38 Proust M (2003) In praise of neurotics [filler]. *BMJ*. **326**: 1455.

39 Thewes B, Meiser B, Duric VM, Stockler MR, Taylor A, Stuart-Harris R *et al.* (2005) What survival benefits do premenopausal patients with early breast cancer need to make endocrine therapy worthwhile? *Lancet Oncol*. **6**: 581–8.

40 Dante Alighieri. *Divina Comedia: Inferno*, canto III, 9.

41 Runco MA and Richards R (eds) (1997) Eminent Creativity, Everyday Creativity, and Health. Ablex, Greenwich, Conn. [reviewed in: (1999) *Am J Psychiatry*. **156**: 2012–13].

42 Levine R, Kinder M and The What Works Working Group (2004) Millions Saved: proven successes in global health. Center for Global Development, Manila. Available at: www.cgdev.org/section/initiatives/_active/millionssaved.

43 Santosham M (2002) Oral rehydration therapy: reverse transfer of technology. *Arch Pediatr Adolesc Med*. **156**: 1177–9.

44 Victora CG, Bryce J, Fontaine O and Monasch R (2000) Reducing deaths from diarrhoea through oral rehydration therapy. *Bull World Health Organ*. **78**: 1246–55.

45 www.gatesfoundation.org/nr/public/media/newsletters/milestones/sum_01.htm.

46 Adam T, Manzi F, Schellenberg JA, Mgalula L, de Savigny D and Evans DB (2005) Does the Integrated Management of Childhood Illness cost more than routine care? Results from the United Republic of Tanzania. *Bull World Health Organ*. **83**: 369–77.

47 El Arifeen S, Blum LS, Hoque DM, Chowdhury EK, Khan R, Black RE *et al.* (2004) Integrated Management of Childhood Illness (IMCI) in Bangladesh: early findings from a cluster-randomised study. *Lancet*. **364**: 1595–1602.

48 Peiró R, Álvarez-Dardet C, Plasència A, Borrell C, Colomer C, Moya C *et al.* (2002)

Rapid appraisal methodology for 'health for all' policy formulation analysis. *Health Policy*. **62**: 309–28.

49 www.gatesfoundation.org/GlobalHealth and www.grandchallengesgh.org.

50 Dhara R (2002) Advancing public health through the assessment initiative. *J Public Health Manag Pract*. **8**: 1–8.

51 Furman JL, Porter ME and Stern S (2002) The determinants of national innovative capacity. *Research Policy*. **31**: 899–933.

52 Gustave Flaubert, in a letter to his friend Madame Roger des Genettes, and then in Marguerite Yourcenar's *Mémoires d'Hadrien*.

53 Ruger JP (2004) Health and social justice. *Lancet*. **364**: 1075–80.

54 Porta M (2006) Things that kept coming to mind while thinking through Susser's South African mémoir. *J Epidemiol Community Health*. **60** (in press).

Chapter 14

Ethical considerations in health systems

Julio Frenk

Every health system reflects a series of ethical assumptions. Consciously or unconsciously, explicitly or implicitly, these assumptions are expressed in the distribution of healthcare benefits and in the organisation of institutions. Before articulating its specific technical proposals, every attempt to reform the health system must begin by asking which values it should promote.[1] In this way, the ethical foundations of reform proposals would be made clear and transparent.[2,3] Such a definition at the systemic level will constrain the ethical choices available at the level of specific organisations charged with financing, providing or managing health services.

In order to develop a normative scheme for system-wide health policy, I propose a hierarchy that includes values, principles and purposes, as shown in Figure 14.1.[4] This Figure should be read from the bottom up, given that the more fundamental concepts are located at the base of the triangle; as one moves towards the apex, increasingly concrete concepts are presented, which are derived from the preceding ones.

Values vary across social groups and over time. Yet health touches such fundamental aspects of human life that there may be grounds to develop a limited set of common values without reducing the rich diversity of human

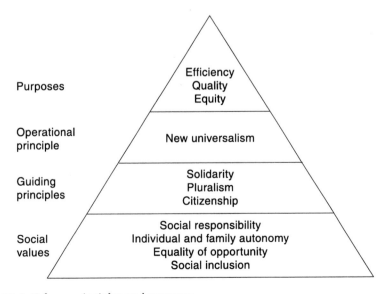

Figure 14.1 Values, principles and purposes.

culture.[5] In this way, the protection of health as a shared value could embody what Václav Havel calls the radical renewal of our sense of responsibility. This new sense of responsibility assumes the acceptance of 'a basic code of mutual coexistence, a kind of common minimum we can all share, one that will enable us to go on living side by side'.[6] Hopefully, the scheme that we will develop here will prove to be sufficiently broad as to offer elements for a shared ethical basis in the analysis of health systems.

Four values

These comprise the most fundamental ethical definitions regarding the model of society that the health system should reflect and reinforce. Four principal values are proposed.

- **Social inclusion:** Based on the premise that all human lives have the same value, the health system must represent an instance where everybody receives similar treatment for similar needs. Since the great majority of health deficits are involuntary, it follows that no type of discrimination in access to health services can be morally valid.[7] Only the need for care should regulate such access. The health system should therefore serve to mitigate differences in need that arise from prior socioeconomic inequalities.
- **Equality of opportunity:** As Sen has argued, inequality can be viewed in terms of differences either in actual achievement or in the freedom to achieve, which is 'the *real opportunity* that we have to accomplish what we value'.[8] Health services should help each generation to enter life with the same opportunities. In this sense, ensuring a basic common floor of healthcare for everyone has the same sense of justice as does primary education. Equality of opportunity offers the ethical foundation for a fair distribution of wealth.
- **Individual and family autonomy:** Every person enjoys the freedom to decide what is most convenient for him or her, a prerogative that the family assumes in the case of minors and of people who are limited in their capabilities to decide. Autonomy is expressed in free choice, which, in the case of health services, has a special meaning that sets them apart from other goods. Indeed, the intimacy entailed by many healthcare situations makes it necessary to empower users to select those professionals in whom they can place their trust. Such empowerment promotes respect for the dignity of the human body.
- **Social responsibility:** This value places limits on the freedom proposed by the former one. This is particularly important in the case of goods such as health services that exhibit what economists call 'externalities', that is to say, the consequences to others of an individual's decisions. Thus, neglect to care for one's own health has effects upon others. This generates a responsibility that limits the freedom to be neglectful. In addition, the involuntary nature of most health deficiencies imposes a shared responsibility to care for the persons who experience them.

Four principles

A series of principles can be derived from the aforementioned values.

1 **Citizenship:** This principle corresponds to the values of social inclusion and equality of opportunity. According to the citizenship principle, healthcare should not be conceived of as a consumer good, a privilege or an object of assistance, but rather as a social right. Under modern definitions of citizenship, this principle arises from an extension of civil and political rights into the social policy arena.[9] One of its premises is that liberty and social justice are empty notions unless all the inhabitants of a country have reached a decent standard of living.[10] It should be clarified that, in this context, the concept of citizenship goes beyond the strictly legal definition, and includes all of the residents in a country. Clearly, this principle has crucial implications for specifying criteria of access to healthcare, as will be explained later.

2 **Pluralism:** This principle is derived from the value of individual and family autonomy. As such, it postulates that the health system must respect personal choices[11] regarding the providers of care. The only restriction is that providers should have demonstrated the required knowledge and skills. Freedom of choice is particularly important with respect to the primary provider of services, who is responsible for the first contact with the health system, as well as for continuity of care. Such a primary provider often acts as the consumer's agent. This complex relationship can only be guided by the trust that free choice allows. In addition to its ethical justification, freedom of choice has the pragmatic advantage of generating incentives for improved performance on the part of providers, who must satisfy users if they wish to be selected. When choice is based on information about performance, it can reduce the asymmetries between producers and consumers that are so characteristic of the healthcare market.[12]

3 **Solidarity:** It corresponds to the value of social responsibility. Solidarity has two meanings. First, it implies sharing the social responsibility for taking care of the most vulnerable groups. Second, it postulates that, at any given time, the healthy should contribute to finance the care of the sick. In this sense, solidarity forms the basis for medical insurance and especially for social security. There is an irreducible uncertainty in health: the risk of falling ill or becoming disabled is unpredictable for an individual, although it can be calculated on actuarial bases for a group. Insurance helps to reduce this uncertainty by pooling the risks across many people. Given that we shall all become sick at some time in our lives, solidarity is essentially fair, since it implies that all of the members of the group will eventually benefit from it. Consequently, the solidarity principle sets limits to the freedom of choice implicit in the pluralism principle, since, when individuals opt to be negligent in the care of their health they impose a financial and pathological burden on the rest of the community.

4 **New universalism:** The three guiding principles described so far converge on a more concrete one that gives them operational expression. A new universalism[13] would solve the dilemma that underlies much of the discussion regarding social policy in the post-World War II era (*see* Figure 14.2).

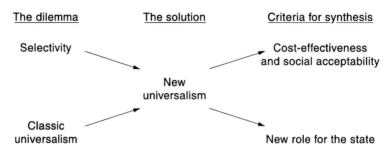

Figure 14.2 Towards a new universalism.

The principle of classical or unrestricted universalism, as formulated in the 1942 Beveridge Report, forms the basis for the contemporary state. In the case of health, classical universalism is expressed as a single system for all citizens, which is free at the time of use. Access is independent of income, and the quality of services is acceptable to the majority of the population. Although this type of system gives great weight to the values of social inclusion, equality of opportunity, and social responsibility, it restricts the value of individual and family autonomy. Furthermore, as healthcare costs escalate, systems based on unrestricted universalism end up resorting to bureaucratic rationing methods, such as queues and waiting lists. Given that these systems have become unaffordable even in the wealthiest countries, as evidenced by the crisis of the European welfare state, they could hardly be offered as a realistic model for developing countries.

At the other end of the dilemma is the principle of selectivity, which proposes that scarce public resources should be focused on the poor. Although it has the advantage of giving priority to the most vulnerable groups, this principle tends to produce stratified systems where the services reserved for the poor are usually of inferior quality. In the words of Richard Titmuss, the famous proponent of classical universalism, services for the poor end up being poor services. Another disadvantage is that administrative procedures for identifying the poor are often cumbersome and stigmatising. For these reasons, selective services hardly ever cover the entire target population, and paradoxically they often end up making inequalities even more profound.

The principle of new universalism offers a way of resolving these ethical dilemmas, and achieving a synthesis of conflicting goods. This principle recovers what is most valuable in classical universalism, since it proposes that the health system be inclusive, but modifies it based on two fundamental criteria that incorporate the positive aspects of selectivity.

As shown in Figure 14.2, the first criterion is the use of cost-effectiveness and social acceptability to decide which services will be accessible on a universal basis. Thus, the system does not guarantee universal access to all the possible interventions available today, but only to those that have demonstrated a favourable cost-effectiveness ratio and that are socially acceptable. It turns out that the most cost-effective interventions currently available tend to deal with the health deficits that disproportionately affect the poor (e.g. infectious diseases, malnutrition, perinatal and maternal morbidity). By preferentially allocating resources to these interventions it becomes possible to give priority to the poor without having to segregate or stigmatise them. Efficiency and equity are thus combined.

In addition, the new universalism suggests a different role for the state. No longer is it required that the state provide the services directly through a public monopoly. Instead, the state limits itself to assuring that there is universal and equitable access to priority services of an acceptable quality and that social inclusion is achieved through a fair fiscal system. Services can then be delivered in a pluralistic system, with a mix of public and private providers, which contains costs and satisfies users.

Three purposes

The values and principles explained above lay the foundation for the three purposes that should guide the health system (*see* Figure 14.1). Every proposal to reform a health system should be evaluated in terms of the extent to which it achieves these purposes.

1 **Equity:** An equitable health system assures that every person has the same opportunity to receive services when confronted with the same health need. Given that the burden of disease and injury is unevenly distributed among social groups and areas of a country, equity implies providing more care for those who suffer the greatest burden. Hence, the health system should not only increase total health levels, but should do so in a way that reduces the gaps among social groups.

2 **Quality:** Expanding access to services would be useless if their quality was not assured. Quality represents the extent to which services effectively improve health. The concept includes two dimensions: technical, which involves following the best healthcare strategy made possible by science; and inter-personal, which consists of achieving the greatest possible satisfaction for the user, respecting his or her autonomy and preferences.[14] A health system that does not place quality at the centre of its concerns runs the risk of spending valuable resources without achieving the desired effect or, which is even worse, of producing malpractice and dissatisfaction.

3 **Efficiency:** This purpose is inseparable from quality. Efficiency means achieving a given health goal by using the minimum possible amount of resources or, conversely, to obtain the maximum possible health gains with the available resources. There are two types of efficiency. The first is *allocative* efficiency, which means that the system defines priorities as a function of the cost-effectiveness and social acceptability of interventions. The second type is *technical* efficiency, which means that, whatever their cost-effectiveness, services are produced with the least waste of resources.[15]

New universalism allows for the optimal combination of equity, quality, and efficiency. However, there can be conflicts between these purposes, particularly between equity and efficiency. For example, people from higher socioeconomic groups are usually in a better position to benefit from services, since they are often more able to resort to them in a timely fashion and to follow professional advice. Because of this, it could be argued that investing in the care of these groups would produce greater aggregate health benefits than would focus on persons from lower socioeconomic status. Any such gains in efficiency, however, would entail a loss in equity. A similar argument could refer to the case of people living in remote rural areas, where the cost of providing services is much higher than that for urban populations.

Given such potential conflicts, I have argued that priority should be given to equity. This is illustrated in Figure 14.1 by placing equity closer to the base of the pyramid and efficiency closer to the apex.

Fortunately, under many circumstances equity, quality and efficiency mutually reinforce each other in a synergistic way. Thus, the delivery of services with good cost-effectiveness and social acceptability generally contributes to all three purposes. Achieving this positive reinforcement is probably the key challenge that every health system must face. How the three purposes are balanced at the systemic level will largely determine the performance of specific healthcare organisations.

Dilemmas and options

Consensus on values, principles and purposes translates into a health-system model that can then reflect societal aspirations. In order to reach such a consensus, it is necessary to address a series of complicating factors that stem from intrinsic characteristics of health phenomena.

Health needs are potentially infinite. Since ultimately we all suffer from disease and die, avoiding or resolving one health problem, by that very fact, increases the risk of suffering from another one. In this sense it can be said that the health system is a victim of its own success, since prolonging life gives rise to new health needs.[16] In addition, growing social expectations determine that an ever-expanding number of situations are defined as health needs. The basic need for simple physical survival and pain relief give way to progressive desires for improvement in the quality of life, including its psychological and social dimensions.

The problem, of course, is that although needs are potentially infinite, the resources to deal with them are not. The resulting shortfall is made even more severe as the demand for health services grows with improved income and education. Furthermore, the technological explosion makes it possible to offer services that may not respond to a need or to a demand, as happens, for instance, when the life of a patient in coma is artificially prolonged. Consequently the ethical discussion about the very definition of human life has become a matter of central importance for health policy.

The foregoing line of reasoning leads to an inescapable conclusion: in healthcare there is always rationing. Every society, even if it is wealthy, confronts the problem of rationing health services. It can do so implicitly, by responding to the economic and political powers that be, or explicitly, by achieving a transparent social consensus. The rationing imperative poses a series of difficult dilemmas. In order to resolve them, a number of criteria, aimed at defining who is to benefit from healthcare, have been proposed.

Indeed, at the ethical and political core of health policy lies the crucial issue of the criteria that determine access to care. These derive directly from the values that guide the health system. It is possible to identify four: purchasing power; poverty; socially perceived priority; and citizenship.[17] The characteristics of each are summarised in Table 14.1. Because resources are always scarce relative to needs, choosing between these criteria will determine the answer to the most fundamental health policy question – 'Who gets what, and at what cost to whom?'

Table 14.1 Bases for the definition of access to health services.

Criterion	Institutional expression	Rationing mechanism
Purchasing power	Unregulated market	Price
Poverty	Public assistance	Bureaucratic barriers
Socially perceived priority	Restricted social insurance	Social exclusion
Citizenship	Universal health system	Cost, effectiveness, and social acceptability

1 **Purchasing power:** This first criterion guides resource allocation in the private market when public regulation and financing are weak. Its ethical basis is the belief that healthcare is no different from other goods and services which are part of the general rewards system. Therefore, this principle postulates that health services can be bought and sold in the private market; the only mechanism for rationing access is price.[18]

For some time now it has been clear that health services, like education, cannot be treated as one more element in the general system of rewards that are obtained through monetary income.[1] To begin with, loss of health is not usually a voluntary act. Nor can it be predicted for a particular individual (although it is predictable, based on probabilities, for groups of people). Furthermore, health services in themselves are not a means of satisfaction, nor can they be considered a 'reward' for social achievement, as in the case of some consumer goods.

In addition, the market for health services exhibits so many imperfections that it might well be characterised as a *perfectly imperfect* market. Perhaps the most important of these are the information asymmetries between producers and consumers.[19] There are several aspects to this. First, information itself is most often the product of many medical care encounters: patients often visit the doctor precisely because they wish to gain access to this information. Second, many health needs arise too infrequently or are too life-threatening to make it feasible to obtain information in order to guide purchasing decisions. Third, ignorance about the technical aspects of healthcare leaves most utilisation decisions in the hands of the provider, thus giving rise to supplier-induced demand.

Another important market imperfection relates to the fact that the benefits of healthcare are not strictly individual, but also extend to the family, the community and the rest of society. This is obvious in the case of the numerous non-personal health services, such as environmental measures, which constitute public goods. In addition, not all the benefits of personal health services accrue to the individual alone, in as much as there are significant externalities. For example, the prevention and treatment of communicable diseases benefit not only the person receiving the service but the entire population. Even in the case of non-communicable diseases, individual health constitutes a social value, for it represents an input for economic development and an investment in human capital.[20] And even in the absence of utilitarian arguments,[21] there can be a social and political preference for not allowing any individual to suffer avoidable deterioration of his or her health.[22] Thus, if the benefits of healthcare are social so should be its costs – they should be distributed among the members of society.

Two critical imperfections in the medical insurance market can be added to the imperfections in the healthcare market: 'adverse selection' and the so-called 'moral hazard'. Adverse selection means that people who plan to use health services, or know that they are likely to require them, have a greater probability of purchasing medical insurance, which leaves underwriters exposed to the costs of future care. Moral hazard means that the very fact of having insurance modifies the behaviour of users of services, as well as of providers. Medical care is not a rigid set of prescribed steps, but in many cases leaves ample room for discretion. In the presence of insurance, patients tend to use more services and providers to prescribe more procedures, given that neither group has fully to bear the costs that derive from their decisions. In order to protect themselves against these two imperfections, insurers attempt to select the risks they will cover, by means of mechanisms such as waiting periods before the policy goes into effect, or the exclusion of coverage for pre-existing conditions. This response, however, leaves without protection pre-cisely those persons who most need it.[23]

Because of their complexity and political value, the mechanisms designed to correct the many market imperfections always entail the participation of some collective mediator – which in the modern world is almost always the state.[24] The resulting mechanisms of collective intervention represent the basis for the remaining three principles of resource allocation in healthcare: poverty, socially perceived priority, and citizenship.

2 **Poverty:** According to this criterion, health services are delivered to those who are indigent or who demonstrate financial need. In many developing coun-tries, it has found its institutional expression in the public assistance sector and especially in conventional ministries of health. Far from establishing a public obligation, it is grounded in political interest and on the moral responsibility of the state to assist the most vulnerable social groups and thereby also protect the rest of society. Poverty is also the criterion that underlies the delivery of services by private charitable organisations. As a rationing mechanism, it relies on bureaucratic barriers, including determination of financial need, queues, waiting lists, restricted hours of service and poor quality of care in both its technical and interpersonal dimensions.

3 **Socially perceived priority:** Allocation of health services according to this criterion has led to the development of social security institutions in many countries, particularly in Latin America. The name of this criterion derives from the fact that it benefits only certain groups whose function or occupation is given priority by the state, either because they have some special merit or because they perform a strategic function – for example, industrial workers, government functionaries and the military. Having recognised the priority of such groups, the state sets a mandatory financial contribution from their members, their employers, and/or the state itself. This special contribution not only finances services but also establishes a right to healthcare, albeit only for limited segments of the population. Thus, the rationing mechanism entails the exclusion of those groups not perceived to be a social priority.

4 **Citizenship:** Until now, the healthcare systems of many countries have been characterised by the simultaneous application of the three criteria already mentioned: purchasing power, poverty and socially perceived priority. Each one has given rise to a different institutional sector: the private sector, public assistance and social security, respectively. In turn, each of these sectors has taken care of some subgroup, though with widely unequal resources. Despite this, there often remains a substantial proportion of the population that is not protected by any of the subsystems. Thus, the coexistence of these three principles not only reflects social inequality, but actually reinforces it.

This problem has made it necessary to develop an alternative form of distributing healthcare, in order to bridge the gap between its potential benefits and actual access to them. This alternative principle is 'citizenship', which was briefly described earlier. It represents a qualitative advance over the others because it is the only one that, by definition, is not restricted to any particular group; on the contrary, its aim is universal coverage by including all the residents in a country.[25] This does not mean that citizenship lacks a rationing mechanism. The difference is that, in this case, such a mechanism is derived from evidence regarding the cost-effectiveness and social acceptability of services, according to the principle of new universalism. If healthcare is considered as a right, then only cost-effectiveness and social acceptability can be used as ethically valid criteria for the distribution of access to services.

In order to ameliorate the uncertainty inherent in the loss of health, correct some market imperfections, and guarantee universal access to cost-effective and socially acceptable services, the criterion of citizenship relies on the solidarity principle that was discussed earlier. Uncertainty regarding loss of health can be approached by pooling individual risks through health insurance. This aggregation of risks makes them predictable, through actuarial calculations, for the whole of the insured. In this way, uncertainty can be managed through the solidarity of the healthy with the sick.

In order to reach a critical mass of insured persons and avoid the adverse selection associated with voluntary insurance, the state may impose a degree of compulsory compliance with enrolment. Its most elaborate expression is social insurance with universal coverage. This degree of compulsion is compatible with the freedom to choose the primary provider of services, which is a central element of the pluralism principle.

The combination of a universal system where all are protected, and are also able to choose their providers, seems to synthesise the aspirations of many modern societies in the search for equitable, high quality and efficient health services.

Conclusions

The adoption of specific policies for health system reform must first achieve societal consensus with respect to the values, principles, and purposes that have been examined in this essay. Policies can then be analysed in terms of their consistency with the preferred ethical framework. Unfortunately, a lot of the debate concerning health reform has not carried out this type of analytical exercise but has instead plunged into the defence of programmatic proposals. I contend that such an approach is often the consequence of an absence of ethical considerations in economic and social policy analysis.[26]

The state has played and will continue to play a very important role in health systems. This is required by ethical imperatives, the wish for social justice, the dynamics of the economy, and the special attributes of healthcare. But this does not imply that the role of the state has to be monopolistic or bureaucratic. Clearly, the citizenship principle emphasises the need to maintain a framework of public leadership in order to attain the purposes of equity, quality and efficiency. Nevertheless, there is nothing in the 'citizenship' principle that would be incompatible with a pluralistic health system where an optimum mix of functions between the public and private sectors is achieved. In fact, the future development of health systems will require that we overcome the old polarisation between what is public and what is private, so that it becomes possible to combine the best of each sphere by introducing choice into a framework of public responsibility and social solidarity.

A broad system-wide ethical framework will determine the adoption of specific codes of conduct for the various groups that are involved in the healthcare industry. At this time of often confusing change, a transparent and explicit consideration of the ethical foundations of policy will be the only way to illuminate the path towards better health.

References

1 Donabedian A (1976) *Aspects of Medical Care Administration: specifying requirements for health care.* Harvard University Press, Cambridge, MA.
2 Daniels N, Light DW and Caplan RL (1996) *Benchmarks of Fairness for Health Care Reform.* Oxford University Press, New York.
3 Priester R (1992) A values framework for health system reform. *Health Affairs.* 11(1): 84–107.
4 Frenk J (1994) Bases doctrinarias de la reforma en salud [Doctrinal basis of health reform]. Series: Economía y Salud: Documentos para el Análisis y la Convergencia, no. 2. Fundación Mexicana para la Salud, Mexico City.
5 Bok S (1995) *Common Values.* University of Missouri Press, Columbia, MO.
6 Havel V (1995) A courageous and magnanimous creation. *Harvard Gazette.* June 15: 9–10.
7 Beauchamp TL and Childress JF (1983) *Principles of Biomedical Ethics* (2e). Oxford University Press, New York.
8 Sen A (1992) *Inequality Reexamined.* Harvard University Press, Cambridge, MA.
9 Bendix R (1964) *Nation-Building and Citizenship: studies of our changing social order.* Wiley, New York.
10 Tawney RH (1961) *Equality.* Capricorn Books, New York.
11 Berlinguer G (1997) Popolazione, etica ed equità. *Genus.* 53: 13–35.
12 Bennett S (1997) Health-care markets: defining characteristics. In: S Bennett, B McPake and A Mills (eds) *Private Health Providers in Developing Countries: serving the public interest?* Zed Books, London.
13 World Health Organization (1998) *World Health Report 1998: making a difference.* WHO, Geneva.
14 Donabedian A (1980) *Explorations in Quality Assessment and Monitoring. Vol I: the definition of quality and approaches to its assessment.* Health Administration Press, Ann Arbor, MI.
15 Ad Hoc Committee on Health Research Relating to Future Interventions Options (1996) *Investing in Health Research and Development.* World Health Organization, Geneva.

16 Gruenberg EM (1977) The failures of success. *Milbank Memorial Fund Quarterly*. **55**: 3–24.

17 This discussion builds upon and expands some of the concepts contained in Frenk J (1993) The public/private mix and human resources for health care. *Health Policy and Planning*. **8**: 315–26.

18 Sade RM (1971) Medical care as a right: a refutation. *New England Journal of Medicine*. **285**: 1288–92.

19 Pauly MV (1978) Is medical care different? In: W Greenberg (ed) *Competition in the Health Care Sector: past, present, and future*. Aspen Systems Corporation, Germantown, MD.

20 Frenk J (1988) Financing as an instrument of public policy. *PAHO Bulletin*. **22**: 440–6.

21 Sen A (1987) *On Ethics and Economics*. Basil Blackwell, Oxford.

22 Steiner PO (1977) The public sector and the public interest. In: RH Haveman and J Margolis (eds) *Public Expenditure and Policy Analysis* (2e). Rand McNally, Chicago, IL.

23 World Bank (1993) *World Development Report 1993: investing in health*. Oxford University Press for the World Bank, New York.

24 Frenk J (1994) Dimensions of health system reform. *Health Policy*. **27**: 19–34.

25 Frenk J and Donabedian A (1987) State intervention in medical care: types, trends and variables. *Health Policy and Planning*. **2**: 17–31.

26 Sen A (1987) *On Ethics and Economics*. Basil Blackwell, Oxford.

Chapter 15

Justice and the allocation of healthcare

Suzanne Rameix and Isabelle Durand-Zaleski

The cohesiveness of a democratic society is founded on a shared feeling that the achievement of health equity is a central consideration for policy makers. However, this ultimate goal over the long term is often too far-sighted for policy makers. Politicians are accountable to their constituents over rather shorter periods of time than would be required to observe the effect of policy on the fair distribution of improvements in health. Society's expectation of justice includes both concerns about the processes by which equity in health is to be achieved, and about the fair distribution of healthcare.[1] In this chapter, although we focus on the distribution of health *services*, we are, of course, mindful that this is only a part of a much broader debate about health and justice in society.

Aristotle stated that justice in the distribution of all material and immaterial goods in society is not based on strict equality, which would result in nonsense or injustice, but on proportional equality.[2] For one person, quantity A of a particular good is the equivalent, for another, of quantity B. This also applies when we come to consider not the allocation of different quantities of the same good, but the allocation of a variety of goods. Translated into the language of modern economic theory this means that the 'marginal utility' of the goods distributed (i.e. the additional benefit one individual gains from using one additional unit of a material or immaterial good) should be equal for all members of society.

The problem is to decide the just criterion for determining the appropriate quantity of that particular good that should go to each individual. Depending on the nature of those goods, and the society, the criteria used to decide the just proportions due to each individual might relate to the individual's work, rank, need, perceived virtue, and so on.

Should this criterion be the same for all goods or should it differ according to the good distributed? If all goods are of the same nature then the same criterion should be used to determine the quantity of goods given to each individual in proportion to work, merit, rank and so on. If they are not of the same nature, then the task is to find a typology of goods that allows us to group them in clusters and to find the appropriate criterion for distributing them in just proportions to each member of society.

The idea that material and immaterial goods belong to different orders was beautifully described by Pascal.[3] Pascal states that tyranny (i.e. the opposite of justice) reigns when one tries to appropriate goods that belong to one 'order' by using means that belong to another. The following are examples of orders (a more spiritual word than 'groups', or 'clusters') of goods, and of the corresponding means to obtain them: love 'corresponds' to beauty; fear to strength, and trust to science. Therefore it is tyranny (unjust) for the strong to demand love, or for the beautiful person to demand fear. Pascal's analysis, the intuition that for each good there is an appropriate means of obtaining it, was the inspiration for Walzer's analysis and description of the spheres of justice.[4] Our objective here is to examine the application of these insights to the provision of healthcare.

In a just society the allocation of goods follows criteria which depend on the 'sphere' the good belongs to. Firstly, for each sphere (Pascal's 'order') there is an explicit and legitimate criterion for obtaining it. In this sense it is just that one obtains love because of one's beauty, or esteem because of one's intelligence. Secondly, in no sphere should there be a monopoly, i.e. one individual or a group of individuals having all the goods belonging to this sphere. Thirdly, there should be no dominant sphere, i.e. people who own the goods belonging to one sphere would be able to own the goods belonging to all the other spheres. Finally, we should not use the criterion that corresponds to one sphere to obtain goods that belong to another sphere (just as the strong cannot obtain love, or esteem, or trust).

In democratic societies we acknowledge four legitimate criteria for the allocation of material goods: strict equality, need, merit and the market. Undemocratic societies apply other rules.

Equality signifies that a good, a service or a right is given to all regardless of their ability to pay, regardless of what they request or what they are deemed to deserve. The same good is given to all without difference or discrimination. The person who benefits from this allocation is not required to pay, the good or service being paid for through some mechanism of social solidarity.

Need signifies that goods or services will be provided only after an independent assessment of what is required. It is the external and objective nature of the assessment that distinguishes need from demand. This point is particularly important in the field of healthcare where demand, which perhaps stems from our desire for immortality, tends to be infinite. The provision of healthcare in response to need is paid for through social solidarity.

Merit signifies that a person can obtain a gratification (for example, a position in public office with an income attached) as a consequence of that individual's achievements recognised by votes, or success in examinations or recognition of past endeavours. The worthiness of the beneficiary must be proven by objective measures and not the whim of princes.

For the sake of simplicity, we consider that any good for which a person is required to pay, either directly or by purchasing insurance, is allocated in accordance with the mechanisms of the fourth criterion, the *Market*. The assumption, implicitly made by society when healthcare is allocated in this way, is that individuals should be free and empowered to make choices about the goods (healthcare among them) that they wish to purchase. In this, society does not concern itself with the justice of final outcomes, only that the processes are considered just. If the market is so organised that the same rules are followed by everyone without cheating, there is no injustice even if, eventually, some persons end up having more than others. Any interference from the state (for example, to ensure some provision of baseline care through taxes or social charges) is held to curtail unjustly individuals' freedom by imposing its own hierarchy of values.

The weight given to these different ideas of justice varies over time in any given country, and, at any one time, varies between different countries. We focus here on the legitimacy (for the allocation of material goods in general, and of healthcare in particular) of the allocation principles or criteria chosen in today's democracies.

Goods in relation to citizenship and politics, such as voting rights that are now allocated on the basis of equality (one person gets one vote), were in earlier times allocated on the basis of net worth. Similarly, care for emergencies and catastrophic illnesses, now provided free of charge in most EU countries on the basis of need, used to require payment – at least from those who could afford it. The allocation of education according to need, and not according to the market (the ability to pay for a private tutor), was proposed by Condorcet during the French Revolution.[5] It took almost 100 years to be fully implemented. Public positions in the civil service or senior positions in the military are now obtained by merit, externally judged on the basis of examinations or performance. In the past such posts were purchased from the king or his representatives.

The point here is that there is no eternally and universally recognised acceptable and proper allocation principle for a given good, only one that is felt just in a given country at a given time, one that reflects how the society translates its ideas about justice.

In a just and democratic society the allocation criteria chosen for a given good or service must be explicit and considered legitimate by all. When such is not the case, for example when public offices are found to be bought or preferentially distributed, or when social housing is traded and not allocated on the basis of need, society demands some form of redress. It follows that, when an allocation principle is considered legitimate for a given good, it should apply to all in society, and should not be changed without due consultation with the stakeholders. For example, decisions about removing medicines from formularies mean that a medicine whose cost was previously reimbursed (i.e. allocated on the basis of need) must now be purchased by patients (i.e. allocated by market mechanisms). While this is indeed the current practice in many countries, its acceptability by the public and the pharmaceutical industry requires explanation and justification from governments.

Lastly, there is an ethical requirement that, whichever criterion is chosen, the distribution of goods must be just and efficient in economic terms. Injustice is experienced at the level of the individual (even by libertarians) when poor sick persons cannot be treated. It is also experienced at the societal level when scarce health resources are wasted in responding to futile demands, and so are foregone for other uses.

The application of these allocation principles to the healthcare sector is not straightforward. Each element has to be considered separately. Because of the current pressure to control health expenditures, we are obliged to consider what inefficiencies may result from the choice of one or another principle. And above all, we need to think about how democratic societies apply the concept of justice to the provision of healthcare.

Medicines, doctor's visits, hospital care, preventive care, dental and eye care are allocated by different principles in different countries. In most EU countries, the dominant principle is allocation on the basis of need. There is however a difference between the so-called Bismarck and Beveridge models. The former was initially liberal, and then evolved into one based on strong social solidarity, while the latter was founded on utilitarian solidarity. These models contrast with that in the USA where the dominant allocation principle is the market.

We have argued that allocation principles or criteria must be explicit, legitimate and also efficient. However, the requirement for both legitimacy *and* efficiency is often difficult to satisfy because of the potential conflicts between them. From the end of the nineteenth century, with Bismarck's reforms in Germany, and then in the mid-twentieth century, with the spread of social health insurance systems and national health services throughout EU countries, most curative healthcare has been allocated according to need. However, a major inefficiency in allocating services in accordance with 'need' is that need is often misunderstood as 'demand'. Since demand for healthcare is only limited by our desire for immortality, it may be thought of as limitless. Any threat to our health triggers this desire, and generates a legitimate demand of healthcare. As a country develops and increases its level of wellbeing, demand for *health* increases, and this is often mistaken for a demand for healthcare. Therefore an allocation of healthcare based on the criterion need ('need' which might actually be 'demand') may use up all of society's resources, to the detriment of the provision of other legitimate social goods. It may also create a moral hazard on the part of patients, who then have no incentive to manage their health responsibly, because they assume that even though they do not participate in preventive care – in respect, for example, of cigarette smoking, alcohol abuse, fast driving – curative or reparative care will be provided. Allocation of healthcare based solely on the criterion of 'need as demand' deprives individuals of responsibility for their own health, resulting in negative effects on both individual and on collective health.

In order to limit the inefficiency of an allocation based on this interpretation of need, the assessment of need is made by a physician or other healthcare professional. This external assessment is intended to differentiate need and demand. In countries where professionals are paid on a fee for service basis, however, this assessment by a professional who stands financially to benefit from confirming 'clinical need' creates an imperfect agency situation. While needs assessment can be carried out by government institutions who do not benefit from that agency, these relate only to classes of need. When it comes to the care of individual patients, a health professional is inevitably involved.[6] The opposite risk also exists and is known as the 'gag rule': here, the assessment of need is made under the control of a payer who stands to benefit from a limitation of the care provided.[7]

'Imperfect agency' is not only the source of inefficiency; it also creates inflationary pressure. Although an allocation based on need may be considered legitimate, and result in positive health outcomes for some, it can also create injustice because resources wasted are lost to others, and inefficiency because those who waste the resources do not achieve good health. This leads us to examine how other criteria can perform in allocating healthcare resources justly and efficiently.

Preventive care is mostly allocated on the basis of equality. In the case of immunisation, the justification is the equal utility for all individuals, and the benefit created for society as a whole, by one of its members not infecting others. In the case of screening, the justification of equal access is more difficult to argue, particularly since identifying particular at-risk groups permits efficient, but selective, targeting. It therefore seems more efficient to restrict screening to such at-risk groups, and to use the resource saved (by screening fewer people) to purchase other desirable health goods. However, although efficient, this approach would meet with opposition from the public on the grounds of justice. There is evidence that populations prefer screening to be allocated equally, even at the price of decreased efficiency.[7,8] In this they would appear to be supported by Aristotelian proportionality that suggests that it must be just to give each individual the same screening test if there is no evidence that some would benefit more than others. And individuals may perceive no evident sign that the utility for some individuals will in fact be greater than for others.[9] For policy makers, however, there is epidemiological evidence that high-risk groups will benefit more, and should therefore receive more.

Merit is seldom used as a criterion in EU countries. Its application to the provision of healthcare would result in goods and services being preferentially allocated to the 'deserving', i.e. to persons who have made some kind of effort or commitment to preserve their health. The negative application of this principle to healthcare would mean that 'reckless behaviour' – such as smoking – would be penalised. Treatments of conditions occurring as a consequence of smoking would not be financed through national solidarity.

Examples of experiments in rewarding virtuous behaviour include full coverage of dental care for patients who attend preventive care clinics in the Netherlands,[10] and better reimbursement for patients who go through the new gatekeeping system recently set up in France (Reform law of the Social Security voted on 13 August 2004). While allocation by merit might be deemed just, and is efficient if it encourages patients to adopt virtuous behaviours and so reduce moral hazard, it can be argued that it is unjust because it favours those in society who have easier access to education, information and so have greater capacity to alter their risk-related behaviour.[11]

Allocation of healthcare through market mechanisms is consistent with the liberal theory of justice. Here healthcare is not considered different from any other sort of good, and can be left to be bought and sold in a competitive marketplace. It is a matter for each individual to order his preferences and devote the resources required to achieve his or her target health status. The amount of resources will depend on where the individual places health relative to other goods, and the price she or he is willing to pay for it.

However, the limitations of this approach were identified as early as the Middle Ages, and resulted in the creation, among craftsmen, of the mutual assistance associations.[12] Later, in the eighteenth, and more actively in the nineteenth, centuries, the state stepped in. While perhaps the first limitation to be identified in the market approach was the injury done to society's sense of justice towards its poorer and more fragile members, latter-day economists too have argued against the market as a sole means of allocating healthcare.

Allocation by the market alone, either directly or via competing insurers, is neither just nor efficient. Arrow points out that market inefficiencies result from the asymmetry of information between professionals, patients and payers.[13] Since patients know more about their own health than do the payers (in this case the private insurance companies) they may tell lies about their actual health risks in order to obtain lower premiums. To cut their potential losses, insurers tend to select patients at lower risk, and to charge premiums for those who are at higher risk, like the elderly. Thus, again, the sicker and more fragile members of society are excluded from coverage.[14]

Empirical evidence from the USA suggests that market mechanisms cannot deal efficiently with the asymmetry between the physician who decides on the provision of services, and the party who is to pay for it – be it the patient or the third party payer.[15] Libertarians argue on moral and political grounds that an imperfect market is better than the state's limitations on the individual's freedom to establish her or his own hierarchy of preferences. The counterargument is that persons with severe chronic (and costly) diseases do not have the freedom to prefer other goods than healthcare if they want to survive.

From this brief review of the filters of 'justice' and 'efficiency' in determining the provision of healthcare in the population, it would appear that no single criterion can fulfil all our expectations. All healthcare systems counterbalance the negative effect of their dominant allocation criterion, by the partial introduction of others. In systems where the dominant criterion is need, co-payment mechanisms (the market criterion) may exist, or patients may qualify for higher reimbursements if they use preventive services (the merit criterion). And where the market predominates, public funding is made available for the poor, the elderly, or patients suffering from severe chronic illnesses, as in Medicaid and Medicare in the USA (the need criterion).

Our conclusion is twofold: healthcare should probably be allocated by a composite of all four criteria and the respective part to be played by each of them is a matter of political choice. Societies, however, may then require from policy makers that the choice of criterion to allocate particular types of care be transparent and legitimate, and that they then build a hierarchy of priorities in order to establish and demonstrate health equity.

Policy makers must pose the following questions for public debate. Does healthcare belong to a sphere apart from other goods, one for which the dominant allocation criterion is need and not the market? If the answer to this question is yes, there remains the problem of how to compensate for any unjust and inefficient outcomes of this criterion. Other allocation criteria can be introduced for goods and services that would *de facto* be withdrawn from the sphere of healthcare: for example, cosmetic surgery, spa therapy, treatment for 'heavy legs' or the common cold could, by political decision, be transferred to the sphere of goods bought and sold on the market. The trade-off is that, on the one hand, no poor person would be denied treatment, and, on the other hand, that there would be ways to limit the opportunity cost resulting from resources wasted on futile care. Establishing the societal preferences for health though public debate means more than the political expediency of accommodating society's whims and desires. It means giving all the members of society the 'fair innings' they deserve, and respecting their human dignity.[1]

References

1 Sen A (2002) Why health equity? *Health Econ.* 11(8): 659–66.
2 Aristotle (384–322 BC) *Nichomachean Ethics*. Book V, 6 (1131a–b) [Bywater (ed)]. Oxford University Press, Oxford (1991) p. 94.
3 Pascal B (1623–62) *Pensées*. Lafuma (ed) Seuil, 1963 Paris, p. 507 (Brunschvicg: Pensée. 322).
4 Walzer M (1983) *Spheres of Justice*. Basic Books, New York.
5 Condorcet, de Caritat MJ, Marquis de (1743–94) French philosopher of the Enlightenment and advocate of educational reform.

6 Saltman RB, Busse R and Figueras J (eds) (2004) *Social Health Insurance Systems in Western Europe*. Open University Press/McGraw Hill, Maidenhead. p. 192.

7 Ball JR (1991) Law, medicine, and the 'gag rule'. *Ann Intern Med*. **115**(5) (Sep 1): 403–4.

8 Ubel PA, Dekay ML, Baron J and Asch DA (1996) Cost-effectiveness analysis in a setting of budget constraints – is it equitable? *N Engl J Med*. **334**(18): 1174–7.

9 Sassi F, Le Grand J and Archard L (2001) Equity versus efficiency: a dilemma for the NHS. *BMJ*. **323**: 762–3.

10 Dufour F (1999) L'analyse comparée des systèmes de santé dentaire dans l'UE. *Inf Dent*. **15**: 1075–90.

11 Popay J, Bennett S, Thomas C, Williams G, Gatrell A and Bostock L (2003) Beyond 'beer, fags, egg and chips'? Exploring lay understandings of social inequalities in health. *Sociol Health Illn*. **25**(1): 1–23.

12 Saltman RB, Busse R and Figueras J (eds) (2004) *Social Health Insurance Systems in Western Europe*. Open University Press/McGraw Hill, Maidenhead. p. 22.

13 Arrow K (1963) Uncertainty and the welfare economics of medical care. *American Economic Review*. **53**: 941–73.

14 Saltman RB, Busse R and Figueras J (eds) (2004) *Social Health Insurance Systems in Western Europe*. Open University Press/McGraw Hill, Maidenhead. p. 181.

15 Bodenheimer T (2005) High and rising health care costs. Part 3: the role of health care providers. *Ann Intern Med*. **142**(12 Pt 1) (Jun 21): 996–1002.

Chapter 16

Health values and the politician

Hans Stein

Theoretical constructs, academic analyses and visionary aspirations about health policy are of little, or at best of only limited, value, if they are not seen to be applicable in real life. Karl Marx, an almost forgotten compatriot of mine, whose ideas are now enjoying some revival of interest, wrote the following about the intentions of politics. 'Die Philosophen haben die Welt nur verschieden interpretiert, es kommt aber darauf an, sie zu verändern.' (The philosophers have only interpreted the world in various ways; the point, however, is to change it.)

Marx is right, and his sentiment applies not least to the world of health polity. On the one hand, there is hardly any other area of public policy where scientific experts have written more evidence based, often even visionary, papers, explaining how and why things went wrong, and how the whole system might be put on the right track. On the other hand, I know of no other area of life, where politics and politicians have done so little to transform these visions into reality. It seems that they prefer to agree with the statement of another German, Helmut Schmidt, a former Chancellor. He is credited with saying, 'If you have visions go and see your doctor.' Possibly this explains why, compared with other German chancellors such as Adenauer, Brandt or Kohl, leaders associated with such great value-laden achievements as European integration or German unification, Schmidt's name will go down in history simply as a pragmatist, a man driven not by vision and values, only by the 'realities' of economics.

Politics, policy and polity

Politicians as decision makers are essential for achieving change. One cannot do without them. Nevertheless we must question whether today they are able and willing to do it, to take the difficult decisions and see them implemented. Good and efficient management is important, but it is certainly not enough if it fails to reflect accepted societal values and beliefs, made visible by creating targets, and transformed into reality by laws, regulations and financial resources.

It is interesting to note that in English, in contrast with most other European languages, it is possible to distinguish between politics, policy and polity. In German, for example, there is only one word for all three meanings – *Die Politik*. Nonetheless I want to look at the ways that *Die Politik* is deconstructed in English.

Politics is defined in Chambers Dictionary not only as 'the art and science of government' but also as 'manoeuvring and intriguing'. This definition includes the whole consensus-building and decision making process connected with political power and influence, and the pursuit of different societal interests. But, as the dictionary definition hints, in common usage 'politics' can have less to do with content, principles and values, and more with the manoeuvring, sometimes even the dirty tricks, of the political power game – those 'manoeuvrings' that seem so necessary to get and stay in power, and to find sufficient majorities in governmental and parliamentarian institutions, in order to legislate.

Policy, the art of government, is concerned with strategy, content, aims, values, principles. To become political realities, policies are often formulated first as strategies, as green papers and then white papers, before being incorporated into national or international law.

Polity describes the institutional structures in which policies are made.

To achieve change this triad of different meanings has to be brought together, so that there is a balance between them that is of practical use to the policy makers. In the foregoing, I intend more than an academic discussion about the meaning of words. I remember a big battle we had in the Health Group of the Health Council of the European Union (EU) when France and Germany demanded the inclusion of a 'Public Health Policy' in a Council Document. They were bitterly opposed by the United Kingdom, on the ground that the EU did not have a sufficient legal base for this. It took me a long time to understand that for the British representative the word 'policy' meant something significantly different from the words being used in German and French.

The question that I want to pose is this. Can the Madrid Framework, with its aim of enabling 'constructive conversations about health policy', contribute to achieving a balance between the demands of politics, policy and polity?

My background

In order to place my views in their historical and political contexts, I should outline the scope of my personal involvement in health policy. I gained my experiences of political and governmental life mainly in Germany, working as a public servant for more than 30 years in the Health Ministry, serving altogether 11 different Ministers from three different political parties, all of them representing quite distinctive (and different) *Weltanschauungen* and societal backgrounds, and worked with innumerable Ministers in Germany's many *Länder* (semi-autonomous Regions). I also had a good 'insider view' (at the highest, as well at more local, levels) of the way in which health policy functioned in the now vanished communist system of the former German Democratic Republic. Moreover, I encountered more than 100 Health Ministers from all EU Member States, when they cooperated, or failed to cooperate, on the Brussels stage. My conclusion is that no matter how different their health systems or political or cultural backgrounds, they were quite similar in their political emotions, actions and reactions.

This essay does not contain the results of empirical studies, and there are no journal references. It is evidential and experiential, not academic and theoretical. It is the subjective summary of many years of personal experience, of time spent mostly in relatively close connection with health policy decision makers in Germany, and in the European Union at large.

There may be any number of reasons that the reader will wish to disagree with my intentionally provocative statements, and it is true that most are grounded in the experience of health policy in Germany, a country, by the way, whose federal structure of government has made it all but ungovernable. However, although some of my views will refer specifically to the specific German situation, others, to my mind, are generally applicable in the wider world of politics and politicians.

There is hardly any other democratic country in the world where the powers of its constituent regional states to veto the wishes of the central government are as strong as they are in Germany. In other countries governments are obliged to achieve some kind of consensus on ethical issues with different groups in society – for example the trade unions, industrial and commercial interests, and possibly religious groups. And of course on health matters they will also consult the health professions. In Germany, however, when the government wants to make a fundamental reform, it has first to get the approval of the majority of the 16 *Länder*. This approval can be very hard to get. To rule in Germany, consensus between the two levels of government is essential. This can only be achieved by making compromises. But can one, should one, compromise on issues concerning values and virtues? I think not.

The issues

The pressures and demands on health policy are increasing because of global relationships – international obligations and commitments. The growing number of EU regulations in other areas having an influence on health could serve as an example. Governments struggle today to address the social and economic pressures stemming from ageing societies, the rising incidence of chronic disease, the progress of technology, greater demands for services and growing inequities in health and access to care. Citizens expect and demand quick answers and even though they may realise the difficulties they are disappointed when political decisions do not sufficiently meet their needs and wants.

Taking long-term perspectives may be the only way out of this present dilemma, but the general public seems unwilling to accept such timescales. People demand instant progress and improvement. They are disillusioned when, as happened in the cases of German unification or European enlargement, their economic as well as their health situations were not improved as quickly as they had expected. Citizens today expect more from governments than governments are able to give them. When they are disappointed they respond with political abstention and apathy. This response is not directed only towards national governments, but towards the European Union, as was shown in 2005 by the negative results of the French and Dutch referenda on the EU Constitution.

The need for continuity

One often underestimated but nevertheless quite important characteristic of health politicians, of all politicians, is their very limited lifespan in office. In terms of the 11 different German Health Ministers I served over 30 years, there was an average stay in office of less than three years. Only one survived more than one legislative period. Generally Health Ministers, in whichever country, have only a four-year term in office – a very short time in which to show success; success so necessary in order to get re-elected. Values-driven reform usually takes a lot longer than this to be conceived, accepted and implemented. And even longer to show positive results.

International cooperation could and should play a bigger role in establishing, formulating and finally implementing values. The role that international institutions such as the EU or the WHO could play is still very much underestimated. But it takes much time for international strategies and conventions to be agreed, and even more to be taken seriously, by the different states.

On the international scale, the rate of turnover of Health Ministers in the EU Member States is quite frightening. The composition of the EU Health Council, which meets at least two or three times a year, changes from meeting to meeting. Within four years at the most, the President and all the Ministers on the Council have usually changed.

There is, however, some stability on the international stage which is lacking in the individual states. If reappointed by the individual's own government, the EU Health Commissioner sometimes survives for more than one period in office. The biggest exception, however, to the general failure of continuity, is the WHO. Here, be it in Geneva or Copenhagen, WHO Heads have in the past stayed in office for quite a long time – a situation made possible because they do not have to stand for popular election.

Such international political actors, because for the most part they depend on the goodwill of their governments to select and reselect them, and not on electorates, have much more time than do national politicians in which to implement change. To bring about reform it is not enough to be a good technocratic manager. There has to be an element of political vision.

Continuity

This pervasive climate of change impedes continuity. It creates quite substantial problems, as health reforms usually take more than four years to be planned and implemented. Sometimes I had the feeling that every new Health Minister wanted to start again from scratch, even when his or her predecessor came from the same political party. I never understood why, when New Labour came into power in the UK after many years in opposition, it could not live and work with the health targets set by the previous Conservative administration, and considered it necessary to produce new ones. Nonetheless, I consider health targets to be a stabilising instrument, enabling long-term strategies and guaranteeing continuity.

The bureaucratic administration as a whole and its civil servants are usually considered to be the decisive elements in guaranteeing continuity of policy. I have my doubts about this. This may be the case in the UK where, despite a change of government, the civil servants remain in office and mostly keep their posts. This does not apply in most other countries where, with a change of government, the Minister and his personal assistants have to leave office. Most often the whole top echelon of the administration is changed.

There is a further reason that civil servants cannot be relied on to implement continuous and sustainable change. Successful implementation requires imagination, experimentation, innovation and flexibility, essential characteristics are not necessarily found among civil servants, who are more often conservative rather than progressive. They prefer conventional, well tried approaches and are wary of the risks of experimentation. They represent the element of stability in the system, not that of change. This stability may be far preferable to hectic change, especially change for change's sake. Civil servants in public bureaucracies consider themselves responsible for the status quo, and very often they are. They are the ones who draw up the laws and regulations of the existing system. Demanding change from them, therefore, can be experienced by them as tantamount to criticism of their past work and achievements.

Loyal and knowledgeable civil servants in a well organised administration are the core element of good government. They represent wisdom, continuity and stability. They are not, and were never meant to be, the driving force for change.

The politician and his values

In any country the best that can be said about the post of Health Minister is that it is a hot seat, possibly the hottest seat in any cabinet. The Minister is permanently at the centre of controversial, critical public debate, and is held to be responsible for anything and everything that goes wrong in the health system. Many things can and do go wrong every day. The Minister has to take the blame, and as often as not the final cost of this universal responsibility is losing his job.

Very few people go into politics with the ambition of becoming Health Minister. This is understandable as it seems to guarantee quite a short term in office, with limited perspectives for a future high-level political career. For only one of the health ministers I served in Germany was this post a stepping stone to bigger things. She became President of the German Parliament, but she was the exception that proves the rule. Most of the others just disappeared from public view.

Top ranking politicians seldom become health ministers. The Foreign Office, the Home Office, the Finance Ministries have political glamour. But Health? No major EU Member State has ever shown any interest in bidding for the post of EU Commissioner for Health. They are happy to leave this position to Greece, Ireland or Cyprus. Nor has health ever played any significant role in the elections to the European Parliament.

More relevant than the future political career prospects of health ministers is where they come from in the first place. Very few come from the medical profession, or have a scientific or academic background. Most are politicians who became health ministers not because they had exhibited any special knowledge of, or interest in, health policy, but because they satisfied the requirements for political balance (male/female, left/right, north/south/east/west, Catholic/Protestant, etc.) in the distribution of cabinet posts. For the most part the only previous contact most of them have had with the health system is a visit to the doctor.

As a rule people become politicians not only to be successful for themselves, but for others; to improve the quality of life, for society as a whole, but especially for their constituents. One visionary, election-winning slogan of the 1970s in Germany was *Mehr Lebensqualität* (More quality of life). It is a sad reflection that were that slogan to be used today, it would immediately prompt the question: 'Who is going to pay for it?'

Of course if Health Ministers wish to be successful, to improve the health system, to make it more effective and efficient, to ensure that it is of good quality, and, most of all, to manage to cut the costs, they must experiment. But they can only do so if they are in power and stay in power. Politicians in opposition can do very little except make suggestions to which no one really listens. To achieve anything, a politician must first be in power, and second, stay in power.

But to be, and stay, in power politicians have to be elected and re-elected. If values and virtues can visibly contribute to this, well and good. But in times dominated by social or economic difficulties, to speak about values can make the politician look like an unrealistic dreamer. The public rhetoric changes from values to warnings – 'the writing's on the wall'; 'the end of the Welfare State'. In difficult economic times expressions of values and virtues can be dangerous for politicians, relics of better times, now best forgotten.

The successful politician should aim to be, and to be seen to be, a pragmatic idealist. In politics it is never enough to do good things. These should be recognised and talked about. Public relations, communications strategy, we used to call it propaganda, all play their part in the politics of health system reform.

The Madrid Framework has postulated eleven dimensions, described as defining the forcefield of health policy making. They are the elements of what are described as constructive conversations. All of them are essential components of such discourse, and here I deal with some of them as they relate to my reflections on policy, polity and politics.

Choice

The actual choices available to the policy maker, as well as to the individual, are very limited indeed. In deciding on the choices that can be made available, politicians attempt some sort of consensus. This implies compromise between different and competing interests. Usually compromise doesn't satisfy anybody, because the compromise cannot fully meet everyone's desires. And often the compromise is seen as a bad solution, because it doesn't solve the problem at all. If the choice you must make is between taking the left or the right road, to compromise by choosing the middle one won't get you anywhere, or at least not to the place that you originally had in mind.

EU measures, and especially its Directives, often provide good examples of bad compromise. The EU, and not only in relation to health policy, could not exist without compromise between big and small, richer and poorer, north and south, and, to be sharply specific and to make the point, compromise between health and other (mostly economic) interests.

Another limitation on choice is the scale of its variety. The beliefs, priorities and wants of the different groups in society, and indeed of the different individuals, are so diverse that a compromise can hardly be negotiated, not least because the choices cannot be funded from the public purse. In the last analysis it is the politicians who make the choices and decide on the winners and losers. Unfortunately, if understandably, they will choose to pursue their votes, and finally lean towards the interests of their own supporters.

Democracy

Democracy is defined as a form of government in which the supreme power is vested in the people collectively, and is administered by them or by officers appointed by them. It is the majority that rules and decides. This situation has been described as a 'two-thirds society', meaning that if a political party pays attention to the desires of two-thirds of the population, it will appear to meet their needs, and it will get their votes. The other third of society can then be forgotten. This is unsatisfactory because, as we know, most people with specific health deficits belong to minorities. To be fully applicable to the requirements of a good health policy, democracies need adequately to safeguard and protect the rights and interests of its vulnerable minorities. A salient example is AIDS. When the virus first emerged, some governments, and the EU itself, had difficulties defining policy because the most endangered section of society was its homosexual minority.

Another question for the democratic politician is the role of health policies in affecting the results of elections. There is a widespread belief that health plays a central role in the social and political agenda at the national and international levels. At least that is the evidence we have from countless political speeches and manifestos. Nevertheless I have the feeling that this is largely just wishful thinking. The policy areas that really do play a decisive role in elections – finances, the economy – do not need to be constantly brought to public attention in party manifestos. They are the really decisive factors, and everybody knows it.

The best indicator of the real political priority accorded to health policy is the role that it plays in elections. Take the German general election in 2005. Before the election the media were so full of health topics that it could be considered that health was going to be one of the decisive issues. But once the party manifestos had been published, the picture looked completely different. I don't really know how seriously one should take party manifestos, but at least they are indicators of what parties think their electorate, or at least two-thirds of them, might want. All the German parties included rather short passages on health in their manifestos, but none of them really addressed health. Rather, they addressed the problems of finance. One party mentioned the growing recognition of the 'responsibility of the citizen'. This did not refer to smoking fewer cigarettes, drinking less alcohol, eating healthier food and taking more physical exercise. It referred to 'responsible citizens' being required to pay a fee of €10 out of their own pockets every time they went to see a doctor.

Consequently the different manifestos said nothing as to how the health system might be improved or could lead to more wellbeing, greater equity, increased efficiency – all the issues referred to in the dimensions listed in the Madrid Framework. Their plans concerned only the way that the health system might be financed in the future, and how to create new sources of finance. They were quite silent about how, and for what purposes, this money was to be spent.

Stewardship

If stewardship has something to do with getting health recognised as a vital national resource, securing the needed financial, human and intellectual re-sources, and implementing change on a long-term basis, then stewardship is very much related to leadership.

Because health is determined by so many societal and political factors outside the health system, leadership is essential in order to influence these other areas, most of which are not within the direct responsibility of the Health Ministry. The implementation of the principle laid down in the Health Article of the EU Treaty –

'A high level of health protection shall be ensured in the definition and implementation of all the Union's policies and activities' – doesn't just happen by carrying out health outcome assessments. Implementation requires great political commitment and political leadership.

It is significant that the areas of policy for which a Health Ministry is responsible differ tremendously from country to country. Some departments cover only a national healthcare services. Others include the education of health professionals and workforce planning, some have pharmaceuticals and health technology within their competence, and some include environmental protection, food and consumer protection, as well as medical and public health research. This colourful picture makes it difficult to find a consensus on Commission proposals, and also on deciding national public health strategies. This muddled situation cries out for strong political leadership.

There are two different kinds of leadership. There is organisational leadership, when a person is responsible for certain issues by law or organisational decrees. At the EU level one powerful example for this is the sole right of the Commission to take the initiative, without which the other EU institutions cannot act. This example contrasts with the rather weak position of the frequently rotating EU Presidency, such that the Presidency can do nothing more than set the immediate agenda for the following six months.

Being able to set the agenda is important, but it is not enough. There is great need for another kind of leadership, a leadership capable of developing new ideas, of shaping the future, and of convincing others – citizens as well as stakeholders – to follow. This sort of leadership needs not only to develop new ideas, but to create trust, societal commitment and engagement. It should provide the kind of orientation often lacking in today's society. This requires charismatic personalities, whose aspirations and ideals are trusted, accepted and shared.

Sometimes I have the feeling that we see fewer and fewer such leaders, that increasingly they are being replaced by well functioning technocrats. Of course governance requires good management, but short-term techno-managerial approaches are not enough. They may guarantee the present-day normal functioning of a health system, but will not provide a longer-term policy grounded in moral intent.

Evidence

Successful governance requires a scientific foundation. 'Evidence based medicine' has become a household word, although whether it is always practised is quite another matter. 'Evidence based *health policy*', however, is still met with doubts and misgivings. Governments seem to be reluctant to base their decisions on evidence. They fear that evidence could be tampered with, might lead to conflicting interpretations, and, most importantly, might not be in line with existing policies.

Nevertheless, policy decisions ought to be more based on facts and less on beliefs. The evidence should come from reliable, valid data, comparable over time and across national borders, able to show trends, and to demonstrate how different policy decisions can produce different results.

It may be that in countries that have adopted health targets, for example in the United Kingdom or the USA, evidence has, to a certain extent, influenced decisions. In Germany this has seldom been the case. Although, especially at the local and regional levels, there may be many examples, at the federal level only one prominent case comes to my mind.

This happened in the mid-1970s at a time when the two parts of Germany, the western Federal Republic and the eastern Democratic Republic, were not only rivals, but enemies. Indisputable data showed that maternal and infant mortality in the East was a lot lower than in the West. As these figures could not be rejected as fakes or propaganda, the situation was unacceptable to the West, and something had to be done. For the first time a quality assurance programme for mothers' and infants' health was implemented. Very soon the West had overtaken the East.

Since then quality assurance has become a firm part of the German healthcare system. Recently the *Institute für Qualität und Wirtschaftlichkeit im Gesundheitswesen* has been founded, quite similar to the UK National Institute for Health and Clinical Excellence (NICE). It remains to be seen how much these, and similar, institutions are able to influence policy.

Politicians don't like to be forced into action by international comparisons, and it is seldom that international comparisons alone trigger action. They are quite sceptical about benchmarking in WHO World Health Reports, or in similar OECD and EU publications. But as these are reports without political consequences, they are simply 'noted'. They have very seldom initiated national activities.

Governments like to keep their total independence in health matters. Their reluctance to being forced into action by data-based international comparisons is shown by their negative attitudes to implementing the EU 'Open Method of Coordination' on health issues. This is a new instrument invented by the EU Commission as a means of structuring and organising cooperation between governments, more effective than a simple exchange of experiences. It consists of a few quite simple elements:

- determination of common guidelines/targets/general aims;
- consensus on quantitative and qualitative data-based indicators, possibly leading to benchmarks;
- implementation of guidelines into national and regional policies;
- regular evaluation of progress.

Governments seem to fear that this could lead to a competition between different national health systems resulting in some attracting bad marks, which would make a bad impression on their own citizens. They appear to overlook the possibility that this instrument could help them influence the content of other policies affecting health, and thereby improve inter-governmental cooperation and collaboration.

Synergy

As many different policy areas influence health, close cooperation between different partners is an essential prerequisite for good policy. This concerns not only cooperation within government, but also within and between different agencies and stakeholders, including the health professions, health insurance, the private sector, patients' and citizens' rights organisations, finance, industry. This interdependency, the Madrid Framework's 'synergy', cannot be exaggerated – for example, activities intended to lead to better health might be seen as damaging to the economy; activities favouring economic growth might be seen to endanger health.

One might think that cooperation within government would be an easy task, simply because they have a common aim. This is not the case. There are so many opposing interests to be accommodated by the different ministries or directorates in the EU Commission, so many conflicts that have to be resolved, that sometimes cooperation within a governmental administration is more difficult than cooperation with institutions outside government.

Quite apart from differences between the aims of different policies, one has to take into account the rivalry between politicians and between different ministries. Seemingly quite simple questions, like which minister or ministry is to represent a country at an international conference, or at the EU Health Council, or which minister is to give a speech at a national congress, suddenly become problematic. Solutions become even more difficult when the media make the differences of opinion known to an interested public.

The fight against tobacco use is a good example in demonstrating the difficulties of inter-governmental cooperation. Tobacco most certainly is a health issue, but at the same time it has economic and financial aspects. The composition of the delegations at the negotiating conferences for the *WHO Framework Convention against Tobacco* demonstrates this. It was not only officials from health ministries who sat at the conference table. There were also officials from the Foreign Offices, from the Finance, Economic and Agriculture Ministries.

Higher taxation of cigarettes is considered to be an adequate measure. The Framework Convention calls for it. But whereas the Health Minister hopes that it will reduce consumption, the Finance Minister is interested in higher revenues – meaning more cigarette sales. Between 2002 and 2004 the annual tobacco consumption in Germany fell by 12% – from 168 billion to 148 billion cigarettes. A health success, but surprisingly not recognised as such in the media, because this didn't contribute to solving the country's pressing financial problems – and these seemed to have priority.

Despite these difference, the interests of health on the one hand, and economic considerations on the other, the successful fight against tobacco has shown how such battles can be won. Even though there remain differing situations in different countries, worldwide the consumption of tobacco is recognised as the greatest threat to health, the attitudes of citizens have changed, and consumption has gone down.

To come that far has not been easy. It didn't happen because laws were passed. It entailed a long and tedious process containing many elements. It began with the scientific evidence about the dangers of smoking, it continued with public pressure, and it ended with a change of attitude in society, as well as among policy makers. This enabled the acceptance of restrictive laws and other measures. Public opinion is often influenced by the often hostile media, and politicians prefer to act only if they have the feeling that public opinion supports them. It seems therefore worthwhile to analyse the process of developments in anti-smoking legislation, to see whether this could serve as an example.

Politics and constructive conversations about health

Although, because of my professional background, I have focused on the role of government and politics in considering health values, it has to be recognised that health policy is not the sole responsibility of the state. The politician certainly has an important role to play as leader, law-maker, moderator. But there are other actors on the stage, villains as well as heroes.

Health is a public task. It is a public, societal and individual concern and responsibility. Cicero said that what concerns everybody has to be discussed by everybody. How can we be assured that these discussions will take place?

We do indeed need constructive conversations about health, as opposed to the destructive debates we experience today – and not only in pre-election times. In our parliamentary institutions, speakers make their points but hardly listen to the arguments of others. Indeed to be seen to agree with the opposition can be considered as a political weakness. We need a climate in which new ideas, even visions, are looked at positively and evaluated with an open mind. Only then can they stand a chance of being applied. At a time when radical changes are taking place, government and politics have to be a part of this process. In many cases they may have to take the lead and get the conversations going.

Long-term concepts, visions instead of short-term political expediencies, need room in which to be discussed and developed. Constructive conversations can provide that room. The participants of that conversation, however, should know and understand the background, the needs and the feelings of the other participants, not least those of the political decision makers. After all, our politicians play an important part in our world, and a very important part at that.

I have tried to paint a realistic and therefore critical picture of politics as I have experienced it. In doing so I hope that I have contributed a little to making the conversations of the future constructive.

Chapter 17

Managing paradox

Josep Figueras, Suszy Lessof and Divya Srivastava

Trade-offs in health reform

In the last three decades, health systems in the European region have gone through a number of major reforms in pursuit of a range of objectives. Since the early 1990s the emphasis of many of these reforms has been on achieving financial sustainability, improving quality and social responsiveness, whilst at the same time maintaining equity and access, which are seen as central tenets of Europe's health systems. Many commentators have argued that these objectives are not complementary, that often they stand in direct contradiction to one another. They identify the need to make explicit trade-offs between them, and assert that these trade-offs should reflect societal values and the relative priority assigned to them.

This chapter starts with the observation that policy makers routinely make trade-offs. With particular focus on the countries of Western Europe, it looks at the nature of the trade-offs between the various objectives of health system reform, implicit and explicit, and explores the salient trends and developments in handling them. The first section seeks to clarify what is understood by health system objectives, and discusses the role of values and ideology in determining their relative importance. Three sections follow, addressing what have been hailed as three main trade-offs for policy makers: between financial sustainability and equity; between responsiveness and equity; and between responsiveness and sustainability. The final section will summarise the main lessons from the review of these three trade-offs, and suggests an approach to managing them.

Health system goals, values and trade-offs

In attempting to assess the trade-offs between different health system objectives we need first to define what these objectives are. This is far from straightforward. There is an ongoing debate about how to define them, and about how to formulate and quantify them. Different policy documents put forward a range of objectives that includes 'health gain', 'improved health outcomes', 'cost containment', 'equity', 'allocative and technical efficiency', 'consumer satisfaction', 'equity', 'access', 'choice', 'quality', 'transparency', 'accountability', 'citizen participation' and 'provider satisfaction', with different priority given to each, and different combinations advocated.

These objectives may all be important but they are not always consistent with one another, nor are they comparable. They exist on different levels – the philosophical, the technical and the operational. They overlap each other and are often difficult to measure. If we are to assign relative values and priorities to them we need a clear and concise framework of objectives.

In this field, a key contribution of WHO's World Health Report 2000 is its definition of health system boundaries. A set of what are termed primary health system goals is postulated: 'improving health', 'enhancing responsiveness to the legitimate expectations of the population' and 'assuring fairness of financial contribution'.[1] The Report argues that all other policy objectives will ultimately affect and feed into these three main goals. Here we suggest a slight adaptation of this approach and propose the following:

- **Health improvement:** The *raison d'être* of the health system and so its primary or defining goal.
- **Responsiveness:** Meeting the population's legitimate expectations and generating satisfaction. This is an important objective in itself, and goes beyond specific health improvements that result from therapeutic intervention. Responsiveness is defined as embodying two major categories, each further subdivided into four domains: *respect for persons*, which includes regard for dignity, confidentiality, communication and autonomy; and *client orientation* which consists of prompt attention, adequate quality amenities, access to social support networks, and choice of institution and care provider.[2]
- **Equity:** The distribution of health and social responsiveness in the population; includes the notions of fairness of financial contribution, and of access, utilisation and treatment according to need.
- **Efficiency:** Both technical efficiency (achieving 'value for money' by minimising costs or maximising outcomes) and allocative efficiency (allocating resources between sectors to maximise overall health levels from within existing resources).
- **Financial sustainability:** An extension of the notion of macroeconomic efficiency to ensure that the appropriate share of society's resources is used. It can be defined simply as the ability of the system to generate sufficient (and sufficiently reliable) resources to allow for the continuing (and improving) provision of healthcare for a growing population, despite increasing costs. It also addresses the need to ensure that the share of society's resources devoted to health is appropriate, and that the demands of meeting present needs do not compromise society's ability to meet future needs.[3] An important implication is the achievement of better value for money in the light of constraints in public financing.

The selection and formulation of the above objectives is by no means universally accepted. There are many debates both about the hierarchy of objectives and about their precise boundaries. There is discussion, for instance, about whether 'quality' constitutes an objective in itself or an intermediate objective, contributing either to the achievement of 'social responsiveness', or to the attainment of the overarching goal of 'health improvement' (a view to which we subscribe). Similarly, 'financial sustainability' is closely linked to 'efficiency', although here, given its importance in policy making, it is singled out as a separate objective. On the whole, however, the above set serves to capture the main objectives of the health system.

Interestingly, these objectives, and the underlying concerns for which they are markers, seem to be shared by diverse health systems in very different countries.

A review of various national policy documents addressing the objectives of health system reforms reveals a striking convergence between them. In practice, however, these national reforms pursue quite different priorities and achieve quite different trade-offs between their objectives.

There seems to be a real reluctance openly to admit and discuss the potential conflicts embedded in the priorities and objectives that are set. It is often very difficult for policy makers, in whatever setting they operate, to be seen to argue that any one of the (very laudable) health system objectives is less or more important than any other: for example, that 'social responsiveness' should be sacrificed in the interests of 'efficiency'. There is a tendency therefore to obscure conflicts, and often the trade-offs, however necessary, are not made explicit. It can be argued that at the outset of any reform process, to keep the precise set of objectives ambiguous, and the possible trade-offs implicit rather than explicit, may avert potentially damaging debate. This ambiguity may allow the creation of a momentum towards reform, and accelerate its implementation. However, in the long run, as the real priorities attached to different policy objectives become apparent, a failure to make explicit the choices that policy makers have to make will be interpreted as excluding the public from the debate, and may thus generate opposition that can undermine and often reverse reform.

Another obstacle to progress is that when the necessary debate on values and trade-offs does take place, it focuses too often on the means and the policy instruments to be applied, rather than on the ends or the objectives of the health system. Moves to introduce elements of privatisation in European health systems serve as a case in point. Often privatisation becomes an end in itself – an ideological goal rather than a means to an end. There is a need to disentangle the evidence on the impact of privatisation on objectives such as responsiveness, efficiency or equity from the values assigned to these objectives by particular social cultures and political philosophies.

Disentangling these elements calls for a clear framework of objectives and demands priority-setting that reflects societal values. Making trade-offs explicit is central to this. An open debate about trade-offs provides for shared ownership of reform and the validation of the choices that policy makers must make, allowing citizens to balance evidence, ideology, culture and policy-judgement. It is also central to the assessment of the impact of reform strategies against goals that have been weighted according to societal values.

This chapter seeks to contribute to that debate by exploring the nature of a number of trade-offs between health system objectives. We focus on three of them, not only because the trade-offs between these three are particularly complex but because they play a central role in the current reform debate (*see* Figure 17.1).

Firstly, we examine the trade-off between financial sustainability and equity – a dilemma rooted in growing healthcare expenditures which challenge governments to question their ability to maintain adequate levels of funding to sustain their health systems. The central question addressed here is whether, in order to ensure financial sustainability, population coverage and benefits from public or statutory sources must be reduced, thus undermining the principle of equity. Secondly, the responsiveness of the health system to citizen expectations (an objective increasingly important in many reforms) is set against financial sustainability. Some strategies aimed at increasing responsiveness may be inefficient and so may undermine the financial sustainability of the system. Thirdly, we explore the trade-off between responsiveness and equity, acknowledging that many strategies aimed at responsiveness do not apply equally to different population groups, and that it is often the younger and the better educated who benefit most from these strategies.

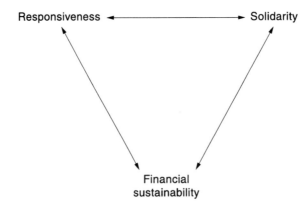

Figure 17.1 Balancing health system objectives.

I Financial sustainability versus equity

The trade-off between financial sustainability and equity is one of the most central in many health system reforms. We focus first on the trend to increasing healthcare expenditure. Then we review strategies aimed at public sector sustainability by shifting healthcare costs to patients, strategies that often have a negative impact on equity. Finally, we question whether the only way to achieve sustainability is to undermine equity.

Health expenditure trends

Much has been written about the pressures on healthcare expenditure. Typically this is ascribed to three factors: the increasing use of more sophisticated and expensive technology, the ageing of the population, and citizens' increased expectations. Figure 17.2 presents the increase in total health expenditure as a percentage of GDP for a selected group of western European countries between 1990 and 2003. In many countries health expenditures have increased at a faster rate than overall economic growth. In 2003, countries of the European Union 15 devoted 8.8% of their GDP to health spending, an increase from 7.1% in 1990. This percentage varies between countries, and in 2003 ranged from 7.4% in Finland to 11.1% in Germany and 11.5% in Switzerland. In most countries the relative ranking as a percentage of GDP was similar to their rankings on a per capita basis. Health expenditures as a share of GDP increased in every EU country except Finland, where health expenditure growth was positive but lagged behind GDP growth.

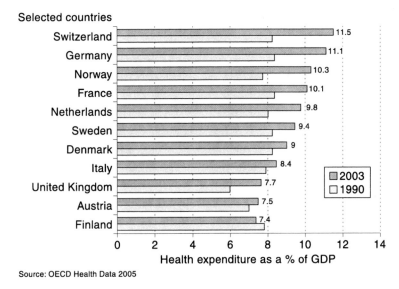

Source: OECD Health Data 2005

Figure 17.2 Total health expenditures as a percentage of GDP (1990–2003).

Shifting costs to individuals

Cost containment in order to ensure financial sustainability has been a major trigger for many reform initiatives, and a central goal of policy. Reforms have focused on a wide range of supply and demand strategies. Supply strategies have aimed at enhancing provider efficiency. They include the introduction of strategic purchasing,[4] market competition between public and private providers, contracting mechanisms, evidence based medicine, performance-based payments systems, putting primary care in the driving seat, and decentralising provider management. These have had varying degrees of impact but on the whole they have resulted in substantial efficiency improvements.

On the demand side, policy makers have been looking at ways to shift costs to the consumers. Initiatives include reliance on out-of-pocket payment by patients, restriction of statutory packages of benefit, increasing cost sharing, and favouring the introduction of voluntary private insurance, which effectively increases the share of private funding in the health system.

We turn now to a more detailed discussion of these strategies. Among Western European countries, health systems rely on a mix of public and private funding. Despite recent increases in the share of private sources, most funding comes from taxation and social health insurance. The main sources of private funding are private (or voluntary) health insurance, and out-of-pocket payments – direct payments, formal cost sharing, and informal payments. In Western Europe, only Austria, Greece, Netherlands and Portugal draw 30% or more of total health expenditure from private sources (*see* Figure 17.3). Apart from France and the Netherlands, out-of-pocket payments form a larger proportion of private health expenditure than private (or voluntary) health insurance.[5]

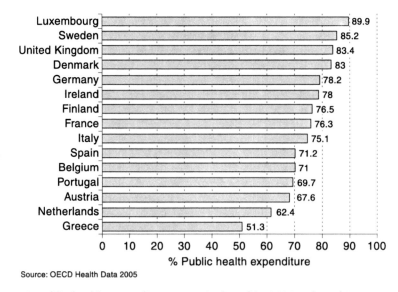

Source: OECD Health Data 2005

Figure 17.3 Public health expenditure as a % of total in 2003, selected Western European countries.

Political and economic difficulties in increasing tax and social insurance payments have contributed to the appeal of cost sharing as a means of raising much needed revenue for the health sector. Data on private sources of financing such as out-of-pocket expenditures (OOP) and private health insurance (PHI) for selected countries are presented in Table 17.1. The numbers are ranked according to OOP and indicate that both sources of expenditure vary considerably between Western European countries. Evidence suggests that cost sharing is a weak instrument for improving efficiency and containing healthcare costs. Providers heavily determine the demand for health services; service intensity, which is provider-driven, has a key impact on healthcare costs. Cost sharing can only reduce consumer-initiated utilisation and is not therefore the most effective tool for cost-containment. Without compensatory administrative procedures, and exemptions, cost sharing undermines equity with respect to financing and access. In spite of these objections, policy makers continue to use cost sharing widely and consider increasing its role in health funding – in part for political and ideological reasons.

Another strategy for shifting costs to consumers is to increase the role of voluntary private insurance. This can substitute for public coverage (substitutive insurance), or supplement current services (supplementary insurance), or cover for benefits not included in the basic package (complementary insurance).

Overall, private health insurance represents less than 6% of total health expenditure for the countries presented in the table. However, there are exceptions. For example, in Germany and the Netherlands private health insurance provides primary coverage for selected groups in the population, and thus is a more important source of financing. While the uptake is still relatively low, there are many voices in the policy arena calling for an increased role of private insurance. However, because insurers engage in a range of strategies to

Table 17.1 Private sources of financing as a share of total health expenditure, 2003.

	Out-of-pocket payment	Private health insurance	Total private
Greece	47	2	49
Switzerland	32	9	42
Spain	24	4	29
Italy	21	1	25
Austria	19	8	32
Finland	19	2	24
Denmark	16	1	17
Norway	16	0	16
Ireland	13	6	22
France	10	13	24
Germany	10	9	22
Netherlands	8	17	38
Luxembourg	7	1	10
Belgium			26
Portugal			30
Sweden			15
UK			17

Source: OECD Health Data 2005.
Note: Sum of private and OOP may not equal total private due to other private funds.
Note: No breakdown available for Belgium, Portugal, Sweden and UK.
Germany (2000) data; Spain (1991) data.

rate or select on the basis of risk, voluntary insurance undermines equity. This is unequivocally demonstrated by experience in the European Region.[6]

Risk rating is used to varying degrees and for different types of voluntary health insurance. Voluntary health insurance premiums are rarely income-related and are usually based on individual health risk, or on an estimate of risk at a community or group level. The methods used to set premiums, and the variables used, may have important implications for cost and access.[7]

Insurers that use health status as a variable for risk rating require applicants to complete a medical questionnaire about their health history. Swedish insurers refrain from obtaining information about family history of disease, whereas this is required in Greece, Luxembourg, Portugal and the UK.[8] As a consequence of such information demanded by insurers, applicants may find their coverage reduced or denied. For instance, most insurers set a maximum age limit, and some cancel contracts when people reach retiring age. Moreover, most voluntary health insurance policies are subject to exclusions. For instance, pre-existing conditions are commonly excluded, although some may be covered for an increased premium.

In sum, in spite of wide European diversity, equity is still at the very core of both taxation and social health insurance systems in the region. While there are concerns with the current levels of equity and equity of access,[9] particularly for minority populations,[10] on the whole European systems exhibit high levels of equity. They have all achieved universal coverage with comprehensive packages of benefit largely maintained. In most countries the role of cost sharing, while increasing, is still limited, with important exemptions on equity grounds. Similarly private voluntary insurance still plays only a minor role in the overall funding of healthcare.

Re-examining sustainability

Many advocate a reduction in the publicly or statutorily provided package of benefits, and an increase in out-of-pocket payments or voluntary insurance, as the only ways to deal with the crisis in health sector financing. Hence the question faced by many health sector policy makers today, and the central trade-off explored here, is whether financial sustainability can be achieved only at the expense of equity. This argument is embedded in a broader political one that advocates limiting the welfare state, and asking citizens to take increased personal financial responsibility. This is advanced both on the ground of economic sustainability and also on ideological grounds. Regardless of the key role played by the societal and political contexts, there is a need for a clearer understanding of the parameters of this trade-off between sustainability and equity. There are four important issues that need further examination.

Firstly, if the notion of financial sustainability is reformulated as 'willingness to pay', new options become available to the policy makers. Equity is a central value in European societies, and evidence indicates that populations are willing to pay more, through statutory sources, for increased services and whole population coverage. There seems here to be a gap between the views of the population and the decisions of political elites.

Secondly, the often cited assumption that increasing public expenditure undermines the economy needs to be carefully revisited. While it is true that increasing taxation, or direct levies on labour by augmenting social health insurance contributions, may have a negative impact on market competitiveness, increases in health expenditure relative to GDP growth, provided there is overall economic growth, are less important than is often assumed. The problem for health funding, particularly in Western Europe, is much more one of sluggish, low-growth economies, than of increasing health expenditures at the macro-economic level.

There is also scope for diversifying funding sources in order to minimise the impact of health spending on unit labour costs. Policy makers can increase sustainability and reduce the pressures on equity by exploring other sources of taxation (for example, from selected use of VAT, so-called 'sin taxes' on alcohol, tobacco, and so on). At the very least they can rebuff the argument that increases in cost sharing and voluntary insurance have no negative impact on the economy. Experience in the United States proves this point.[11] Unregulated increases in private insurance undermine employment markets, increase labour costs and reduce workforce mobility due to risk-related premiums for pre-existing conditions.

Thirdly, policy makers need to differentiate between financial and social sustainability, and consider the implications of the latter, including the implications for economic viability. For example, in terms of social stability, the benefits of covering 'marginal' populations are considerable. There is ample evidence from across Europe of the corrosive effect of excluding minority groups from social provision.[12]

Health coverage contributes to social cohesion. It is an enabling factor which ultimately fuels increases in economic productivity, and links with the next consideration.

Fourthly, in assessing trade-offs between sustainability and equity, the hidden costs of failing to maintain full and equitable coverage must be factored into decision making. There has long been a recognised link between health status and economic productivity in developing countries.[13] It is now increasingly clear that this link applies also in developed countries.[14] To concentrate on mechanisms for increasing financial sustainability that reduce coverage for the poor may therefore prove to be economically short-sighted.

In the light of all these considerations, the trade-off between sustainability and equity may not be as problematic, nor pose as serious a threat, as policy makers envision. They need to factor in the consequences of failing to invest socially and as well as economically.

2 Social responsiveness versus financial sustainability

Responsiveness has become an increasingly important objective in many health systems since the early 1990s. In many countries in the Region there is a noticeable trend towards increasing social responsiveness, part of a broader reform movement concerned with citizen empowerment. However, social responsiveness can be seen to present challenges to financial sustainability because in some instances giving greater weight to patient preferences, whether through improving the physical environment of health service provisions, or by increasing provider choice, may result in higher health service costs. This section reviews the evidence for an unavoidable trade-off between financial sustainability and social responsiveness.

Firstly, we need to re-emphasise that the intentions of responsiveness go beyond those of health gain or efficiency. For instance, there are many interventions not deemed to be effective with respect to health gain, or efficient with respect to value for money, that nonetheless respond to citizens' expectations. Prioritising responsiveness sometimes means opening the door to such interventions. The choice becomes more critical when their cost, unsupported by scientific evidence, begins to threaten the financial sustainability of the system itself. Increased pressure on resources associated with increased responsiveness may also put the spotlight on interventions whose appropriateness previously went largely unquestioned. This raises the spectre of increased cost and diminished financial sustainability, positing a direct trade-off between responsiveness and sustainability.

Clearly how the trade-off is resolved depends on the extent to which different societies and policy makers are willing to allocate limited resources to interventions that respond to the wishes of citizens, but that cannot be shown to impact on either health or cost-effectiveness. On the whole, there is evidence that policy makers are prepared to invest in these areas. In a recent comparison between social health insurance (SHI) and National Health Service (NHS) systems, Figueras *et al.* illustrate this, showing what seems to be higher satisfaction/ responsiveness in SHI countries. The central question for policy makers is this: 'Is greater social responsiveness worth the additional costs?' The study concludes that 'this requires a societal rather than a technical judgment', noting that 'SHI systems respond to a way of understanding the world' and calls for 'a framework for making policy based on that societal perspective'.[15]

One should be cautious about oversimplifying the decisions policy makers face in these circumstances. There is a wide and diverse range of strategies available, and scope for improving responsiveness for little or no additional expenditure – for example, by ensuring that cost-effective interventions are delivered in a way that responds to users' expectations. Responsiveness can be enhanced by better staff training, by improving amenities, increasing choice, or reducing waiting lists.

The challenge for policy makers is to disentangle the various elements as they interact in particular contextual circumstances, and as they relate to the values of a given society. Policy makers may struggle to decide between the marginal cost benefit of investing in better hospital rooms, or user-friendly information systems, and that from putting the same resources into proven clinical interventions. To explore some of these tensions we now focus briefly on one particular strategy which has been central to enhancing responsiveness in recent years – increasing the choice of insurer and provider.

Increasing choice

The right to exercise a degree of choice when accessing healthcare is often seen to play an instrumental role in increasing responsiveness. In practice, however, the implementation of choice strategies is rather complex and has often resulted in unintended consequences. In some cases the two objectives of social responsiveness and efficiency are at odds with one another, and trade-offs are required.

During the 1990s a relatively new dimension of choice emerged in a number of SHI countries such as Germany and the Netherlands, where citizens were given the right to choose between competing insurers or sickness funds. Admittedly, the focus of this reform was not only to increase responsiveness but also to unleash the perceived benefits of market forces. The degree to which consumers now change their insurance funds, the impact of these changes on economic efficiency in the overall system, and the impact on equity (which we address in the section below) remains a contentious political issue.

There is clear evidence that countries with a multiplicity of sickness funds have higher administrative costs, and that these increase significantly with the introduction of choice and competition between sickness funds.[16] This appears to be linked to the costs of marketing and advertising, to risk selection and to management costs. With respect to the impact on economic efficiency (and so on the sustainability side of this trade-off), the question of whether the increased costs resulting from competition between insurers will be offset by the hoped for (but not yet proven) efficiency savings from market competition remains unanswered.

Consumers in most Western European countries have the right to choose primary care providers. In SHI systems, consumers can also choose ambulatory specialists and hospitals, albeit in some cases through a gatekeeper system (e.g. the Netherlands). In NHS countries, the choice of hospital provider has traditionally been relatively restricted, although this has changed recently in many countries. Norwegian, Danish and Swedish patients, for example, are now allowed to choose any hospital outside their county of residence. Similarly in other NHS type systems such as the UK and Spain, patients have seen their choice of hospital greatly increased. The introduction of choice in these countries was aimed at increasing competition among providers, encouraging them to operate more efficiently, and also to be more responsive to patients.

Evidence on the impact of these various strategies to increase choice is still incomplete. While there has been an increase in provider responsiveness, the extent to which this has been accompanied by efficiency is unclear. For instance, there are concerns about the degree to which information given to consumers can sometimes lead to provider capture. The evidence is clearer when looking at choice of primary and ambulatory doctors in countries without a primary care gatekeeper function. In countries such as France and Germany, the absence of a gatekeeping mechanism often results in high levels of unnecessary service use. This is even worse when free choice of ambulatory provider is combined with fee for service schemes: this creates perverse incentives and encourages provider-induced demand. Consequently many of these countries have been trying to bolster sustainability by putting in place systems aimed at curtailing choice and reducing moral hazard.

In Germany, while most citizens are said to have a family physician, they frequently choose directly to consult office-based specialists. With the implementation of user charges for physician and dentist visits in 2004, the number of physician visits decreased by 10% and the rate of direct consultations with specialist fell by 7% (60 to 53%). In contrast, the rate of referred consultations (from family physician to specialist) increased from 40% to 47%.[17]

Similarly, in France, recent reforms are aimed at increasing cost-effective choices of treatment, and seek to control costs by reducing patient choice of specialists by the introduction of a gatekeeping function.[18] Incentives are provided to GPs (annual payment for each patient registered) and patients are exempted from any co-payment for a doctor visit. By contrast, patients receive a lower reimbursement if they visit a specialist without a referral, and specialists can charge higher fees for such direct consultations. So far, in 2004 only 1.8% of patients have consulted via a referring physician, and only 10% of GPs have joined the scheme.[19] The extent to which this approach will have a significant effect in curtailing inefficient utilisation, once the programme goes into full force in 2006, is unclear.

In Denmark, disincentives are introduced to reduce choice. Residents can choose to belong to one of two groups. In the first group residents are registered with a GP in their geographical area, have free access to both GPs and specialists, but are required to have a referral from their GP to see a specialist.[20] If they visit a specialist directly they are liable to pay the full fee. Changing to another GP is allowed every six months, but in some counties a small fee for this is required. Official figures are unavailable but switching between doctors is considered to occur infrequently. In the second group residents have a free choice of GP and specialist, but are subject to a co-payment. Less than 2% of the population has opted to be in this group.[21]

Many countries in the Region have also introduced strategic purchasing reforms, with the aim of increasing provider efficiency. In these schemes purchasers, such as insurance funds or regions, may contract with providers selectively in the light of cost-effectiveness and quality criteria. Although, as noted above, many countries also encourage consumer choice of provider, in practice choice available to the consumer and the purchaser cannot be equally met. Strategic purchasing shifts the balance of power to the purchaser agent, thereby reducing or even removing the choice available to the consumer.

Evidence suggests that in all these reforms the trade-off is resolved in favour of financial sustainability. The choice of provider is curtailed by purchasers, or linked to some financial disincentives, with social responsiveness taking a back seat. In many instances, the consumer has to set the utility derived from choosing her or his provider, against the out-of-pocket costs incurred. There is, then, a money barrier to the exercise of choice that will clearly affect the poorest service users. This raises fundamental equity issues, and leads us to the third trade-off we consider in this chapter.

Responsiveness versus equity

The third set of trade-offs closes our conceptual triangle (*see* Figure 17.3 above) – it counterpoises responsiveness and equity and argues that strategies to increase social responsiveness, now at the centre of so many reforms, will have a negative impact on equity. In no small part this is because of the inequitable way health systems respond to users' expectations. We now discuss whether strategies to improve responsiveness benefit all population groups equally, or some more than others.

Studies of healthcare utilisation reveal that higher-income groups utilise services more often than low-income groups, although the latter have greater health needs.[22] There may be several reasons for this. For instance, access to services may be relatively more costly both in time, and in earnings forgone, for those in lower income groups, who are therefore less able to obtain good services.[23] In Sweden, those who financially assessed their situation as being poor were ten times more likely to forgo care as those who assessed their financial situation as being good.[24] In Denmark, the probability of obtaining dental care is positively related to household income.[25]

Evidence also shows that those more active in exercising choice are usually younger, healthier, more affluent and better educated.[26] This is demonstrated by the introduction of choice of insurers in Germany and the Netherlands.[27] The evidence shows that healthier, younger and higher-earning individuals not only shift funds more often, but also into funds that are cheaper or offer better benefit packages.[28,29] This is further illustrated in a recent report in the UK which argues that current measures to increase patients' choice favour 'the healthy, wealthy and demanding' and those who have access to information and transport.[30] The report notes that people from lower socioeconomic groups had 20% fewer hip replacements than people from other groups, despite an estimated 30% higher need. Also people from social classes IV and V had 10% fewer consultations about preventive care than those from social classes I and II.

It is not only that those from lower socioeconomic groups experience less social responsiveness than those from higher status groups (who have higher expectations and the confidence and negotiation skills to pursue their entitlements). The poor also have access to fewer services, which tend to be of poorer quality and seem to result in relatively poor health outcomes. The suggestion is that, given the scarcity of resources, system changes aimed at increasing social responsiveness, and particularly choice, may result in better and more expensive amenities for some, while reducing the level of essential clinical services available to others.

On one hand, the principle of equity is at the core of the European social model. On the other, choice is enshrined in the European internal market and the freedom of movement of people, services and goods. This dilemma is well illustrated by the current debate about patient cross-border mobility between EU countries.[31] While the number of patients crossing borders is still relatively small, there is a trend towards progressively greater mobility with respect to both the volume and the range of services involved. This recent trend has been underscored by the rulings of the European Court of Justice to protect freedom of movement, and the discussions around the formulation of the new services directive. Although health services fall under the principle of subsidiarity, increasing cross-border entitlement is seen by many national governments as jeopardising the sustainability of their own health systems. They fear that the costs of treating their more mobile citizens in other European countries will undermine cost control, because reimbursing patients treated abroad will use up a large part of their budget. Permitting cross-border entitlement could result in limiting services available for those unlikely to seek care in this way – usually the older, poorer and sicker citizens. This threatens both financial sustainability and equity.

One policy response to this trade-off is to reduce responsiveness to the population's lowest common denominator in line with 'the equity in poverty' argument, i.e. offering equally unresponsive services to everyone. Arguably this would meet the equity principle, but it would surely encounter resistance in most of our societies, particularly given the strategies in place to empower citizens. Also, as noted by den Exter in a recent analysis of patient empowerment in Europe, '. . . these developments may incur increased costs, threatening social equity and financial stability, but they are a consequence of a democratic evolutionary process in many health systems and cannot be ignored.'[32]

Perhaps a more acceptable response to this trade-off is to focus efforts on achieving wider access to information about services, and on tailoring support through positive discrimination strategies that increase access and choice for the underprivileged. There is a wide range of measures to make healthcare choices more effective for the poorest. These aim to overcome those barriers that prevent people exercising full choices, including lack of information and knowledge, language problems, inadequate transport and information technology, and disability. There are also many examples of strategies to prevent discriminatory practices. For instance, some countries with free choice of insurer, such as Germany and the Netherlands, use active regulation to prevent risk selection, including open enrolment and financial redistribution formulae between insurers.

In all these cases addressing this trade-off involves investing substantial additional financial resources. It begs the question: 'Are societies prepared to pay for equity in responsiveness?' Interestingly this brings us back to the first set of trade-offs discussed here – that between sustainability and equity.

Can we have it all? Managing the paradox

This essay has selected and explored three of the many sets of trade-offs that policy makers have to face. They have been chosen because of their key role in the healthcare reform debate and because they illustrate the complexities and difficulties of managing paradox.

Trade-offs take place all the time and on a range of levels. Sometimes they are implicit, sometimes explicit, but ultimately at least some of them are necessary. It is scarcely surprising that we have failed to identify any magic recipe that will manage all the paradoxes or deliver all our competing demands for fair, responsive and affordable health systems. Rather we have attempted to offer some insights into their nature, and the nature of the task of balancing competing demands.

Our most compelling conclusion is that this is fundamentally a debate based on values which will vary between different populations. If that debate is to be inclusive and effective, policy makers should avoid confusion between the choices that are value laden, and the choices that hinge on technical debate. There is a need, therefore, for an explicit framework that sets out the evidence and the options, that facilitates an open debate about the true nature of the trade-offs to be made. This will allow public participation in decision making and public ownership of the preferences expressed.

Our close look at the three trade-offs dealt with here has revealed interesting, and perhaps some unexpected, dimensions of choice for policy makers, and something about the true nature of choosing between health policies. In many instances specific trade-offs are poorly understood and overly politicised. This exposes policy makers to unnecessary pressures. The degree to which policy makers really have to exercise absolute choice, or the extent to which trade-offs are entirely necessary, may be much smaller than we thought.

The first trade-off that we considered demonstrates this clearly. Improvements in the efficiency of service delivery may not be sufficient to address cost pressures and secure financial sustainability. It is hard to contest that equity is likely to suffer if measures to control demand and achieve substantial savings are introduced as the core response to cost pressures, when these depend heavily on shifting costs to patients. This suggests the need for trade-off between sustainability and equity, one which is central to the political debate in most reforms. However, the premise that the only way to address financial sustainability is to reduce levels of equity is a false one which requires some fundamental qualifications.

Financial sustainability is not about absolutes. It reflects a population's 'willingness to pay' – in this case for equity. This perception allows for more flexibility than is sometimes thought. Some societies may be willing to devote increased resources to healthcare in order to pay for equity, either by shifting funds from other areas of public expenditure (such as defence) or by increasing contributions. These strategies need not threaten a society's broader economic viability. Further, the imperative of financial sustainability should be set against that of social sustainability and the wider societal implications of excluding poorer populations. Finally, the benefits of equity with respect to economic productivity may ultimately offset the costs of universal population coverage. We suggest that policy makers need always to question the absolute of any trade-off, to look for the relative, and to take into account the wider societal context in which they make choices.

The requirement for the second trade-off is based on the argument that measures aimed at increasing responsiveness, so central to many reforms, decrease efficiency, and will therefore undermine financial sustainability. Again, however, there are a number of important qualifications to be considered.

Sustainability is in many respects about willingness to pay rather than about given financial limits. Arguably, if citizens are willing to pay collectively for social responsiveness, responsiveness ceases to threaten sustainability. The use of resources for responsiveness ceases to be seen as 'inefficient' if, in addition to improved health status, it is fully valued for itself, and recognised as a core health system goal. What is more, responsiveness includes a wide range of measures many of which may require relatively few additional resources in order to have a potentially significant impact. Ensuring dignity, confidentiality and effective communication can in part be addressed by reforming medical curricula and training. We argue that there is much scope for improving responsiveness without jeopardising sustainability.

However some elements of responsiveness must entail some cost. In particular the dimension of choice of provider and insurer poses very clear trade-offs with financial sustainability. Here, again, policy makers can benefit from a detailed examination of the trade-off. The core issue is not simply the right to choose, but how appropriately that choice is exercised. It is hard to defend an arrangement that demonstrably gives rise to inappropriate, unnecessary and therefore inefficient utilisation of services. Better education, more outreach to, and dialogue with, the public, and more explicit statement of benefits, can all help tackle inappropriate demand. Such efforts may be more effective, and more equitable, than measures to introduce disincentives through cost sharing, since these inevitably hurt the poor and threaten equity. Similarly, focusing on ways of ensuring appropriate levels of access to good quality general practitioners as gatekeepers may be enough to satisfy the demand for choice in many societies. These efforts may prove just as acceptable as, and more efficient than, offering choice of specialists for each episode of care. Policy makers are already aware that there are different perceptions of choice and different importance ascribed to it in different countries, contexts and cultures.

Consideration of the third trade-off leads to similar conclusions about the danger of considering trade-off in absolute terms. While there are legitimate concerns that increases in health system responsiveness, particularly the ability to choose, can sometimes have a negative impact on equity, the link is not an inevitable one. Given that limiting social responsiveness for all in order to achieve greater equity would not be acceptable in most of our societies, the policy maker must look to invest and target resources at the less privileged, so as to ensure 'equal responsiveness for equal need'. This does however, brings us back to the first trade-off, and to ask whether society is willing to pay for equal responsiveness across all social groups. This trade-off is a function of society's willingness to pay for equity. As with the other examples addressed here, there are no simple answers. However, it is clear that an explicit discussion of the options, the values and implications of any given trade-off, can reduce the complexity of any decision, remove some of the artificial barriers to managing the paradoxes, and pave the way for solutions that can be owned by the whole of society.

References

1 World Health Organization (WHO) (2000) *World Health Report 2000: health systems: improving performance.* WHO, Geneva.
2 Valentine NB, de Silva A, Kawabata K, Darby C, Murray CJL and Evans DB (2003)

Health system responsiveness: concepts, domains and operationalization. In: CJL Murray and DB Evans (eds) *Health Systems Performance Assessment Debates, Methods and Empiricism*. World Health Organization, Geneva.

3 McIntosh T, Forest P-G and Marchildon GP (2004) *The Governance of Health Care in Canada: selected papers from The Commission on the Future of Health Care in Canada, Volume III*. University of Toronto Press, Toronto.

4 Figueras J, Robinson R and Jakubowski E (eds) (2005) *Purchasing to Improve Health Systems Performance*. Open University Press, Maidenhead.

5 Mossialos EA and Thomson S (2004) *Voluntary Health Insurance in the European Union* (1e). WHO Regional Office for Europe on behalf of the European Observatory on Health Systems and Policies, Copenhagen.

6 Mossialos EA and Thomson S (2004) *Voluntary Health Insurance in the European Union* (1e). WHO Regional Office for Europe on behalf of the European Observatory on Health Systems and Policies, Copenhagen.

7 Mossialos EA and Thomson S (2004) *Voluntary Health Insurance in the European Union* (1e). WHO Regional Office for Europe on behalf of the European Observatory on Health Systems and Policies, Copenhagen.

8 (2004) *Health Care Systems in Transition: HiT Country Profiles*. WHO Regional Office for Europe on behalf of the European Observatory on Health Systems and Policies, Copenhagen. Available from: www.euro.who.int/eprise/main/WHO/Progs/OBS/Hits/20020525_1.

9 Judge K, Platt S, Costongs C and Jurczak K (2005) *Health Inequalities: a challenge for Europe. An independent expert commissioned report by, and under the auspices of, the UK Presidency of the EU*. Produced by COI for the UK Presidency of the EU.

10 Healy J and McKee M (eds) (2004) *Accessing Health Care: responding to diversity*. Oxford University Press, Oxford.

11 Enthoven AC (2003) Employment-based health insurance is failing: now what? *Health Affairs*. May 28 2003. Web exclusive available from: www.healthaffairs.org/.

12 (2005) European lessons from the French riots. *The Economist*. November 10 2005.

13 WHO (2001) *Report of the Commission on Macroeconomics and Health. Macroeconomics and Health: Investing in Health for Economic Development*. World Health Organization, Geneva.

14 European Commission (2005) *The Contribution of Health to the Economy in the European Union*. Office for Official Publications for the European Communities, Luxembourg.

15 Saltman RB, Busse R and Figueras J (eds) (2004) *Social Health Insurance Systems in Western Europe*. Open University Press, Maidenhead.

16 Figueras J, Saltman RB, Busse R and Dubois HFW (2004) Patterns and performance in social health insurance systems. In: RB Saltman, R Busse and J Figueras (eds) *Social Health Insurance Systems in Western Europe*. Open University Press, Maidenhead.

17 Busse R and Reisberg A (2004) *Health Care Systems in Transition: Germany*. WHO Regional Office for Europe on behalf of the European Observatory on Health Systems and Policies, Copenhagen.

18 Dourgnon P (2005) Choice in the French health care system. *Euro Observer*. 6(4): 9–10.

19 Sandier S, Paris V and Polton D (2004) *Health Care Systems in Transition: France*. WHO Regional Office for Europe on behalf of the European Observatory on Health Systems and Policies, Copenhagen.

20 Vallgårda S, Krasnik A and Vrangæk K (2001) *Health Care Systems in Transition: Denmark*. WHO Regional Office for Europe on behalf of the European Observatory on Health Systems and Policies, Copenhagen.

21 Bech M (2004) Choice in the Danish health care system. *Euro Observer*. 6(4): 5–6.

22 Wagstaff A and van Doorslaer E (eds) (1993) *Equity in the Finance and Delivery of Health Care: an international perspective*. Oxford University Press, Oxford.

23 Le Grand J (1982) *The Strategy of Equality: redistribution and the social services*. Allen & Unwin, London.

24 Elofsson S, Unden AL and Krakau I (1998) Patient charges – a hindrance to financially and psychosocially disadvantage groups seeking care. *Social Science and Medicine.* **46**(10): 1375–80.

25 Schwarz E (1996) Changes in utilization and cost sharing within the Danish National Health Insurance dental program, 1975–90. *Acta Odontologica Scandinavica.* **54**(1): 29–35.

26 Thomson S and Dixon A (2004) Choices in health care: the European experience. *Euro Observer.* **6**(4): 1–4.

27 Schut F, Gresz S and Wasem J (2003) Consumer price sensitivity and social health insurance choice in Germany and the Netherlands. *International Journal of Health Care Finance and Economics.* **3**(2):117–38.

28 Busse R and Reisberg A (2004) *Health Care Systems in Transition: Germany.* WHO Regional Office for Europe on behalf of the European Observatory on Health Systems and Policies, Copenhagen.

29 den Exter A, Hermans H, Dosljak M and Busse R (2004) *Health Care Systems in Transition: Netherlands.* WHO Regional Office for Europe on behalf of the European Observatory on Health Systems and Policies, Copenhagen.

30 Institute for Public Policy Research (IPPR) (2005) Patient choice should reduce health inequalities. Press Release [online] [cited 16 November 2005]. Available from: www.ippr.org/pressreleases/?id=1790.

31 Bertinato L, Busse R, Fahy N, Legido-Quigley H, McKee M, Palm W, Passarani I and Ronfini F (2005) *Policy Brief Cross-Border Health Care in Europe.* WHO Regional Office for Europe on behalf of the European Observatory on Health Systems and Policies, Brussels.

32 den Exter AP (2005) Purchasers as the public's agent. In: J Figueras, R Robinson and E Jakubowski (eds) *Purchasing to Improve Health Systems Performance.* Open University Press, Maidenhead.

Chapter 18

The future

Martin McKee

Prediction is both art and science. US Secretary of Defence Donald Rumsfeld famously observed that, 'there are known knowns; there are things we know we know. We also know there are known unknowns; that is to say we know there are some things we do not know. But there are also unknown unknowns, the ones we don't know we don't know. And if one looks throughout the history of the UK and other free countries, it is the latter category that tend to be the difficult ones.'[1]

Although the prose is less than elegant, and the grammar faulty, Rumsfeld summarises almost exactly the challenge posed to anyone seeking to predict the future. Prediction is something that many have attempted, using a variety of approaches.[2] Perhaps the longest established method is prophecy. One of its most famous exponents, Nostradamus, may have been emulating the oracle at Delphi when he penned his collection of quatrains,[3] ensuring that there was so much scope for interpretation that it would be possible to argue, albeit by means of often highly tortuous logic, that they had eventually been fulfilled.[4]

By seeking to predict events far in the future, Nostradamus had the reassurance that if he was wrong he would not be around to answer for his mistakes. Others have been more adventurous, predicting events in the near future, even though they risk being called to account if they are mistaken. This is easiest if one can see where the train of events is leading. Given events in Rome in 44BC, the soothsayer who advised Julius Caesar to 'beware the ides of March'[5] had a reasonable certainty that *something* would happen at that time. His advice would have been much more useful if he had said 'beware the ides of March (and keep an eye on Brutus)'. Alternatively he might have predicted a certainty, such as advising Caesar that he would die, but omitting to mention when. While this advice would obviously have been correct it would have had little predictive value.

There are, however, many prophets who have ignored these lessons and insisted on predicting events in sufficient detail for it to become apparent to all that they have failed to occur. One common example is the prediction that the world was to end on a particular day, now long since past. These have been around throughout recorded history. The fact that you are reading this chapter today provides objective proof that these countless would-be prophets have been entirely mistaken. Prophecy has undergone many refinements, including the inspection of chicken entrails, tea leaves and the movements of heavenly bodies. Yet, whatever the method, the results seem less than impressive.

A second approach is based on the belief that the development of the world is proceeding along some pre-ordained course. Perhaps the most extreme adherent to this theory was the Marquis de Laplace, who contended that, if one had complete knowledge of the state of the universe and the laws of nature, every detail of the future could be predicted.[6] In this he went further than Newton, who believed that divine intervention was required to prevent the perturbations in planetary orbits leading to instability. Laplace responded to Napoleon's complaint that he had left God out his system, by averring that he had 'no need of that hypothesis'.[7]

This determinist approach is not limited to the physical sciences. It also occurs in 'scientific' Marxism based on the notion that the world moves on a pre-determined path – in Marx's case, towards the victory of the proletariat.[8] The limitations of this interpretation were apparent to many long before the collapse of the Soviet system. Yet, just as Marx's vision of the march of history was becoming no longer tenable, an alternative vision was emerging, in which the end of history was no longer the communist state but the liberal democracy, a view advanced most compellingly by Francis Fukuyama.[9]

A third approach is based on faith in technological progress. In several past epochs, for example during the Renaissance and the Industrial Revolution, the rapid pace of change inspired individuals to anticipate what might one day be possible. However, as with other prophets, their predictions often lacked suffi-cient detail to make them useful. Leonardo da Vinci may have drawn something that can now be interpreted as a precursor of the helicopter. However, even with today's technology, it is difficult to envisage how his design could ever be turned into something that would fly. Similarly, while Jules Verne is often extolled as someone who, in his depiction of the vessel Nautilus,[10] anticipated modern submarines, he was somewhat less than accurate when he foresaw the possibility of a journey to the centre of the earth.[11]

All of these approaches have their contemporary manifestations. It is arguable that the passing fad for what became known in the 1990s as the 'Third Way'[12] had about as much substance as some of Nostradamus' predictions. It was certainly subject to as many different interpretations. The historical determinism of Marx has its counterpart in the widespread view that health systems of all types are inevitably converging on some model based on the concept of a quasi-market.[13] Faith in technological determinism, the notion that scientific and technological progress is pre-ordained by the nature of things, is a further example. There have been countless exhortations of what information technology can do to revolu-tionise healthcare, yet the evidence for this is still missing.

Fundamental to all of these approaches is a belief in determinism, in other words that what has happened in the past can predict the future. Where these approaches differ is in their identification of the determinants of change, a deity, the influence of the stars, the progressive increase in knowledge, deep-seated social forces, or something else.

In contrast, there is a view of the world that holds that things simply cannot be predicted. The world is far too complex, with many factors interacting in a non-linear fashion. Chaos and complexity theories, based on this view, have had considerable success in explaining the behaviour of a wide variety of phenomena, ranging from weather patterns to movements in the stock market, and in populations of animals.[14] These patterns can be observed from the sub-atomic to the global levels, offering insights to disciplines as diverse as physics, biology and economics. A key element is the way in which a small difference in the starting conditions within a system can make a massive difference to the progress of the system. A frequently cited example is how a butterfly flapping its wings in West Africa might give rise to a hurricane in the Caribbean. However, the crucial feature of complexity and chaos theories is that while they can explain the existence of patterns, such as stock market crashes and hurricanes, they cannot predict them.

There are, of course, many intermediate positions. Karl Popper introduced the concept of conditional predictions. These are possible in relation to situations that are stationary or repetitive, such as planetary orbits. However, this is emphatically not the case with human systems, in which conditions change with the accumulation of new, and as yet unknown, knowledge.[15] Thus, some things can be predicted with virtual certainty. I can be quite confident that if I turn on the switch beside me that the light will come on (although I cannot be certain because the bulb or the electrical power may have failed) – offering an example of Rumsfeld's 'known knowns'. On the other hand, I have sufficient insight into my lack of predictive abilities never to have purchased a lottery ticket – an example of acting on a 'known unknown'.

One concept offering useful insights is that of path dependency. This sees a system as having the potential to go in many directions at the outset but then, as a result of what may be seen as one or more minor decisions, the future pathways becomes increasingly circumscribed.[16] The path that is eventually followed may be far from optimal, as was the case with the decisions that led to the dominance of the QWERTY keyboard on which I am now typing.[17] The success of the Matsushita Corporation in securing distribution rights for its VHS format videocassette through the large Hollywood studios ensured its subsequent dominance of the market despite the technical superiority of its competitor, Betamax.[18] Path dependency offers a means of placing boundaries around the unpredictability of the world in which we live. However those boundaries are rarely inviolable. While it would have been difficult to imagine how an alternative type of videocassette could penetrate a market dominated by the VHS format, it was entirely possible that a completely new, and previously unforeseen, way of viewing moving pictures in the home might emerge, as it did in the form of the DVD. As Kuhn noted,[19] such a shift may also occur in relation to our understanding of the rules that govern the world around us. When these are seen no longer to provide the answers we need, an alternative set of rules, a new paradigm, may emerge offering greater explanatory power. Although the new paradigm will initially be contested, in time it will become established wisdom until it in turn is replaced.

Kuhn was looking at changes in scientific knowledge. However, we can also identify points in time when events change the fundamental assumptions about how the world works. An example is the French revolution, which overturned the then widespread views about the relationship between rulers and those they ruled.

There are many approaches based on the notion that failures of prediction are in part a consequence of inadequate information. These seek to draw on a much wider pool of knowledge than is usually the case when attempting to forecast. They include formal consensus methods, such as the Delphi techniques that have been found to outperform more traditional ways of assimilating expertise, for example the functioning of standard committees.[20] A more recent approach is based on the notion that the market is the most efficient way of pooling the available knowledge on a subject. Developed at the University of Iowa, this employs a system based on futures trading to predict not just the behaviour of the stock market but also such phenomena as the box office receipts of new film releases, or the share of votes in presidential elections.[21] Ongoing research is examining the scope of this approach to predict outbreaks of influenza. However, the proposal to apply it to the prediction of possible terrorist attacks was rejected as being unacceptably macabre. While some of the more recent proposals to use this method seem to verge on fantasy, there is a serious underlying message that there is a lot of evidence that can be drawn upon that goes far beyond the much more restrictive limitations imposed by the requirements of the peer review system.[22]

For someone charged with looking to the future, this brief and admittedly superficial review of some selected theories can, I think, offer some useful insights. Most importantly, the review indicates the need for caution, as history is littered with the discredited reputations of those who sought to predict the future and have been proven wrong. Thus, it is reasonable to suppose that a significant number of military leaders who died in battle did not do so because of a desire to join their troops in collective suicide. Rather, many fell victim to their over-confidence in their ability to triumph over the intrinsic unpredictability of the world.[23]

Nonetheless this review suggests that, given that we maintain a degree of caution, it is possible to predict some things with reasonable certainty, while incorporating systems to detect and respond to unexpected changes. In this it is vital, at all times, not to get caught up in the details. This is the approach that I will take in the remainder of this chapter, in which I will propose a mechanism that can to some extent help us to anticipate and respond to change.

'Known knowns' and 'unknown unknowns'

While bearing in mind the many caveats already noted, there are some things that can be predicted with a degree of certainty, although in all cases, their consequences are less than certain, largely because of the wide scope of different responses to them. Perhaps the most discussed example is the ageing of populations, as life expectancy continues to lengthen. Of course, this is not the case everywhere. The toll exacted by HIV/AIDS is driving the current decline in life expectancy seen in sub-Saharan Africa and some Caribbean islands, and the societal fragmentation that accompanied the break-up of the USSR explains the worsening life expectancy there.[24] These are reminders that the upward trajectory in life expectancy experienced in the industrialised world cannot be taken for granted. However, there is a reasonable likelihood that it will continue for several decades to come. Indeed, as the OECD has noted, most population projections in the industrialised world assume substantially lower rates of growth in life expectancy than those seen in recent decades, so it is likely that populations in these countries will age more rapidly than is currently assumed.[25]

At the same time, across the industrialised world, birth rates are falling rapidly and, in many countries, are substantially below replacement level. Coupled with ageing populations, this can be expected markedly to increase the dependency ratio (the ratio of those aged 0–14 and 65+ to those aged 15–65). This, in turn, has implications for many public policy areas including labour supply and pensions. Here I want to look at the consequences of these changes for healthcare.

All else being equal, these projections might be expected to result in an increase in the costs of healthcare, because as there are more older people needing treatment, the revenue base from which the money needed can be raised is reduced, and the pool of health professionals and others working in the health system that can be drawn upon to provide the care is similarly reduced. Yet 'all else is not equal'. The dependency ratio as presently calculated assumes a retirement age of 65. This has remained unchanged throughout a period that has seen substantial increases in life expectancy. OECD calculations show that, in most countries, relatively modest increases in the retirement age, and thus in the age threshold for calculating the dependency ratio, would be sufficient to prevent that ratio from rising.[25] If the retirement age is to increase, then the pool of labour supply will also increase, providing both additional tax revenue and more people to be employed in the delivery of healthcare. Of course, the first challenge is to reduce markedly the large proportion of people in their fifties who, in most European countries, have withdrawn from the labour force.[26] The way that they are classified varies according to the mix of social and fiscal policies in each country, with some labelled as 'early retirees', others as 'disabled' or 'unwell', and others as 'unemployed'. However, there are many policies that could substantially increase the labour force participation among this age group.

The declining birth rate clearly poses a problem, by reducing the pool of recruits into health systems. Of course this is an issue for the labour force as a whole. There are, however, a number of possible responses. One is the adoption of family-friendly policies that encourage higher birth rates (or at least remove family-unfriendly ones that discourage them). The other, although not without its problems, is the encouragement of migration from other parts of the world. One of the challenges this poses is how to mitigate the damaging effects of such movement of people on the countries from which they come. In this it is important to recognise the complex balance between the loss to those countries of skilled professionals, and the benefits of financial remittances from abroad. In some countries these constitute a substantial proportion of national income.[27]

A second challenge is how to ensure that the emergence of multi-ethnic and multicultural societies does not undermine Europe's system of social solidarity. In the USA, racial divisions have contributed to the unwillingness of many to accept a system of universal healthcare coverage that would require them to pool their healthcare resources with all their fellow citizens.[28]

Then there is the increased burden of disease associated with an older population. Yet, once again, the past is a poor guide to the future.[29] There is now considerable evidence that it is not age but rather proximity to death that determines health expenditure.[30] Many people aged 75 today are substantially healthier than those of the same age two decades ago.[31] This observation has led some analysts to look at the benefits that might be achieved by investing in policies that will enhance the health of populations so as to reduce future expenditure on health systems. One example is provided by the British Treasury, whose arguments are set out in the report written by Sir Derek Wanless.[32] Employing three scenarios, differing mainly in terms of what happens to the health of the British people, the report estimated the likely financial requirements of the UK NHS in 2030. These estimates ranged from €195 to €235 billion, a difference of €40 billion. In similar vein, a report for the European Commission has demonstrated the importance of investing in health as a means of boosting the economy of the European Union, extending earlier work that showed the importance of health as a driver of economic growth in low income countries.[33] Thus, effective investments in population health offer the prospect of creating a virtuous cycle of economic growth and better health. In summary, while there is considerable certainty that Europe's population will be older in the future than it is now, there are many plausible scenarios describing how society might respond to this challenge. This makes the overall consequences much more difficult to predict.

What about the future of healthcare? Again, it is possible to discern a number of clear trends. The present systems in most countries are based on a network of hospitals into which patients flow, typically from health professionals working in primary care facilities or as community-based specialists. The modern hospital was fashioned in the nineteenth century in response to changing technology.[34] The development of aseptic techniques and anaesthesia gave rise to the operating theatre. Until then, the few procedures undertaken by surgeons, such as amputations, could equally well be undertaken on a kitchen table. Roentgen's discovery of x-rays, offering a means of seeing inside the intact human body, made necessary the creation of radiology departments. Countless chemists, microbiologists, and other scientists made discoveries that paved the way for a variety of clinical laboratories. This combination of developments argued strongly for concentration of facilities. It made more sense for the patient to visit the medical specialist in the hospital, where all the equipment was in place, than for the specialist to visit the patient in his or her house, where little could be done. At the same time the development of a coherent and comprehensive approach to medical education and clinical training, linked to the expansion of the medical curriculum to incorporate the rapid growth in knowledge, argued for a means to ensure that the most interesting patients were brought together under one roof.

Yet things move on. By the end of the twentieth century, many of the arguments for concentrating facilities were being contested. New, less invasive forms of surgery using laparoscopes and endoscopes meant that many procedures once only carried out in hospital could be safely performed in community facilities. Short-acting intravenous anaesthetics greatly shortened recovery times so that patients who would once have stayed in hospital to recover from inhalation anaesthesia could return home on the day of their surgery. Cumbersome laboratory equipment was being replaced by silicon chips bearing micro-arrays able to accomplish multiple analyses in minutes. Increasingly sophisticated portable ultrasound machines have provided new ways of seeing inside human bodies.

At the same time, the conditions in which people live have changed beyond recognition. In the 1950s it was entirely justified to keep someone in hospital until they were fully recovered in order to protect them from the burden they would face in a home bereft of labour-saving devices. It is much less justifiable when they return to a kitchen in which microwave ovens, washing machines and other equipment offer the productive capacity of a small Victorian factory. For all these reasons, the rationale for the major hospital is being questioned, as an increasing share of its traditional workload is taking place in other settings.[35] Once again, the situation is far from simple. Hospitals do much more than treat people.

They are major providers of training and research. For these reasons there are still powerful arguments for the concentration of resources in them. Furthermore, while individual investigations and treatments can be carried out in multiple settings outside hospital, a patient with a complex disorder who must navigate a complicated path between these settings may find it easier if they are brought together in one place. To add further to the complexity, there is one factor that could lead to the complete reconfiguration of the delivery of healthcare. That is the emergence of antibiotic resistant infections. There is a real danger, in some countries, that the rise of resistant infections could take us back to the days of Florence Nightingale, when being admitted to hospital significantly increased one's risk of death. So once again, while we may be quite clear about the changes that are taking place, their eventual consequences are much less clear.

Then there are the 'unknown unknowns'. What will be the impact of knowledge that is not yet available? Here we are on shaky ground. As Karl Popper noted, knowledge that does not currently exist cannot be predicted.[15] Yet this has not prevented many from trying. Unsurprisingly, the enthusiasm for prediction is most common where the prophet concerned is trying to sell us something. Among the most enthusiastic are those selling health information technology systems. Unembarrassed by ever growing examples of expensive failure,[36] they continue to hold out a vision of a world in which files are never lost, and where information is available instantly to those who have need of it. Promises of a brave new world are made with equal enthusiasm by the biotechnology industry. Yet, as a recent review has noted, this industry has consistently failed to live up to these promises.[37]

This rather gloomy analysis should not be seen as a denial of the many benefits that scientific and technical developments have brought. There have been numerous achievements in health research. One need do no more than look back to the situation in the eighteenth century. Healthcare was essentially limited to first aid, or to providing a place of tranquillity where people could either recover spontaneously or die in peace. It is now possible to cure many previously fatal disorders. Survival of low birthweight babies has improved dramatically, with especially rapid changes in the countries of central Europe since 1990, where the gap in the quality of their neonatal care that had opened up with the West during the years of communism was quickly closed.[38] Deaths from childhood infections are now extremely rare, whereas a century ago parents in many of the new industrialising cities could expect to lose up to a third of their children. New drugs to treat cancers have considerably improved survival, and others only now being introduced hold out future promise. More active policies on revascularisation have contributed significantly to the decline in deaths from ischaemic heart disease.[39] So in many areas of healthcare, conditions that were once fatal are now routinely cured.

Healthcare can now make a real contribution in prolonging and enhancing life and it can be shown that about half of the improvement in life expectancy in western European countries over the past three decades can be attributed to the impact of healthcare. There is every reason to believe that advances in scientific knowledge and in the application of evidence based practice will continue to improve the probability of survival following the onset of disease, and that ways of alleviating conditions that are currently untreatable will continue to emerge. However, it is also likely that this progress will be uneven. Many developments fail to live up to their initial promise.[40] While there are many truly innovative and effective products, these are substantially outnumbered by a plethora of 'me-too' preparations that offer little advantage over what already exists.[41]

What of the potential contribution of genomics? Unsurprisingly, given the vast resources that have been expended on genetic research, our knowledge of our genetic make-up and its relation to human disorders is expanding rapidly. Yet this has not been matched by a corresponding advance in the ability to prevent or treat disease. Even where genetic factors play a significant role in the development of disease, they often do so by means of a complex set of interactions with environmental factors.

Misplaced heroics? Predicting the future of healthcare

Given the considerable uncertainty outlined above, what can be concluded about the future of healthcare? There is one aspect that is common to all the scenarios set out previously. This is that the delivery of healthcare will be much more complex in the future than it was in the past. This is a problem that is common to almost all aspects of our lives. The simple village school, with its spartan rooms equipped with little more than a blackboard and a few books, has given way to an educational resource centre filled with multimedia resources accessed through the Internet. The infantry soldier in the trenches of Flanders has been succeeded by the high-tech warrior in his Apache helicopter seeing clearly through the fog of battle to pick off the enemy with his 'fire and forget' missiles. In each case there have been profound consequences for those in charge, whether Ministers of Education or army generals. What they now face is the exponential growth in complexity – the same key challenge that faces healthcare in the future.

None of the foregoing is to deny that many achievements in past decades have been accomplished with what now appear to us to be very basic interventions, such as immunisation, simple antibiotics and basic cardiovascular drugs, all of which have saved countless lives. However the newer interventions, in particular those responsible for the improved outcomes of cancer and neonatal care, require very complex systems of care.

To a considerable extent because of our ability to enable people with a range of previously fatal disorders to survive into middle and old age, today the greatest challenge is posed by the increasing burden of chronic diseases.[42] These conditions require effective care to be delivered in many different settings over very prolonged periods of time.

The case of juvenile onset diabetes well illustrates this. The discovery of insulin transformed this condition from an acute, rapidly fatal disease of childhood into a lifelong chronic disorder affecting many body systems, whose management requires the integrated skills of a broad range of specialists. Diabetes is a good example of the challenge to be faced because it is possible to see the consequences of failing to get it right.[43] Integration of services is crucial. Outcomes are much worse in countries where health services are fragmented (for example, most notably in the United States) than in those countries, such as Finland or the United Kingdom, where they are much more fully integrated.[44,45]

The implications of complexity

Whether it is the complexities of managing diabetes, AIDS, cancer, heart failure or any of the many conditions that affect individuals – or groups (involving even greater complexities) – the key to success is the creation of commensurately complex, integrated systems. These will involve numbers of different professionals and specialists working as teams to ensure that the right patient gets the right type of care at the right time. Unfortunately, there is no preordained set of rules to ensure that this will happen.

There are two implications, not only for healthcare but also for education, warfare, or almost any aspect of modern life. The first is that if society is to respond effectively to these challenges, it must take a long-term perspective and undertake sustained investment in the resources that will be needed in the future, a task that is made difficult by the unpredictability of that future. The second is that these resources must be managed effectively, with a particular emphasis of the management of the complex interactions between them.

Investment for health

This complexity of healthcare means that it is necessary to go beyond the traditional production function, in which output is maximised by the optimal combination of labour and capital. An alternative model sees the optimal outcome of healthcare as involving sustained investment in the optimal combination of people (or human capital) of facilities and equipment (or physical capital) of knowledge (or intellectual capital) and of human relationships (or social capital).

Over the next few decades a key challenge will be to ensure that there is the appropriate mix of skills in the healthcare workforce. In the past, most countries have taken a *laissez faire* approach, hoping that individuals will read the signals from the market and adapt their career aspirations appropriately. This has not been successful in the past, and with increasingly mobile populations it is even less likely to succeed in the future. Some countries in Europe have trained far too many physicians, and some, like the UK, too few. Ideally, in a perfectly functioning single market, in which free movement is actually guaranteed, these imbalances would correct themselves. Yet they have not, for many reasons.

Looking ahead, one can anticipate some major difficulties. Projections across the EU, simply on the basis of anticipated retirements, indicate that there will be a substantial overall deficit of physicians by around 2010.[46] However, this does not take account of the shift, in many countries, to early retirement, with many physicians feeling burnt-out by the growing pressures they face in a healthcare environment that is ever more complex and demanding. Nor does it take account of the consequences of an increasing number of women in the medical workforce, whose chosen balance between families and careers may be different from those in earlier male-dominated generations. Finally, in the European Union, the implementation of the Working Time Directive will have profound consequences for the ability to staff many small hospitals.[47]

The situation is even more problematic for nurses and other paramedical professionals. The need for people with basic nursing skills is diminishing as nurses take on increasing specialised roles, whether in hospitals, providing more intensive levels of care, or in the community, providing tailored disease management programmes.[48] Yet many countries have consistently under-invested in nursing skills, often because in the past there were surpluses of (often poorly paid) junior doctors, and they, rather than nurses, were expected to undertake the more technical aspects of healthcare.

It would, however, be a mistake to think that the health professionals whose training programmes must be developed now will be carrying out these same tasks in the future. The range will be very different, and many tasks now undertaken by doctors will be the responsibility of nurses and other health professionals.[49] The most significant change in the training of all of them, however, will be the enhancement of their ability to absorb the increasing volume of knowledge that will emerge throughout their professional lives, preparing them to engage in a process of lifelong learning.

As to physical capital, it is very obvious from even a superficial inspection that some countries have seriously under-invested in healthcare facilities.[50] In strictly numerical terms they may have enough buildings and equipment, but this is often woefully inappropriate for the healthcare needs of tomorrow. Earlier in this chapter I considered some of the ways in which the hospital is changing. Building on these developments, it is possible to deconstruct the potential functions of a hospital and explore plausible scenarios as to how they might change.[35] The results of such an exercise bear little resemblance to the hospitals that are being built today. In the hospital of the future the ratio of operating theatres to beds is likely to be much greater than now, patients will be grouped not by specialty but by intensity of treatment, and by body system, and the Emergency Department, now a chaotic clinical melting pot, will be comprehensively reconfigured, with many of those who now attend it being diverted to more appropriate facilities. However, planning for Emergency Departments will need to be based on a constantly changing scenario. Whatever is to be constructed must be sufficiently flexible to adapt to the evolving patterns of clinical care. This has always been necessary, for example when some of the tuberculosis sanatoria transmuted into cardiac hospitals, when the thoracic surgeons they employed learned new skills to replace the old ones that were no longer needed once effective chemotherapy was introduced. However, that change required relatively little reconfiguration of facilities. The changes that are likely to be needed in the future may be much more radical. Yet, ironically, in some countries governments are introducing new forms of capital financing, such as the ill-fated British Private Finance Initiative, which will make the necessary future changes prohibitively expensive and difficult.[51]

There will also be a need to take a much more strategic approach to health technology. The challenge being faced is how to determine what the implications of new technology are for patient pathways, and thus what reconfigurations of facilities and services are needed.

The further need is for investment in intellectual capital. This goes far beyond the health technology assessment programmes that most countries now have. It will require a knowledge system in which generation of information, synthesis and implementation are integrated in the healthcare system. This will involve sustained investment in three linked communities – researchers, disseminators of research (or knowledge brokers), and research-aware practitioners who have the skills to interpret the research and to apply it to clinical practice.

Finally, there is a need for investment in social capital, a term that is widely used, but poorly understood. In its present, rather narrow, context it means investment in relationships between healthcare staff, ensuring that these are based on trust and are facilitated by good means of communication. There is now compelling evidence, in particular from the work on American 'magnet hospitals' (so called because they attract and retain staff) that good staff relations are associated with lower costs and improved outcomes.[52]

If the challenges of the future are to be confronted, there will have to be programmes of sustained investment in the inputs to healthcare, with an emphasis on the word *sustained*. Healthcare is not the place for 'just in time' procurement. There are no factories that can gear up production of doctors and nurses to meet a sudden surge in demand. Hospitals do not come in flat packs, to be assembled overnight. Knowledge of what works, and what does not, requires more than sitting under a tree and thinking for a few days. It is essential to look at these issues over a long timescale, linking the efforts of many different sectors, but most obviously of education.

This investment must incorporate great flexibility. There is no benefit in spending substantial resources to train people to undertake a task that will be obsolete by the time they have completed their training. Instead they need transferable skills and, in particular, the ability to review critically the evidence that will accumulate over their professional lifetimes, and adapt it to the problems they face. By the same token, those planning healthcare facilities must ensure that they have the ability to be reconfigured continuously over the course of their lifespan.

Optimising existing resources

Investment alone is not, however, enough. It is equally important to manage those resources that are available, in a way that maximises health gain. Drawing on Kuhn's analysis, the present paradigm, based on the interaction between an individual seeking healthcare and a health professional who can offer it, is in crisis. In many countries those who pay for healthcare, such as sickness funds, simply act to ensure that the patient can get treatment and that the professional will be paid. This is little different, in conception, from the sort of funds established in the nineteenth century by small retailers. Throughout the year families would pay a small amount into the fund in order to have enough credit to pay for presents at Christmas. As with our present day sickness funds, this was simply a means of ensuring that the money was available when it was needed. The fund took no interest in what the family bought at Christmas, assuming that they were the best judges of what they wanted, and that retailers would respond to their wishes.

This may have worked relatively well when healthcare providers had little to offer, and what was available was fairly easily understandable, although of course this did not stop many charlatans from engaging in what would now be described as supplier-induced demand, subjecting poorly informed patients to treatments that ranged from bleeding and cupping to the sale of snake oil. In the much more complex healthcare environment that now exists, this model is clearly obsolete. Instead what is now needed is that organisations which have so far limited their role to providing money – for example, sickness funds and county or regional health authorities – take active steps to decide what they want to buy, on behalf of those whom they represent, a process that has been termed strategic purchasing.[53]

The pace of change: a caveat

A consistent theme throughout this chapter has been the accelerating pace of change. The speed with which people, information, and ideas move around the world is increasing all the time. Whether investing in people, facilities or organisational structures, it is essential to incorporate sufficient flexibility to adapt to changing circumstances. Yet if this is to happen, it will also be important to establish zones of stability, in which those charged with responding to these changing circumstances have the space and the time to look beyond the horizon and construct the varying scenarios that may unfold.

I make this point because, in some places, the pursuit of change has become an end in itself, rather than an adaptation to changing circumstances. One of the most extreme examples is England (the other parts of the United Kingdom have to some extent been spared the worst effects of this ideology), where a stream of government ministers seek to ascend to what Disraeli called the top of the greasy political pole[54] on the basis of their ability to come up with ever more rapid reconfigurations of health, education and criminal justice symptoms. Safe in the knowledge that they will have moved on before the consequences of their actions become apparent, they have managed to discredit totally the word 'modernisation', which in England has become a byword for fundamental but short-lived structural disruptions. While these policies have the benefit of providing a rich catalogue of mistakes (although, among them, a few successes) that others can learn from, they exact a severe toll on those seeking to make the system work.

Conclusion

The history of prediction cautions against attempting to define a blueprint for the future of healthcare. Just as chaos theory can explain why the weather is as it is, yet cannot predict what the temperature will be on a given day one month hence, so it can be predicted with some confidence that whatever the details, the delivery of healthcare in the future will be much more complex than it is at present. The systems currently in place are simply not adequate to respond to the challenges posed. It is not feasible to leave healthcare to the invisible hand of the market, hoping that providers will recognise and respond to the signals generated by individual patients. First, the scope for opportunistic behaviour, combined with the difficulty in defining the inputs and the product, means that, except in strictly circumscribed circumstances, the creation of a market will simply add expense[55] and, worse, create incentives that may damage the interests of the patient. Second, the delays inherent in assembling effective packages of care, including the acquisition of technology, the training in its use, and the reconfiguration of facilities, mean that even the most efficient market will be unable to respond in a reasonable time. This becomes apparent each year when governments actively intervene to ensure that influenza vaccines will be available.

Instead governments must take an active role, anticipating the changing nature of disease and the responses to it, and taking a long-term perspective to ensure that decisions to invest in what is needed have been made in a timely manner.

Furthermore, there is a need to move away from models of healthcare concerned with only brief, clearly defined interactions between individual patients and providers. This model may seem reasonable when planning for a patient who consults a doctor because of an acute respiratory infection, or is admitted for a cataract extraction. A combination of ageing populations and new therapeutic opportunities mean that an increasingly large volume of healthcare will be for people with chronic disorders, requiring coordinated interventions by different professionals and specialists over a prolonged period of time. Yet paradoxically, many reforms of health services go in the opposite direction, trying to package illnesses into discrete, easily measurable commodities. The inexorable spread of *Diagnosis Related Groups* is an example. The fragmentation of care that a DRG system promotes does little to facilitate the integrated care of patients with, for example, the multiple complications of diabetes.

However future health systems are going to be organised, there will be a need for a major investment in the acquisition of skills and infrastructure, such that governments, and those acting on their behalf, will be enabled to anticipate, to the extent that this is possible, generating plausible scenarios and continuously revising them as new information becomes available. Unfortunately, it is the lack of this expertise that may be the main constraint that we face in meeting the challenges of health services in the future.

References

1 Rumsfeld D (2002) Department of Defense Press Briefing. Washington DC, 12 February 2002.
2 McKee M (1995) 2020 Vision. *J Publ Health Med.* **17**: 127–31.
3 Nostradamus (1999) *The Complete Prophecies.* Wordsworth, Ware.
4 Loire P (2005) *Nostradamus 2003–2025: a history of the future.* Simon Schuster International, New York.
5 Shakespeare W (2005) *Julius Caesar.* Penguin, London.
6 Holden ES (ed) (2002) *Essays in Astronomy.* University Press of the Pacific, Honolulu, HW.
7 Honderich T (1995) *The Oxford Companion to Philosophy.* Oxford University Press, Oxford.
8 Marx K (1992) *Capital: a critique of political economy, Vol 1.* Penguin, London.
9 Fukuyama F (1993) *The End of History and the Last Man.* Penguin, London.
10 Verne J (1994) *Twenty Thousand Leagues Under the Sea.* Penguin, London.
11 Verne J (1994) *Journey to the Centre of the Earth.* Penguin, London.
12 Giddens A (1998) *The Third Way: renewal of social democracy.* Polity Press, London.
13 Nolte E, McKee M and Wait S (2005) Research on health, health system and service evaluation. In: A Bowling and S Ebrahim (eds) *Handbook of Health Research Methods: investigation, measurement and analysis.* Open University Press, Milton Keynes.
14 Gell-Mann M (1994) *The Quark and the Jaguar: adventures in the simple and the complex.* Little, Brown and Company, London.
15 Popper K (2002) *Conjectures and Refutations: the growth of scientific knowledge.* Routledge, London.
16 Tissot L and Veyrassat B (2002) *Technological Trajectories, Markets, Institutions. Industrialized Countries, 19th–20th Centuries: from context dependency to path dependency.* Peter Lang, Brussels.
17 David PA (1985) Clio and the economics of QWERTY. *Am Ecom Rev.* **75**: 332–7.

18 Cusumano MA, Mylonadis Y and Rosenbloom RS (1992) Strategic maneuvering and mass-market dynamics: the triumph of VHS over Beta. *Business History Rev.* **66**: 51–94.

19 Kuhn T (1996) *The Structure of Scientific Revolutions.* University of Chicago Press, Chicago, IL.

20 Rowe G and Wright G (2001) Expert opinions in forecasting: The role of the Delphi technique In: JS Armstrong (ed) *Principles of Forecasting.* Kluwer Academic Publishers, Boston, MA.

21 Forsythe R, Nelson F, Neumann G and Wright J (1992) Anatomy of an experimental political stock market. *Am Econ Rev.* **82**: 1142–61.

22 European Advisory Committee on Health Research (Banta HD, Dab W, Gabrielyan ES, Jonsson E, Martin-Moreno JM, McKee M, Rantanen JH, Raspe H-H, Svensson P-G, Edejer T, Lopez A and Varavikova E) (2003) Considerations in defining evidence for public health. *Int J Technol Assess Health Care.* **19**: 559–73.

23 Perry JM (1996) *Arrogant Armies: great military disasters and the generals behind them.* John Wiley & Sons, Chichester.

24 McMichael AJ, McKee M, Shkolnikov V and Valkonen T (2004) Mortality trends and setbacks: global convergence or divergence? *Lancet.* **363**: 1155–9.

25 Martins JA, Gonand F, Antolin P, de la Maisonneuve C and Yoo K-L (2005) The impact of ageing on demand, factor markets and growth. *Economics Working Papers No 420.* OECD, Paris.

26 Commission of the European Communities (2002) *Report from the Commission to the Council, the European Parliament, the Economic and Social Committee and the Committee of the Regions. Report requested by Stockholm European Council: 'Increasing labour force participation and promoting active ageing'.* COM (2202) 9 Final. European Commission, Brussels.

27 Stilwell B, Diallo K, Zurn P, Dal Poz MR, Adams O and Buchan J (2003) Developing evidence based ethical policies on the migration of health workers: conceptual and practical challenges. *Human Resources for Health.* **1**: 8.

28 Kunitz SJ and Pesis-Katz I (2005) Mortality of white Americans, African Americans, and Canadians: the causes and consequences for health of welfare state institutions and policies. *Milbank Q.* Brussels: 5–39.

29 Robine JM and Michel JP (2004) Looking forward to a general theory on population aging. *J Gerontol A Biol Sci Med Sci.* **59**: M590–7.

30 McGrail K, Green B, Barer ML, Evans RG, Hertzman C and Normand C (2000) Age, costs of acute and long-term care and proximity to death: evidence for 1987–88 and 1994–95 in British Columbia. *Age Ageing.* **29**: 249–53.

31 Fries JF (2003) Measuring and monitoring success in compressing morbidity. *Ann Intern Med.* **139**: 455–9.

32 Wanless D (2002) *Securing our Future Health: taking a long-term view.* HM Treasury, London.

33 Suhrcke M, McKee M, Sauto Arce R, Tsolova S and Mortensen J (2005) *The Contribution of Health to the Economy in the European Union.* European Commission, Brussels.

34 McKee M and Healy J (eds) (2002) *Hospitals in a Changing Europe.* Open University Press, Milton Keynes.

35 McKee M, Edwards N and Wyatt S (2004) Transforming today's hospital to meet tomorrow's needs. *Revista Portuguesa de Saúde Púlica.* **4**: 21–7.

36 Kleinke JD (2005) Dot-gov: market failure and the creation of a national health information technology system. *Health Aff (Millwood).* **24**: 1246–62.

37 Joppi R, Bertele V and Garattini S (2005) Disappointing biotech. *BMJ.* **331**: 895–7.

38 Koupilová I, McKee M and Holčik J (1998) Neonatal mortality in the Czech Republic during the transition. *Health Policy.* **46**: 43–52.

39 Tunstall-Pedoe H, Vanuzzo D, Hobbs M, Mahonen M, Cepaitis Z, Kuulasmaa K and Keil U (2000) Estimation of contribution of changes in coronary care to improving

survival, event rates, and coronary heart disease mortality across the WHO MONICA Project populations. *Lancet*. **355**: 688–700.

40 Twombly R (2005) FDA Oncology Committee debates Iressa's status following negative trial results. *J Natl Cancer Inst*. **97**: 473.

41 Croghan TW and Pittman PM (2004) The medicine cabinet: what's in it, why, and can we change the contents? *Health Aff (Millwood)*. **23**: 23–33.

42 World Health Organization (2005) *Preventing Chronic Disease: a vital investment*. WHO, Geneva.

43 Hopkinson B, Balabanova D, McKee M and Kutzin J (2004) The human perspective on health care reform: coping with diabetes in Kyrgyzstan. *Int J Health Planning Management*. **19**: 43–61.

44 Matsushima M, LaPorte RE, Maruyama M, Shimizu K, Nishimura R and Tajima N (1997) Geographic variation in mortality among individuals with youth-onset diabetes mellitus across the world. DERI Mortality Study Group. Diabetes Epidemiology Research International. *Diabetologia*. **40**: 212–16.

45 Laing SP, Swerdlow AJ, Slater SD, Botha JL, Burden AC, Waugh NR, Smith AW, Hill RD, Bingley PJ, Patterson CC, Qiao Z and Keen H (1999) The British Diabetic Association Cohort Study, I: all-cause mortality in patients with insulin-treated diabetes mellitus. *Diabet Med*. **16**: 459–65.

46 European Commission, DGXV (2004) *Committee of Senior Officials on Public Health. Statistical tables relation to the migration of doctors in the Community from 1977 to 2000*. European Commission, Brussels.

47 Paice E and Reid W (2004) Can training and service survive the European Working Time Directive? *Med Educ*. **38**: 336–8.

48 McKee M and Nolte E (2004) Responding to the challenge of chronic disease: ideas from Europe. *Clin Med*. **4**: 336–42.

49 Sibbald B, Shen J and McBride A (2004) Changing the skill-mix of the health care workforce. *J Health Serv Res Policy*. **9**(Suppl 1): 28–38.

50 Thompson CR and McKee M (2004) Financing and planning of public hospitals in the European Union. *Health Policy*. **67**: 281–91.

51 Atun RA and McKee M (2005) Is the private finance initiative dead? *BMJ*. **331**: 792–3.

52 Aiken LH, Smith HL and Lake ET (1994) Lower Medicare mortality among a set of hospitals known for good nursing care. *Med Care*. **32**: 771–87.

53 McKee M and Brand H (2005) Purchasing to promote population health. In: J Figueras, R Robinson and E Jakubowski. *Purchasing to Improve Health Systems Performance*. Open University Press, Maidenhead.

54 Monypenny W and Buckle G (1929) *The Life of Benjamin Disraeli, Earl of Beaconsfield*. John Murray, London.

55 Williamson O (2000) The New Institutional Economics: taking stock, looking ahead. *J Econ Lit*. **38**: 595–613.

Index